Meningiomas: Biology, Pathology, and Differential Diagnosis

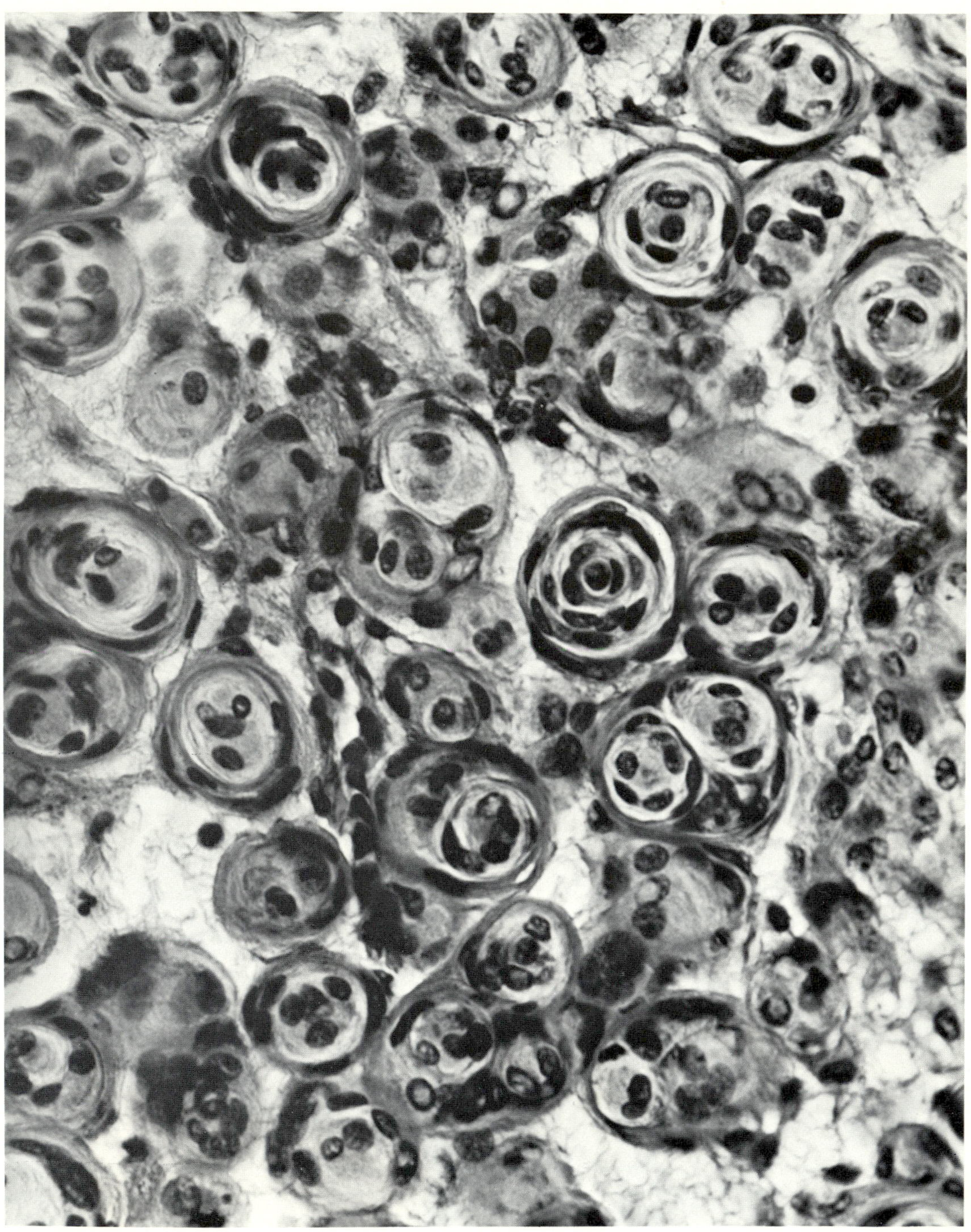

Meningiomas

Biology, Pathology, and Differential Diagnosis

JOHN J. KEPES, M.D.

Professor of Pathology
Department of Pathology and Oncology
The University of Kansas
College of Health Sciences and Hospital
Kansas City, Kansas

Distributed by
YEAR BOOK MEDICAL PUBLISHERS • INC.
35 EAST WACKER DRIVE, CHICAGO

Library of Congress Cataloging in Publication Data

Kepes, John J.
Meningiomas, biology, pathology, and differential diagnosis.
(Masson monographs in diagnostic pathology; v. 4)
Bibliography:
Includes index.
1. Meningioma. I. Title. II. Series.
RC280.M4K46 616.99'28107 81-18659
ISBN 0-89352-136-1 AACR2

ISBN 0-89352-136-1
Library of Congress Catalog Card Number: 81-18659
Printed in the United States of America

Masson Monographs in Diagnostic Pathology

Series Editor: **Stephen S. Sternberg, M.D.**

1. *Tumors and Proliferation of Adipose Tissue: A Clinicopathologic Approach*

   By Philip W. Allen (1981)

2. *Diagnostic Immunohistochemistry*

   Edited by Ronald A. DeLellis (1981)

3. *Diagnostic Transmission Electron Microscopy of Human Tumors*

   By Robert A. Erlandson (1981)

4. *Meningiomas: Biology, Pathology, and Differential Diagnosis*

   By John J. Kepes (1982)

5. *Pathology and Clinical Features of Parasitic Diseases*

   By Tsieh Sun (1982)

6. *Pathology of Radiation Injury*

   By Luis F. Fajardo (1982)

Foreword

It is not without trepidation that a new monograph on meningiomas is being presented. The monumental historic work of Harvey Cushing and Louise Eisenhardt, *Meningiomas. Their Classification, Regional Behaviour, Life History, and Surgical End Results*, first published in 1938 and reprinted in 1962, provided so comprehensive a storehouse of knowledge of, and insight into, this subject that any additional monograph on meningiomas may seem superfluous and even somewhat disrespectful. In the preface of the 1962 second printing, Dr. Eisenhardt said, "It is almost a quarter of a century since the monograph was completed. Dr. Cushing would have been pleased to know that this work is regarded as a continued source of information and inspiration." She could have made this statement with equal justification today, 43 years after the first edition was published.

Still, a great body of knowledge and practical experience has accumulated with regard to meningiomas since 1938. Dr. Cushing himself said in the Introduction to their monograph, "Our knowledge of intracranial tumors of all sorts has advanced greatly, and yet it is only the beginning of what another generation will in all certainty come to know."

Since 1938, techniques of histopathology have improved. New investigative tools of histochemistry, electron microscopy (both the transmission and scanning variety), tissue and organ cultures, and immunocytology have been applied to the structural study of brain tumors. Neuropathology of this field did not remain untouched by developments in related disciplines, for example, the radionuclide and computerized axial tomography (CAT) scan studies of the brain, as well as the vastly improved technology of brain surgery itself. In addition, the discovery of estrogen followed by that of progesterone receptors in meningiomas and the use of drugs to combat these sex hormones may, in the future, have a profound effect on the treatment of meningiomas that are inaccessible for total surgical removal.

Therefore, an attempt not to substitute, but rather to update, previous comprehensive works on meningiomas led to the present publication. It is another reflection on Harvey Cushing's genius that he personally contributed details on pathology, radiology, as well as clinical aspects of meningiomas in his book with Dr. Eisenhardt, whereas today members of at least three specialties—pathology, neurosurgery, and neuroradiology—would be needed to create a work of this type.

This monograph is being published as part of the series, *Masson Monographs in Diagnostic Pathology*. It is intended to become, at a later date, part of a more comprehensive work, one dealing with the neuroradiological and neurosurgical approaches to meningiomas as well. I sincerely hope that this volume will be of practical use to my fellow pathologists, but also to neurologists and neurosurgeons in diagnosing and combating this sometimes benign, but all too often dangerous and treacherous, tumor, the meningioma.

JOHN J. KEPES, M.D.

Gratefully dedicated to the memory of
two of my great teachers:

James W. Kernohan, M.D.
Professor of Neuropathology
Mayo Clinic
Rochester, Minnesota

and

László Zoltán, M.D.
Professor of Neurosurgery
National Institute of Neurosurgery
Budapest, Hungary

Contents

CHAPTER 28. Tissue Culture 185
CHAPTER 29. Metastases of Meningiomas 190

Introduction

The term pathology may be used to describe the gross and microscopic features of a given disease or abnormal condition, or it may be applied in a broader sense to include other characteristics as well. In the case of meningiomas the latter include chemical components, enzyme activity of tumor cells, statistical data about the occurrence of meningiomas in various age groups, and the geographic aspects of their incidence in the Western world and other parts of the globe, genetic aspects, familial occurrence, and chromosomal patterns. Inquiries directed toward the possible etiology, histogenesis, the study of meningiomas occurring spontaneously in some animals, and experimental production of such tumors in others, are all rightfully included in the discussion of pathology. Accordingly, an attempt is made to provide up-to-date information regarding knowledge that has accumulated in these areas. Of all the foregoing, however, the largest and the most extensively illustrated part of this work deals with microscopic characteristics of meningiomas, particularly as they relate to the numerous variants of this tumor. This is probably as it should be, since the author of this monograph is primarily a practicing diagnostic neuropathologist who has had more exposure to, and first-hand experience with, the histology than with the other aspects of the pathology of meningiomas.

It is quite true that most meningiomas are rather easy to diagnose under the microscope. This is made possible by well-known features seen in many of these tumors, such as cellular whorls with psammoma bodies, which provide clues for an easy diagnosis in many instances. The more meningiomas one examines, however, the more obvious it becomes that quite a number of these tumors are among the most difficult to diagnose histologically, and such difficulties are naturally increased by the need to render a frozen section diagnosis in many instances. A sometimes uncanny similarity to tumors that are vastly different in their biology and prognosis characterizes some meningiomas. Conversely, some tumors of a nonmeningiomatous nature may have histological features that closely imitate meningiomas. Clues to prognosis, that is, predictability of future recurrences or of distant metastases, or both, are also to be found in the histological makeup of many meningiomas. Any neuropathologist who has reviewed large numbers of meningiomas will have developed a heightened sense of the need for detailed analysis of such diagnostic problems. Electron-microscopic, immunopathologic, and other studies can be of great further assistance in elucidating problems raised at the light-microscopic level. It is hoped that the examples of histologic variants of meningiomas provided in this book will be of help to practicing pathologists as well as to their neurosurgical colleagues in identifying a doubtful tumor as a meningioma, as well as in gaining some insight regarding its prognosis.

The portion of this work dealing with histologic variants of meningiomas was presented in an abridged version as a poster at the 8th International Congress of Neuropathology in Washington, D.C.[1] This review of the histopathology of meningiomas was based on a study of 600 cases seen at the University of Kansas Medical Center as local material or consultations between 1959 and 1980 and on 700 cases operated upon in the Department of Neurosurgery of the University of Vienna, Austria, between 1964 and 1974. I owe my gratitude to Professors Franz Seitelberger and Kurt Jellinger, who welcomed me to the Neurologisches Institut of Vienna and gave me every possible assistance in reviewing their material. It follows from the preceding that our material predominantly represents surgically removed meningiomas, rather than autopsy cases. Of the latter, we had relatively few. I am grateful to Dr. Haruo Okazaki of the Mayo Clinic for having permitted us to use some of his excellent gross material. I am also greatly indebted for advice and helpful comments over the years from Dr. J. W. Kernohan and Dr. L. J. Rubinstein. Dr. Dante O. Garrido was of great help in compiling this material for the 8th International Congress of Neuropathology. For submitting cases and photographs used in this volume, I would like to express my sincere thanks to the following: Dr. A. Barabas, Budapest; Dr. V. R. Challa, Winston-Salem, N.C.; Dr. R. A. Clasen, Chicago, Ill.; Dr. G. F. Froio, Drexel Hill, Pa.; Dr. D. Horoupian, New York, N.Y.; Dr. S. Lipper, Chapel Hill, N.C.; Dr. B. Liwnicz, Cincinnati, O.; Dr. S. S. Mirra, Atlanta, Ga.; Dr. C. Pena, Pittsburgh, Pa.; Dr. B. N. Pham, Kansas City, Mo.; Dr. L. Price, Omaha, Neb.; Dr. S. Rengachary, Kansas City, Mo.; Dr. H. V. Rizzoli, Washington, D.C.; Dr. B. Scheithauer, Rochester, Minn.; Dr. W. Schoene, Boston, Mass.; Dr. N. Schuman, Kansas City, Mo.; Professors I. Virtanen and J. Wartiovaara, Helsinki; Dr. I. Watanabe, Kansas City, Mo.; and Professor H. Zankl, Homburg, Saarland. I am also indebted to the Photography Department of Kansas University Medical Center and to Mr. C. Sittler for developing and printing the photomicrographs and electron micrographs, respectively, and also to the tireless work of Mrs. D. Roembach in typing the manuscript.

Reference

1. Garrido, D. O., and Kepes, J. J.: Histologic variants of meningiomas: Interrelations between subgroups. (*8th International Congress of Neuropathology, Washington, D.C.*) *J. Neuropathol. Exp. Neurol. 37: 616, 1978.*

CHAPTER 1

The Origin of the Term Meningioma: A Concept and Its Boundaries

At this writing, the term *meningioma* is 58 years old. Harvey Cushing, in his 1922 Cavendish Lecture, gave this name to tumors of the meninges that have been known for many decades before that time, but were called by a variety of names—some of them reflecting the gross appearance of these tumors, for example, *fungus* of the dura mater, and others the fact that they frequently contain calcium deposits: *psammoma*. Still other names represented an attempt to reflect histogenesis and character of the main tumor cell (e.g., *meningoexothelioma*, *endothelioma*, *mesothelioma*, *arachnoidal fibroblastoma*). Such names usually also implied an understanding of the basic histogenesis of the tumor in question, and yet, even today, one cannot be absolutely certain about the embryologic derivation of the cells that compose meningiomas. It was to avoid such unnecessary commitment regarding histogenesis that Cushing[1] coined the name *meningioma* for this neoplasm and for what he considered its variants. Cushing and Eisenhardt[2] believed that there exists a basic cell within meningiomas that sometimes appears in pure form, whereas in other instances it undergoes morphological changes, creating the variants of meningiomas. They stated, "and if we are to judge from the variable histology of the tumors in question, granting their origin from meningocytes (or meningoblasts, if preferred), these cells appear capable of transformation, not only into fibroblasts but (admittedly with less frequency) into cells of other types." Since that time, some very important ultrastructural characteristics of the basic tumor cells have been elucidated by electron microscopy, and it became possible to recognize the presence of the same basic cell in a number of variants of meningiomas, as well as transitions from "pure" meningiomas to ones with more complex cellular composition.

However, there are still areas of controversy regarding certain primary tumors involving the meninges, which are thought by some to represent variants of meningiomas and by others to be really quite unrelated, their true nature being neoplasms developing in and involving the meninges, but without any histogenetic kinship to meningiomas as such. This question is currently being debated with regard to the following tumors:

1. *Primary melanotic tumors of the leptomeninges:* Are they meningiomas with cells that contain melanin pigment, or do they represent a very different tumor, that is, melanocytomas involving the meninges with no relationship to meningiomas?
2. The group of *angioblastic meningiomas:* Some of these undoubtedly simply represent highly vascularized but otherwise conventional meningiomas. A problem exists, however, with meningeal examples of hemangioblastoma or Lindau tumor, believed by some to represent a form of angioblastic meningioma, whereas others consider it a meningeal example of the same hemangioblastoma we find in the cerebellum, brainstem, or spinal cord. The same problem, and a very lively controversy, exists regarding a much more malignant type of meningeal tumor that has a hemangiopericytomatous pattern. Arguments have been put forward to the effect that this tumor is a variant of meningioma—albeit with disturbing prognostic implications—whereas others are equally convinced that this tumor is identical with hemangiopericytomas elsewhere in the body, and its occurrence in the leptomeninges is merely a matter of chance.
3. During the last few years, benign as well as malignant *fibrous histiocytomas* have been observed with increasing frequency in the meninges with implied questions as to their relationship to meningiomas.
4. Whereas *chondroblastic meningiomas* have been known for a long time and are considered otherwise typical meningiomas with focal

chondroblastic changes or differentiation, recently a number of much more primitive tumors of the chondroid series have been encountered in the meninges. Such neoplasms have the same morphology as *mesenchymal chondrosarcomas* elsewhere in the body, and their relationship, if any, to meningiomas has yet to be established.

These controversial problems are illustrated and discussed in greater detail in Chapter 25 of this book.

References

1. Cushing, H.: The meningiomas (dural endotheliomas). Their source and favoured seats of origin. (Cavendish lecture.) *Brain 45: 282–316, 1922.*
2. Cushing, H., and Eisenhardt, L.: *Meningiomas. Their Classification, Regional Behaviour, Life History and Surgical End Results.* Springfield, Ill., Charles C Thomas, 1938.

CHAPTER 2

The Nature of Meningothelial Cells (Meningocytes, Meningoblasts) as Reflected in the Nomenclature of Meningiomas

It is probably not an exaggeration to say that no other neoplasm in human pathology has caused so much difficulty for those who tried to coin an appropriate name for it. This is because meningiomas are derived from cells of the arachnoid membrane—in particular, the external covering cell layers of the membrane (arachnoidal cap cells)—which, in many ways, are unique in structure and function. True, there are other areas in the body where basically nonepithelial cells assume the role of covering a surface or lining a cavity: mesothelial cells covering serous membranes, and synovial cells lining joints, bursae, and tendon sheaths, come to mind. What all these cells have in common is that although they are not truly epithelial cells, by covering a surface as a continuous layer, they perform the functions of epithelium. Mesothelial and synovial cells maintain their contact with the underlying mesenchyme. When they form neoplasms (mesotheliomas, synoviomas), such tumors, not surprisingly, often show a mixture of mesenchymal and "epithelial" characteristics, hence the well-known fibrous and papillary mesotheliomas and the synovial sarcomas, which have a biphasic pattern.

In many respects, the arachnoidal cap cells have similar characteristics. Disregarding for the moment polemics about alternate origins from the neural crest or mesoderm, by the time the pia and arachnoid membranes are fully formed, they represent essentially well-vascularized connective tissue. In the outer zone of the arachnoid, the cells are more closely packed (epithelial function), but in deeper layers of that membrane the intercellular connections are looser and between the pia and arachnoid one finds septa with fibroblasts.Not surprisingly, therefore, many meningiomas are also biphasic, containing mixtures of meningothelial and fibroblastic elements, often with no sharp demarcation between these components (transitional meningiomas). Here, however, the similarity to mesotheliomas and synoviomas ends, because the arachnoidal cap cells also have some special characteristics unparalleled in other organs or tissues of the body. First, the epithelia of the body cavities as well as the mesothelium of the serous membranes and the synovia of joints form the *innermost* lining cell layer of their respective cavities. This does not apply to arachnoidal cells. If one can talk of a cavity at all, with respect to the meninges, the subarachnoid space in which the cerebrospinal fluid (CSF) circulates comes to mind. Yet, the arachnoidal cap cells do *not* form the inner lining of that space; rather, they seal it off from the outside, while they themselves are facing the dura mater. This is certainly different from lining a cavity, as under normal circumstances there is hardly such a thing as a subdural space unless it is expanded or created under pathologic conditions by hemorrhage, serous fluid, or pus. As a matter of fact, recent studies have shown that the outermost arachnoidal cells are contiguous with the inner cell layer of the dura mater. Electron microscopic studies of normal meninges by Andres,[1] Klika and Zajicova,[2] Rascol and Izard,[3] among others, and more recently by Schachenmayr and Friede,[4] clearly indicate that when *in situ* fixation of the cranial contents is carried out, the cranial meninges of humans do not include a subdural space. The dura and leptomeninges are said to be connected by a tight layer of cells called the interface layer—the neurothelium of Andres and of Rascol and Izard—itself composed of two layers—the arachnoid barrier layer and the innermost portion of the dura mater, the so-called dural border cells. These latter two layers are very intimately fused. But because no collagen fibers connect them, they can easily be ripped apart when manipulated, the tear usually occurring within the layer of the dural border cells. Such separation of cell layers may occur at autopsy or surgery when the dura is being reflected from the brain, or under pathologic conditions, for example, in subdural hematomas. Of the two layers forming the interface between the dura and arachnoid, the inner arachnoid barrier layer usually has electron-lucent cells with many tonofibrils and there are many tight junctions, with desmosomes and gap junctions between them. Such junctions are felt by Schachenmayr and Friede to correspond in tightness to interendothelial junctions of cerebral capillaries, and indeed they seem to be most responsible for sealing in the spinal fluid within the subarachnoid space. By contrast, the dural border cells have much fewer tight junctions.

The arachnoidal barrier cells are separated from the rest of the arachnoid tissue by a thin basal lamina (Fig. 167). No such lamina exists between the dural border cells and their zone of transition to the less cellular and more collagenous portions of the dura.

The arachnoidal cells are also different from mesothelium and synovium in other respects. Their job is not only to seal the subarachnoid space—from the outside—but in certain strategic areas, namely, the arachnoid villi, they serve as conduits for the CSF into the venous circulation of the dural sinuses. No such function is needed in serous cavities, joints, bursae, or tendon sheaths. The most the lining cells accomplish there is to produce a lubricating fluid to facilitate motions involving the cavity walls.

In addition to this different—one might safely say unique—function and differentiation of arachnoidal cap cells, their cellular morphology, as perceived by light and electron microscopy, is also essentially unparalleled. No other cell known to histologists has the tendency to form cellular whorls to the extent that meningothelial cells do. It is an inherent characteristic of these cells, not forced on them by pressures of spatial requirements or other external causes. They form whorls in tissue cultures and, if provided appropriate three-dimensional scaffolding in culture,[5] these whorls will also be three-dimensional, that is, globular. Such whorls may be found in the normal meninges, not just in meningiomas, and even in the non-neoplastic stage, they often undergo hyalinization and calcification, a feature easily seen in normal arachnoidal villi. When viewed under the electron microscope, many meningothelial cells, both in the normal state and in neoplasms, display an exaggerated interdigitation of cell membranes that is also unparalleled in other tissues, and which, because of its intricacy, cannot always be resolved by the light microscope, causing an apparent blurring of cell membranes[6–8] that has led, in neoplastic forms, to the term *syncytial meningioma*. The above-mentioned biphasic nature of some meningiomas, and particularly the fact that in some the fibroblastic component dominates the histologic appearance, created an additional difficulty in coining an appropriate name for these tumors. Pre-Cushing investigators tried valiantly to express the nature of this neoplasm, using familiar histologic terms. They found, however, that this tumor was an apparent hybrid between a known component, for example, fibroblasts, and another cell, the arachnoidal cap cell, which, as stated earlier, basically has no real counterpart in human or animal histology. Trying to fit such a neoplasm into the existing categories of tumor nomenclature truly amounted to the proverbial attempt to force a square peg into a round hole. For example, to call the tumor *meningothelioma* would at least recognize the unique and special character of one of its most important constituents, but such a term would be insufficient if applied to a variant that, for the most part, is of a fibroblastic or vascular character. These difficulties were there from the beginning; names for meningiomas were chosen on the basis of the particular histologic feature that seemed most important to those trying to coin an appropriate name. Cushing and Eisenhardt provide a magnificent historic review of the kaleidoscopic development of terms in historic sequence, beginning with early papers on the subject when meningiomas were thought to derive from the dura mater[9,10] until two anatomists (Cleland[11] and Robin[12]) and a pathologist (Schmidt[13]) recognized the histologic similarities between meningiomas and normal arachnoidal villi.

The histologic diversity of these tumors, and the above-mentioned difficulty in finding terms analogous with names of tumors elsewhere in the body, resulted in Cruveilhier's[14] considering them carcinomas, and in Virchow's[10] hedging, "Ein gewisser Theil zum Krebs gehört, aber es gibt auch 'unzweifelhafte Sarkome'." [A certain part belongs to cancer, but there are also unquestionably sarcomas among them.] The preoccupation with the calcifying element in the tumor was reflected in Virchow's *Gehirnsandgeschwülste* (*Brain-sand tumors*, for psammomas). Golgi[15] called them endotheliomas, but Hortega del Rio[16] believed that because the cells of origin were external to a membrane, the tumor should be called a meningo*exothelioma*. Emphasizing their presumed fibroblastic character, Mallory[17] called them arachnoidal fibroblastomas, while Penfield[18] preferred meningeal fibroblastomas. Other interesting names in the list include the one proposed by Cornil and Ranvier,[19] sarcome angiolithique, and finally a somewhat bizarre example, Hansemann's[20] subclassification of this tumor into such entities as sarcoma endotheliale, carcinoma endotheliale, carcinoma sarcomatodes endotheliale, and adenoma endotheliale.

Under these conditions, there can be no question that Cushing rendered an enormous service to pathologists and clinicians alike by coining the term meningioma for primary tumors of the meninges, whether they seemed predominantly to involve the dura, the leptomeninges, or both. Whereas this term may not be the answer to all questions of ultimate histogenesis, it appropriately describes and identifies these tumors for neurosurgeons and pathologists alike. The term meningioma is *not* an oversimplification of the problem as some critics of Cushing have suggested. On the contrary, it does what none of the previous terms did: it recognizes the special character and uniqueness of these meningeal tumors as contrasted with all the other known tumors of the body and leaves histologic classification within this group of tumors a subsequent, but different, task. As is well known, Dr. Cushing did not spare his efforts in this second task either, and together with Dr. Eisenhardt, described and discussed nine major types and no less than 22 variants of meningiomas, on the basis of histological appearances.

From the review of the history of nomenclature, it is clear that one of the important developments was the recognition of the relationship between meningiomas and the arachnoid mater. It follows, then, that the understanding of the ultimate derivation of meningiomas must necessarily tie in with the embryology of the leptomeninges, and in particular with that of the arachnoid membrane. The next section, therefore, reviews the conflicting views that still exist regarding this subject.

References

1. Andres, K.H.: Ueber die Feinstruktur der Arachnoidea und Dura mater von Mammalia. *Z. Zellforsch. Mikrosk. Anat. 79: 272–295, 1967.*
2. Klika, E., and Zajicova, A.: The development of meninges in chicken embryos. *Anat. Anz. 140: 379–386, 1976.*
3. Rascol, M.M., and Izard, J.Y.: The subdural neurothelium of the cranial meninges in man. *Anat. Rec. 186: 429–436, 1976.*
4. Schachenmayr, W., and Friede, R.L.: The origin of subdural neomembranes. I. Fine structure of the dura-arachnoid interface in man. *Am. J. Pathol. 92: 53–61, 1978.*
5. Kersting, G., and Lennarzt, H.: In vitro cultures of human meningioma tissue. *J. Neuropathol. Exp. Neurol. 16: 507–513, 1957.*
6. Luse, S.A.: Electron microscopic studies of brain tumors. *Neurology (Minneapolis) 10: 881–905, 1960.*
7. Kepes, J.: Electron microscopic studies of meningiomas. *Am. J. Pathol. 39: 499–510, 1961.*
8. Napolitano, L., Kyle, R., and Fisher, E.R.: Ultrastructure of meningiomas and the derivation and nature of their cellular components. *Cancer 17: 233–241, 1963.*
9. Louis, A.: Mémoire sur les tumeurs fongeuses de la duremère. *Mem. Acad. R. Chir. (Paris) 5: 1–59, 1774.*
10. Virchow, R.: *Die krankhaften Geschwülste.* Berlin, Hirschwald, 1864, Vol. II, p. 343.
11. Cleland, J.: Description of two tumours adherent to the deep surface of the dura mater. *Glasg. Med. J. 11: 148–159, 1864.*
12. Robin, C.: Recherches anatomiques sur l'epithelioma des séreuses. *J. Anat. 6: 239–288, 1869.*
13. Schmidt, M.: Ueber die Pacchionischen Granulationen u. ihr Verhältniss zu den Sarcomen und Psammomen der Dura mater. *Virchows Arch. [Pathol. Anat.] 170: 429–464, 1902.*
14. Cruveilhier, J.: Anatomie pathologique du corps humain. Paris, J.B. Baillière, 8, 1829–1835.
15. Golgi, C.: Sulla struttura e sullo sviluppo degli psammomi. *Morgagni, Napoli 11: 874–886, 2869.*
16. Hortega del Rio, P.: Para el mejor conocimiento histologico de los meningoexotheliomas. *Arch. Esp. Oncol. 1: 477–570, 1930.*
17. Mallory, F.B.: The type cell of the so-called dural endothelioma. *J. Med. Res. 41: 349–364, 1920.*
18. Penfield, W.: Tumors of the sheaths of the nervous system. *In Penfield's Cytology and Cellular Pathology of the Nervous System*, New York, Hoeber, 1932, Vol. 3, pp. 953–990.
19. Cornil, A.V., and Ranvier, L.A.: Manuel d'histologie pathologique. Paris, Germer-Baillière, 1881–1884, p. 756.
20. Hansemann, D.: Ueber Endotheliome. *Dtsch. Med. Wochenschr. 22: 52–53, 1896.*

CHAPTER 3

Embryology of the Meninges and Its Relationship to Concepts of Meningiomas

If one examines the extensive literature on the development of the cranial and spinal meninges, it becomes immediately apparent that a large consensus exists. Nevertheless, there are also questions being debated.

The consensus relates the fact that in the early development of the human embryo a layer of mesenchymal tissue comes to surround the neural tube, later condensing to form the coverings (primitive meninx) of the brain and spinal cord.

Whereas there seems to be general agreement about this primitive mesenchymal mass located between the neural tissue and ectoderm, being the source of all the meninges—dura as well as pia-arachnoid—a controversy exists about participation of neural crest elements in the formation of this primitive meninx.

This debate, reviewed in detail by Sensenig,[1] is an old one: Bischoff[2] suggested in 1852 that all the meninges—dura mater as well as pia-arachnoid—are derived from neural elements, whereas Kölliker[3] believed in an origin from a mesenchymal mass similar to Wharton's jelly. Reichert[4] favored a compromise; he regarded the dura and outer arachnoid as being derived from the mesenchyme, the inner arachnoid, and pia from the neural crest. Harvey and Burr[5] and later Harvey *et al.*[6] conducted interesting transplantation experiments on amblystoma, frog, and chicken embryos. They found that homo- as well as heterotransplants of developing brains without neural crest elements failed to have leptomeninges formed around them, whereas if the brains were transplanted together with neural crest tissue, the leptomeninges did develop appropriately. But even these investigators stressed that they thought only a part of the leptomeninges developed from the neural crest and they considered the dura entirely as mesodermal in origin. The notion that neural crest elements are involved in the formation of leptomeninges was supported by Hörstadius.[7] Spinal meninges, according to Sensenig,[1] arise predominantly from paraxial somatic mesenchyme with neural crest cells primarily involved in the formation of the pia mater. As recently as 1973, Gil and Ratto[8] observed what they believed were leptomeningeal membranes, developing directly from the everted lips of the neural tube in a human embryo. Some recent texts in embryology, however, seem to favor mesenchymal origin of the meninges: neither Allan[9] nor Snell[10] mentions neural crest elements in the formation of the definitive meninx, and Bodemer[11] does not include the meninges in the list of neural crest derivatives. On the other hand, Moore[12] holds out the possibility that the innermost layer of the primitive meninx "may be derived from the neural crest," and Harrison[13] simply states that the primitive meninx is composed of mesoderm entangled with cells from the neural crest.

It would seem, then, that even the proponents of neural crest participation in the formation of the meninges believed that this was most pronounced in the layer closest to the surface of the brain and spinal cord—the future pia mater. Yet, to the observer of the normal mature meninges, it must be obvious that the pia mater is composed of rather conventional loose vascular connective tissue—it is the *outer* layers of the arachnoid, located much farther away from the cerebral surface, that do not resemble, either by light or electron micoscopy, conventional mesenchymal elements.

The histomorphology of the arachnoidal cap cells or meningothelium is so unique that it does not provide clues to its developmental origins, since, as was pointed out earlier, it simply has no totally analogous counterpart among tissue either of neuroectodermal or of mesenchymal derivation. In an attempt to apply data from embryology to our understanding of meningiomas, it should not be neglected that, at least in terms of variants of meningiomas, all these tissues seem to follow mesenchymal lines (such forms as fibroblastic, xanthomatous, chondroblastic, angioblastic, and so forth). No transformation either to neuronal or glial cells has been observed in meningiomas, nor has electron microscopy as yet demonstrated the presence of neurosecretory granules in meningiomas on record, as one might see in some other tumors of supposed neural crest derivation. One case, however, has been reported by Gabriel and Harrison,[14] in which a meningioma apparently had functional characteristics of a pheochromocytoma and caused elevated urinary vanillylmandelic acid (VMA) levels. There is also a case of an orbital neoplasm observed by Amemiya and Kadoya[15]; this tumor contained membrane-bound granules, but otherwise had the light and electron microscopic features of a mengioma. The authors considered this tumor a paraganglioma, but the neurosecretory nature of the few granules in the tumor cells needs further documentation.

From the pathogenetic standpoint, a relationship between meningiomas and neural crest derivates is suggested by the occurrence of meningiomas, often in the multiple form, in von Recklinghausen's neurofibromatosis. Also, occasional tumors with features suggesting derivation of both meningeal and Schwann cell elements have been described.[16] (Interestingly, however, Feigin[16] thought this could best be explained by considering both the meningothelial and the Schwann cell elements of such tumors to be derived from a common *mesenchymal* origin.) The precise reason of participation of meningiomas in von Recklinghausen's disease is not known. Whereas it appears that the abnormal growth potential of neuroectodermal elements has an effect on meningeal tissues, this fact by itself does not establish a histogenetic relationship between the neural crest and meninges and awaits further explanation. One must remember that, while patients with neurofibromatosis often display abnormalities of ectodermal elements (e.g., café-au-lait spots, gliomas of the optic nerve, ependymomas, syringomyelia), some also have nonectodermal neoplasms (e.g., rhabdomyosarcomas, liposarcomas),[17] tumors clearly of mesodermal origin composed of blood vessels or striated muscle cells and fat cells.*

Since in many respects meningiomas and their variants behave as mesodermal tumors, Rubinstein[18] did not hesitate to include them under the heading of mesodermal neoplasms of the nervous system. The present author agrees with this overall view of the nature of meningiomas, regardless of the possibility that neural crest elements might have contributed to the development of the meninges.

* This does not, of course, rule out nonmesenchymal origin entirely. Smooth muscle cells of the iris, of ectodermal origin, do not appear different from "ordinary" smooth muscle cells of mesenchymal origin found in other organs. The iris, interestingly, may give rise to a tumor with mesectodermal characteristics,[19] a tumor having muscle and neural elements, which, however, has no counterpart among meningiomas.

References

1. Sensenig, E.C.: The early development of the meninges of the spinal cord in human embryos. *Contrib. Embryol. 34: 145–157, 1951.*
2. Bischoff, Th. L.W.: Entwicklungsgeschichte der Säugethiere and des Menschen. 575, Leipzig 1842.
3. Von Kölliker, A.: Entwicklungsgeschichte des Menschen und der höheren Thiere, Leipzig, 1861, p. 468.
4. Reichert, K.B.: Der Bau des menschlichen Gehirns durch Abbildungen mit erläuterndem Texte dargestellt. Leipzig, 1859, p. 192.
5. Harvey, S.C., and Burr, H.S.: The development of the meninges. *Arch. Neurol. Psychiatry 15: 545–567, 1926.*
6. Harvey, S.C., Burr, H.S., and Van Campenhout, E.: Development of the meninges. Further experiments. *Arch. Neurol. Psychiatry 29: 683–690, 1933.*
7. Hörstadius, S.: *The Neural Crest. Its Properties and Derivatives in the Light of Experimental Research.* London, Oxford University Press, 1950.
8. Gil, D.R., and Ratto, G.D.: Contribution to the study of the origin of leptomeninges in the human embryo. *Acta Anat. (Basel) 85: 620–623, 1973.*
9. Allan, F.D.: *Essentials of Human Embryology.* London–Toronto, Oxford University Press, 1973, p. 310.
10. Snell, R.: *Clinical Embryology for Medical Students.* Boston, Little, Brown, 1972, p. 234.
11. Bodemer, C.W.: *Modern Embryology.* New York, Holt, Rinehart, 1968, p. 234.
12. Moore, K.L.: *The Developing Human.* Philadelphia, W.B. Saunders, 1973, p. 310.
13. Harrison, R.G.: *Clinical Embryology.* London, Academic Press, 1978, p. 58.
14. Gabriel, R., and Harrison, B.D.: Meningioma mimicking features of a phaeochromocytoma. *Br. Med. J. 2(194): 312, 1974.*

15. Amemiya, T., and Kadoya, M.: Paraganglioma in the orbit.
J. Cancer Res. Clin. Oncol. 96: 169–179, 1980.

16. Feigin, I.: Mixed mesenchymal tumors: Meningioma and nerve sheath tumor.
J. Neuropathol. Exp. Neurol. 37: 459–470, 1978.

17. D'Agostino, A.N., Soule, E.H., and Miller, R.H.: Sarcomas of the peripheral nerves and somatic soft tissues associated with multiple neurofibromatosis (von Recklinghausen's disease).
Cancer 16: 1015–1027, 1963.

18. Rubinstein, L.J.: Tumors of the central nervous system. *Atlas of Tumor Pathology.* Washington, D.C., Armed Forces Institute of Pathology, 1972, Vol. 6, p. 169.

19. Jakobiec, F.A., Font, R.L., Tso, M.O.M., and Zimmerman, L.E.: Mesectodermal leiomyoma of the ciliary body.
Cancer 39: 2102–2113, 1977.

CHAPTER 4

Meningiomas Occurring in Animals

Meningiomas are not exclusively human tumors. Quite apart from experimentally induced neoplasms (*vide infra*), the spontaneous occurrence of meningiomas in a wide variety of animals, large and small, has been well documented in the veterinary literature. Among the large animals, meningiomas have been found in horses, cattle, sheep,[1] and even in bullock.[2] McGrath[3] in 1956 reported his observations on five meningiomas in dogs aged 7–10 years. Three of the animals were females, two males. Another particularly useful clinical pathologic review of meningiomas in dogs was provided by Andrews,[4] who added three cases to 28 from the literature. Meningiomas in dogs can occur at various intracranial sites, but as in their human counterparts, most of them are found on the surfaces of the brain.[5] Blanton[6] observed a male Golden Retriever whose meningioma encircled the brainstem and infiltrated the nervous parenchyma. Intraorbital meningiomas also occur in dogs. In Buyuhmikci's[7] case, the tumor behind the eyeball contained islands of cartilage as well. Langham *et al.*[8] described a more conventional retrobulbar meningioma of the optic sheath that had not penetrated the eyeball, but in one of Andrews's[4] cases, the tumor invaded the globe through the optic disk precisely as it happens in some human cases. Canine meningiomas are not restricted to the cranial cavity. Zaki *et al.*,[9] in a study of six spinal tumors in dogs, found two of them to be meningiomas, and Vuletin[10] found a meningioma in the subcutaneous tissue of the shoulder in a dog. Cats also develop meningiomas. Luginbuehl's[11] careful autopsy study of 165 cats demonstrated meningiomas in eight. Interestingly, seven were located in the tela chorioidea of the third ventricle, and two had, in addition, multiple meningiomas on the convexity. In cats spinal meningiomas occasionally develop as in the case reported by Jones.[12]

Even small rodents can have meningiomas, although not commonly. Fitzgerald *et al.*[13] found three instances of meningeal tumors in 7803 autopsies of albino rats. These were quite fibroblastic and mostly plaquelike, apparently lacking a meningothelial pattern.

References

1. Innes, J.R.M., and Saunders, L.Z.: *Comparative Neuropathology*, New York, Academic Press, 1962, pp. 728–731.
2. Yadgirker, G., Rao, P., and Naidu, N.R.: Meningioma. A case report in bullock. *Indian Vet. J. 47: 561–562, 1970.*
3. McGrath, J.T.: Neurologic examination of the dog, with clinicopathologic observations. Philadelphia, Lea & Febiger, 1956, pp. 109–110, 115.
4. Andrews, E.J.: Clinicopathologic characteristics of meningiomas in dogs. *J. Am. Vet. Med. Assoc. 163: 151–157, 1973.*
5. Simon, J., and Stone, A.B.: A psammous meningioma in a dog. *J. Am. Vet. Med. Assoc. 156: 1574–1576, 1970.*
6. Blanton, L.H., Jr.: Epilepsy due to infiltrating meningioma in a dog. *J. Am. Vet. Med. Assoc. 166: 448, 1975.*
7. Buyukmihci, N.: Orbital meningioma with intraocular invasion in a dog. Histology and ultrastructure. *Vet. Pathol. 14: 521–523, 1977.*
8. Langham, R.F., Bennett, R.R., and Zydeck, F.A.: Primary retrobulbar meningioma of the optic nerve of a dog. *J. Am. Vet. Med. Assoc. 159: 175–176, 1971.*
9. Zaki, F.A., Prata, R.G., Hurwitz, A.I., and Kay, W.J.: Primary tumors of the spinal cord and meninges in six dogs. *J. Am. Vet. Med. Assoc. 166: 511–517, 1975.*
10. Vuletin, J.C., Friedman, H., and Gordon, W.: Extraneuraxial canine meningioma. A light and electron microscopic study. *Vet. Pathol. 15: 481–487, 1978.*
11. Luginbuehl, H.S.: Studies on meningiomas in cats. *Am. J. Vet. Res. 22: 1030–1040, 1961.*
12. Jones, B.R.: Spinal meningioma in a cat. *Aust. Vet. J. 50: 229–231, 1974.*
13. Fitzgerald, J.E., Schardein, J.L., and Kurtz, S.M.: Spontaneous tumors of the nervous system in albino rats. *J. Natl. Cancer Inst. 52: 265–273, 1974.*

CHAPTER 5

Experimental Meningiomas

Induction of tumors in experimental animals, with the purpose of studying the development and biological behavior of neoplastic tissue under laboratory conditions, was first accomplished with extraneural tumors. Later, using similar carcinogenic methods, tumors of the nervous system in animals were produced. These methods include chemical carcinogens, oncogenic viruses, and irradiation. Another way in which experimental animals are used for the study of tumors is through heterotransplantation of human neoplasms into animals.

CHEMICAL CARCINOGENS

The first highly effective agents whereby neoplasms were induced in laboratory animals were members of the aromatic hydrocarbon series. One such chemical, styril-430—formerly used in the chemotherapy of trypanosomiasis—was injected intracerebrally in white rats by Weil.[1] This resulted in the first successfully produced brain tumors using this method. Of the five tumors thus induced, one was a meningeal neoplasm with meningioma-like formation containing whorls and collagen. Seligman *et al.*[2] were able to produce various kinds of brain tumors, including two meningeal sarcomas through intracranial implantation of 20-methylcholanthrene pellets in mice. Sweet and Bailey[3] used intracerebral injection of 20-methylcholanthrene to induce a meningeal fibroblastoma in a white rat, and Greenwood (cited in Sweet and Bailey[3]) in the same year also induced a meningioma in a rat using the same substance. Similar results were achieved in mice with the use of methylcholanthrene in 1941,[4] and with 3,4-benzpyrene in 1943 by Zimmerman and Arnold,[5] and with 1,2,5,6-dibenzanthracene by Arnold and Zimmerman,[6] also in 1943. The latter experiments also induced gliomas while the meningeal tumors were of a sarcomatous nature. Vazquez-Lopez[7] in 1945 was the first to produce a brain tumor (glioma) by *feeding* a carcinogenic substance (2-acetylaminofluorene) to an albino rat, and Hoch-Ligeti and Russell[8] succeeded in producing, in addition to numerous gliomas, a rather typical meningothelial meningioma in a Wistar rat through the feeding of the same substance. Oyasu *et al.*,[9] using the same method, induced two malignant meningeal tumors in rats.

ONCOGENIC VIRUSES

Some of the viruses previously known for their general carcinogenic effect have also been found capable of inducing the formation of intracranial tumors, including meningeal neoplasms. The Rous sarcoma virus was used by Rabotti *et al.*[10] to produce gliomas and meningeal sarcomas in dogs. Later, meningothelial as well as sarcomatous tumors were also induced in dogs by intracranial inoculation of Rous sarcoma virus. Haguenau *et al.*[11] produced 64 brain tumors, 44 of which were meningiomas, in a total of 74 dogs. Using guinea pigs, Ahlstrom *et al.*[12] injected Rous sarcoma virus and produced 10 meningiomas and meningosarcomas. Bucciarelli *et al.*,[13] who induced meningiomas and sarcomas in 11 dogs, were also able to show the presence of viral particles in tumor cells by electron microscopy. Using bovine papilloma virus (BPV), an agent known to produce skin papillomas as well as fibroblastic tumors of soft tissues, Gordon and Olson[14] produced meningiomas in cats and Robl *et al.*[15] in hamsters. Lancaster *et al.*[16] examined meningiomas produced by BPV in calves; no virus particles were seen using electron microscopy, but they could nevertheless detect the BPV viral genome in diploid tumor cell nuclei after labeling viral DNA with ^{32}P and ^{3}H.

IRRADIATION

There is much evidence pointing to the role of irradiation as a cause for the development of meningiomas in humans (*vide infra*). Dimant *et al.*[17] succeeded in inducing meningeal tumors in rabbits by the use of irradiation. They implanted cobalt-60 (15 μCi) in the spinal intradural space and were able to produce three tumors: two fibroblastic meningiomas and one sarcoma.

HETEROTRANSPLANTATION OF MENINGIOMAS

Another facet of the experimental work with meningiomas relates to growing human meningioma cells outside the human body. The two main avenues used are 1) explantation into tissue and organ cultures (see Chapter 28), and 2) xeno- or heterotransplantation into animals. The first to transplant human brain tumors into the anterior chamber of the guinea pig's eye were Greene and Arnold,[18] whose material included meningiomas. These investigators found that endothelial meningiomas were transferable, but that fibroblastic meningiomas were not. They wondered if this might be related to the possible neural crest origin of endothelial meningiomas. Greene[19] also transplanted human brain tumors, including meningiomas, into the brains of laboratory animals, using guinea pigs and mice. Transplanted meningiomas can have quite a devastating effect on the recipient animal. Ueyama *et al.*[20] transplanted human brain tumors into nude mice. The intracranial tumor they used was a peritorcular meningioma having a storiform pattern and fibroblastic characteristics. The transplant in the nude mice began growing in 3 weeks. The animals died in 16 weeks as a result of the enlarging tumor mass if it was not removed by that time. In those animals in which the tumor was surgically excised prior to 16 weeks, the animals lived longer, but in 50% pulmonary metastases developed. The tumor was more cellular in the transplant. Not only mature animals can be used for heterotransplants: the chorioallantoic membrane of the chick embryo has also been used to grow meningiomas; for example, Vogel and Berry[21] found it easy to grow meningiomas as well as other tumors in this tissue.

References

1. Weil, A.: Experimental production of tumor in the brains of white rats. *Arch. Pathol. Lab. Med. 26: 776–790, 1938.*
2. Seligman, A.M., Shear, M.J., and Alexander, L.: Studies in carcinogenesis. VIII. Experimental production of brain tumors in mice with methylcholanthrene. *Am. J. Cancer 37: 364–399, 1939.*
3. Sweet, W.H., and Bailey, P.: Experimental production of intracranial tumors in the white rat. *Arch. Neurol. Psych. 45: 1047–1049, 1941.*
4. Zimmerman, H.M., and Arnold, H.: Experimental brain tumors. I. Tumors produced with methylcholanthrene. *Cancer Res. 1: 919–938, 1941.*
5. Zimmerman, H.M., and Arnold, H.: Experimental brain tumors. II. Tumors produced with benzypyrene. *Am. J. Pathol. 19: 939–956, 1943.*
6. Arnold, H., and Zimmerman, H.M.: Experimental brain tumors. III. Tumors produced with dibenzanthracene. *Cancer Res. 3: 682–65, 1943.*
7. Vazquez-Lopez, E.: Glioma in a rat fed with 2-acetyl-amino-fluorene. *Nature 156: 296–297, 1945.*
8. Hoch-Ligeti, C., and Russell, D.S.: Primary tumors of the brain and meninges in rats fed 2-acetylaminofluorene. *Acta Union Int. Contr. Cancer 7: 126–129, 1951.*
9. Oyasu, R., Battifora, H.A., Clasen, R.A., McDonald, J.H., and Hass, G.M.: Induction of cerebral gliomas in rats with dietary lead subacetate and 2-acetylaminofluorene. *Cancer Res. 30: 1248–1261, 1970.*
10. Rabotti, G.F., Grove, A.S., Sellers, R.L., and Anderson, W.R.: Induction of multiple brain tumors (gliomata and leptomeningeal sarcomata) in dogs. *Nature 209: 884–886, 1966.*
11. Haguenau, F., Rabotti, G.F., Lyon, G., and Moraillon, A.: Tumeurs cérébrales experimentales d'étiologie virale chez le chien. Leur similitude histologique avec les tumeurs humaines démontrée par une épendymome. *Rev. Neurol. (Paris) 126: 347–370, 1972.*
12. Ahlstrom, C.G., Olin, T., and Smitterberg, B.: Intracranial tumors induced in guinea pigs with Rous sarcoma virus. *Acta. Pathol. Microbiol. Scand. [c] 82: 326–336, 1974.*
13. Bucciarelli, E., Rabotti, G.F., and Dalton, A.J.: Ultrastructure of meningeal tumors induced in dogs with Rous sarcoma virus. *J.Natl. Cancer Inst. 38: 359–31, 1967.*
14. Gordon, D.E., and Olson, C.: Meningiomas and fibroblastic neoplasia in calves induced with the bovine papilloma virus. *Cancer Res. 28: 2423–2431, 1968.*
15. Robl, M.G., Gordon, D.E., Lee, K.P., and Olson, C.: Intracranial fibroblastic neoplasms in the hamster from bovine papilloma virus. *Cancer Res. 32: 2221–2223, 1972.*
16. Lancaster, W.D., Olson, C., and Meinke, W.: Quantitation of bovine papilloma viral DNA in viral-induced tumors. *J. Virol. 17: 824–831, 1976.*
17. Dimant, I.N., Loktionov, G.M., and Sataev, M.M.: Induction of spinal cord meningeal tumor in rabbits with radio-active cobalt. *Vopr. Onkol. 11: 46–53, 1965.*
18. Greene, H.S.N., and Arnold, H.: The homologous and heterologous transplantation of brain and brain tumors. *J. Neurosurg. 2: 315–331, 1945.*
19. Greene, H.S.N.: The transplantation of human brain tumors to the brains of laboratory animals. *Cancer Res. 13: 422–426, 1953.*
20. Ueyama, Y., Morita, K., Ochiai, C., Ohsawa, N., Hata, J., and Tamaoki, N.: Xenotransplantation of a human meningioma and its lung metastasis in nude mice. *Br. J. Cancer 37: 644–647, 1978.*
21. Vogel, H.B., and Berry, R.G.: Chorioallantoic membrane heterotransplantation of human brain tumors. *Int. J. Cancer 15: 401–408, 1975.*

CHAPTER 6

Theories on the Etiology of Human Meningiomas

It is probably safe to say that the etiology of most naturally occurring meningiomas, as with other intracranial neoplasms, is yet unknown. Nevertheless, there are some factors that have been and are being considered as playing a role in causation, either by themselves or in association with unknown factors: genetic factors, trauma, irradiation, and oncogenic viruses.

GENETIC FACTORS

The occurrence of meningiomas in several members of the same family, with or without von Recklinghausen's disease, suggests the presence of a genetic factor promoting the development of meningiomas. This subject is discussed in Chapter 11.

TRAUMA

The role of trauma in the formation of neoplasms in general, and of meningiomas in particular, has been the subject of lively debate over the years—one that is likely to provoke a heated controversy even today, particularly as it may be the subject of litigation in the case of patients with a history of head trauma in whom a brain tumor of any type develops at a later time. But it seems that there is more evidence suggestive of trauma playing a role in the development of meningioma than in the case of other brain tumors.

Keen[1] suggested as early as 1888 that head trauma at birth might be responsible for the development of meningiomas later in life. Cushing and Eisenhardt[2] observed that no less than 101 of their 313 patients with meningiomas had a history of some sort of head trauma, 24 of whom had actual physical evidence of previous trauma in the form of a scar, depressed fracture, or other signs. This may be regarded by some as an unconvincingly high incidence; many of the cases are said to fall under the *post hoc ergo propter hoc* argument. Indeed, some investigators, such as Dunsmore and Roberts,[3] expressed strong skepticism for any suggested relationship between trauma and meningiomas. Boldrey[4] observed wryly, "It is certainly no compliment to our civilization that a tumor more commonly encountered in women than in men should be regarded to have trauma as a major etiologic factor."

Having given skepticism its due, there are nevertheless a number of impressive cases in the literature in which the relationship between trauma and subsequent meningioma appears quite convincing. Such is the famous case of Reinhardt,[5] which involves a 58-year-old man who was injured in a boiler explosion. A flying piece of a water gauge had wounded him above the left eye. Twenty years after the accident, a calcified meningioma developed in the same area, and the tumor contained two pieces of wire within its substance. There are also a number of cases in the literature in which the patient suffered a skull fracture either from a blunt blow or from a gunshot wound, and in whom a meningioma later developed in the area that included the healed fracture line. Such patients were reported by Walshe,[6] Lanigan,[7] Turner and Laird,[8] Walsh *et al.*,[9] and others. Several attempts have been made to establish acceptable criteria for a relationship between previous trauma and the development of a tumor. Auster[10] believed that the role of trauma in oncogenesis should be verified for juridical consideration. He suggested six criteria that should be applied before such relationship can be accepted:

1. The site of injury must correspond to the region in which the tumor develops.
2. The trauma should be authentic and of sufficient importance.
3. The previous integrity of the wounded part must not be in doubt, and there must be proof

that neither primary nor metastatic malignant disease was present before injury.

4. The time interval between injury and the development of the neoplasm must be significant.
5. There must be continuity in the pathologic changes or symptoms in the wounded part from the time of injury to the appearance of the tumor.
6. There must be microscopic proof of the existence of the tumor, its character, and structure.

The above listed criteria were used, for example, in an editorial concerning trauma and tumors in *Lancet*[11] in accepting a case reported by Whatmore and Hitchcock.[12] Trauma of the spine was invoked as the cause of meningioma by Von Holländer *et al.*[13]: A 38-year-old female patient had sustained a traumatic fracture of her twelfth thoracic vertebra; 19 years later, a meningioma developed at the same site.

The third requirement of Auster, "that the previous integrity of the wounded part must not be in doubt," is often difficult to fulfill because there is always the possibility that a very early meningioma was already present at the site that accidentally became traumatized. In this respect, the case of Hung *et al.*[14] is of interest. Their patient, a 44-year-old woman, was hit over the head with a stick of wood, and later a subdural hematoma developed. This was evacuated through a frontal craniotomy, and the underlying brain was exposed. Other than some bruising, it showed no pathologic changes, specifically, no tumor was found in the area on gross inspection. Three years later, a meningioma developed in the same territory, which was then surgically removed.

In the present era of computerized axial tomography (CAT scans), Gardeur *et al.*[15] reported two cases in which a CAT scan detected a meningioma in a previously traumatized area. One of the patients was a 60-year-old man who, at the age of 20, suffered a motorcycle accident with fracture of the skull and an extradural hematoma that had to be evacuated. The CAT scan showed a meningioma just anterior to the old craniotomy wound. The second patient also had fractured his skull, and a meningioma developed 10 years later that included the fracture line.

Up to this point, the possible role of a single traumatic episode in the development of meningioma had been considered. Somewhat different is the situation in which, as a result of trauma, a subdural hematoma develops, is not evacuated, and becomes chronic, and later a meningioma forms at the same site. Such was the case described by Cusick and Bailey,[16] a patient with a bilateral ossified subdural hematoma since early childhood, in whom a meningioma later developed underlying one of the hematomas. In such a situation, the ongoing chronic irritation by pressure, and perhaps by chemical changes of the chronic subdural hematoma, rather than the injury of the original trauma, may play an etiological role.

IRRADIATION

There are several cases of meningiomas in humans wherein prior irradiation appears to have played a role in the development of the neoplasm. These reports can be roughly divided into two groups: those cases in which irradiation was necessitated by the presence of another type of brain tumor, and those in which it was done for other causes. The first report belonging to the first category was by Mann *et al.*[17] The patient, a 4-year-old boy, received 6500 rads for the treatment of a left optic nerve glioma. Five years later, a left supraorbital ridge meningioma developed, which was histologically malignant. Norwood *et al.*[18] saw a meningioma develop 25 years after irradiation of an optic nerve glioma. The tumor initially radiated was a medulloblastoma in a second case of Norwood *et al.*[18] and in the case of McCormick *et al.*[19] Gauthier-Smith[20] described a 10-year-old boy with a cerebellar astrocytoma, who was irradiated, only to develop a parasagittal meningioma 15 years later. In a patient described by Tanaka *et al.*,[21] the irradiated tumor was a frontal oligodendroglioma, with a meningioma developing 23 years later. Ependymoma was the first tumor in the case described by Bojsen-Moller and Knudsen[22] and Katakura *et al.*,[23] whereas irradiation of a pituitary adenoma preceded the development of the meningioma in a patient of Lawrence *et al.*[24] A 23-year-old female patient of Waga and Handa[25] received radiation for a craniopharyngioma. Twelve years later, she was found to have a tentorial meningioma.

In the second category (i.e., irradiation for reasons other than brain tumors), the most common indication for irradiation of the head appears to have been mycotic infection of the scalp, particularly microsporiasis. Horanyi[26] described a case of a 5-year-old girl who received 2000 rads to the scalp for tinea capitis (microsporiasis) in whom a malignant meningioma developed 2 years later. Meningiomas developed in cases of scalp irradiation in five patients of Munk *et al.*[27] in 16 patients of Beller *et al.*[28] (all for tinea), and a patient each of Waterson and Shapiro[29] and of Russell and Rubinstein.[30] Following these impressive case reports, it was not surprising that Modan *et al.*[31] found in an epidemiological study that 11,000 immigrant children in Israel, who received irradiation of the scalp for tinea at the time of their arrival, had a rate of subsequent intracranial meningiomas of 0.4/1000, as compared with an incidence of only 0.1/1000 in the control group.

There are also cases in the literature wherein the primary reason for irradiation was neither brain tumor nor skin infection. In a 32-year-old female patient of Patronas *et al.*[32] an enlarged thymus was irradiated during infancy. She was later found to have carcinoma of the thyroid, and this, too, was irradiated. Still later, three spinal meningiomas developed, all within the field of the previous irradiation. Kandel's[33] patient had a meningioma 10 years after irradiation for skin cancer of the head. Port wine stains of the face were the reason for irradiation in the cases described by Feiring and Foer[34] (using radium) and of Watts[35] (using x-rays). Meningiomas developed on the side of the treatment in both patients. The same was true for one of the three patients of Bogdanowicz and Sachs,[36] who also received radiation therapy for port wine stains (the other two patients were irradiated for acromegaly and medulloblastoma, respectively). It is possible, of course, that the presence of port wine stains on the skin may be related to future development of an underlying meningioma on the same side, even without irradiation, perhaps indicating a relationship as seen in the Sturge-Weber syndrome, in which vascular malformations of the leptomeninges parallel the presence of port wine stains on the face on the same side. Naturally, such a relationship cannot be invoked in the case of irradiated fungal infections of the scalp.

A special kind of radiation effect has been attributed to Thorotrast (thorium dioxide suspension). This substance was at one time used in diagnostic radiology. Injected intraveneously, it was phagocytized by cells of the reticuloendothelial system, thus enabling visualization of the spleen, among other organs. Thorotrast has also been used in diagnostic neuroradiology for ventriculograms and myelography. Its use was later discontinued because the agent was found to cause meningeal irritation and adhesions. Apparently in some instances it was also responsible for inducing intracranial neoplasms. Kyle *et al.*[37] reported a 25-year-old man who, as a 1-year-old child, had had ventriculography with thorium dioxide for projectile vomiting, but no abnormalities were detected at that time. Twenty-four years later, a meningioma of the sphenoid ridge developed. It was removed, and Thorotrast was found within the tumor by light microscopy as well as autoradiography. Meyer *et al.*[38] had a 56-year-old male patient who, at age 23, had Thorotrast myelography for sequela of a back injury. Thirty-three years later, a meningioma developed at the tip of the temporal bone as well as a neurilemmoma of the cerebellopontine angle, both tumors containing Thorotrast in their substance. The effect of Thorotrast, of course, has to be viewed somewhat differently from irradiation therapy, which, even if extensive, is a one-time event, whereas the Thorotrast itself was left within the CSF close to the meninges and was able to exert a prolonged effect, partly as a foreign body, but also as a source of continuous radiation.

It has also been mentioned, under experimental induction of meningiomas, that Dimant *et al.*[39] were able to induce spinal meningiomas in rabbits by subdural implantation of cobalt-60.

ONCOGENIC VIRUSES

As indicated in Chapter 5, several successful attempts have been made to induce meningeal tumors in animals with the use of oncogenic viruses. Viral agents have been suspected by some to have a role in the formation of human meningiomas as well. Both DNA and RNA viruses have been implicated. As to the former, Weiss *et al.*[40] found simian virus 40 (SV 40)-related antigens in two out of seven meningiomas examined. Weiss *et al.*[41] found such antigens in three out of eight meningiomas; the particles of this antigen were rescued, which on further examination corresponded to papovaviruses. Zang and May[42] examined the cell cultures of 27 meningioma tumor biopsies; in 11 of them, these investigators found SV 40-related T antigen by immunofluorescence. Fibroblast cultures from the same patients, and of other tumors, were always negative. These findings were not confirmed by all workers, however. Merletti *et al.*[43] analyzed eight meningiomas, finding all negative for SV 40 antigen.

As to RNA viruses, Cuatico *et al.*[44] found particles of RNA with high molecular weight and RNA-directed DNA polymerase in 3 out of 11 meningiomas. These were felt to correspond to tumor viruses in animals. Bendheim and Dinowitz[45] cultured cells from a spinal meningioma of a

17-year-old boy and found particles fulfilling standard criteria for RNA virus particles with density similar to Rous sarcoma virus.

Whereas these findings are naturally of great interest, the presence of such particles within, and their isolation from, tumor cells does not necessarily indicate an etiological relationship.

Some speculation has arisen as to the possible role of prior human viral disease in the formation of meningiomas. For example, Soo[46] described the case of a 7-year-old boy in whom a spinal epidural meningioma developed at the level of C4-5. The young patient had poliomyelitis at age 4. The patient of Ohry and Rozin[47] also had polio at age 4, which left him with substantial paralysis of the lower limbs. At age 30, a meningioma developed at D10. Again, although these appear to be noteworthy cases, caution must be exercised in assuming any causal relationship between the early viral disease and the subsequent meningioma in these patients.

References

1. Keen, W.W.: Three successful cases of cerebral surgery including: 1) the removal of a large intracranial fibroma; 2) exsection of damaged brain tissue; and 3) exsection of the cerebral center for the left hand; with remarks on the general technique of such operations. *Am. J. Med. Sci. 96: 329–357, 1888.*
2. Cushing, H., and Eisenhardt, L.: *Meningiomas: Their Classification, Regional Behaviour, Life History and Surgical End Results.* Springfield, Ill., Charles C Thomas,1938, pp. 71–73.
3. Dunsmore, R.H., and Roberts, M.: Trauma as a cause of brain tumor. A medicolegal dilemma. *Conn. Med. 38: 521–523, 1974.*
4. Boldrey, E. The meningiomas. *In Pathology of the Nervous System*, J. Minckler (ed.). New York, McGraw-Hill, 1971, pp. 2125–2144.
5. Reinhardt, G.: Trauma-Fremdkörper-Hirngeschwulst. *Münch. Med. Wchschr. 75: 399–401, 1928.*
6. Walshe, F.: Head injuries. Trauma as a factor in the aetiology of intracranial meningioma. *Lancet 2: 993–996, 1961.*
7. Lanigan, J.P.: Can a head injury cause a meningioma? *J. Irish Med. Assoc. 56: 12–13, 1965.*
8. Turner, O.A., and Laird, A.T.: Meningioma with traumatic etiology. Report of a case. *J. Neurosurg. 24: 96–98, 1966.*
9. Walsh, J., Gye, R., and Connelley, T.J.: Meningioma: A late complication of head injury. *Med. J. Aust. 1: 906–908, 1969.*
10. Auster, L.S.: The role of trauma in oncogenesis. A juridical consideration. *JAMA 175: 946–950, 1961.*
11. Editorial: Trauma and tumours. *Lancet 2: 545–546, 1973.*
12. Whatmore, W.J., and Hitchcock, E.R.: Meningioma following trauma. *Br. J. Surg. 60: 496–498, 1973.*
13. Von Holländer, H., Kosmaoglou, V., and Sturm, W.: Intraspinales Meningeom nack Wirbelfraktur. Kasuistische Mitteilung. *Zentralbl. Neurochir. 32: 179–185, 1971.*
14. Hung, C.C., Chang, W.Y., and Yao, Y.T.: Post-traumatic intracranial meningioma. *J. Formosan Med. Assoc. 71: 214–219, 1972.*
15. Gardeur, D., Allal, R., Sichez, J.P., and Metzger, J.: Post-traumatic intracranial meningiomas: Recognition by computed tomography in three cases. *J. Comput. Assist. Tomogr. 3: 103–104, 1979.*
16. Cusick, J.F., and Bailey, O.T.: Association of ossified subdural hematomas and a meningioma. Case report. *J. Neurosurg. 37: 731–734, 1972.*
17. Mann, I., Yates, P.C., and Ainslie, J.P.: Unusual case of double primary orbital tumor. *Br. J. Ophthalmol. 37: 758–762, 1953.*
18. Norwood, C.W., Kelly, D.L., Jr., Davis, C.H., and Alexander, E., Jr.: Irradiation-induced mesodermal tumors of the central nervous system: Report of two meningiomas following x-ray treatment of gliomas. *Surg. Neurol. 2: 161–164, 1964.*
19. McCormick, W.F., Menezes, A.H., and Grin, O.D., Jr.: Meningioma occurring in a patient treated for medulloblastoma. *J. Iowa Med. Soc. 62: 67–71, 1972.*
20. Gautier-Smith, P.C.: *Parasagittal and Falx Meningiomas.* London, Butterworths, 1970, p. 350.
21. Tanaka, J., Garcia, J.H., Netsky, M.C., and Williams, J.P.: Late appearance of meningioma at the site of partially removed oligodendroglioma. Case report. *J. Neurosurg. 43: 80–85, 1975.*
22. Bojsen-Moller, M., and Knudsen, V.: Radiation-induced meningeal sarcoma. A case report with review of the literature. *Acta Neurochir. 37: 147–152, 1977.*
23. Katakura, R., Ohara, H., and Sakurai, Y.: Malignant meningioma following irradiation therapy for ependymoma. *No Shinkei Geka 6: 935–939, 1978.*
24. Lawrence, J.G., Tobias, C.A., Linfoot, J.A., Born, J.L., Lyman, J.T., Chong, C.Y., Manougian, E., and Wei, W.L.: Successful treatment of acromegaly. Metabolic and clinical studies in 145 patients. *J. Clin. Endocrinol. Metab. 31: 180–198, 1970.*
25. Waga, S., and Handa, H.: Radiation-induced meningioma: With review of literature. *Surg. Neurol. 5: 215–219, 1976.*
26. Horányi, B.: Röntgen besugárzás hatására keletkezett meningeoma gyermekben. *Magy. Radiol. 17: 1–7, 1961.*
27. Munk, J., Peyser, E., and Gruszkiewica, J.: Radiation induced intracranial meningiomas. *Clin. Radiol. 20: 90–94, 1969.*
28. Beller, A.J., Feinsod, M., and Sahar, A.: The possible relationship between small dose irradiation of the scalp and intracranial meningiomas. *Neurschirurgia (Stuttg) 15:135–143, 1972.*
29. Waterson, K.W., Jr. and Shapiro, L. Meningioma cutis: Report of a case. *Int. J. Dermatol. 9: 125–129, 1970.*
30. Russell, D.S, and Rubinstein, L.J.: *Pathology of Tumours of the Nervous System*, 4th ed. Baltimore, Williams & Wilkins, 1977, p. 67.
31. Modan, B., Baidatz, D., Mart, H., Steinitz, R., and Levin, S.G.: Radiation induced head and neck tumor. *Lancet 1: 277–279, 1974.*

32. Patronas, N.J., Brown, F., and Duda, E.E.: Multiple meningiomas in the spinal cord.
Surg. Neurol. 13: 78–80, 1980.
33. Kandel, E.I.: Development of meningioma after x-ray irradiation of the head.
Vopr. Neurokhir. 1: 51–53, 1978.
34. Feiring, E.H., and Foer, W.H.: Meningioma following radium therapy. Case report.
J. Neurosurg. 29: 192–194, 1968.
35. Watts, C.: Meningioma following irradiation.
Cancer 38: 1939–1940, 1976.
36. Bogdanowicz, W.M., and Sachs, E., Jr.: The possible role of radiation in oncogenesis of meningioma.
Surg. Neurol. 2: 379–383, 1974.
37. Kyle, R.H., Oler, A., Lasser, E.C., and Rosonoff, H.L.: Meningioma induced by thorium dioxide.
N. Engl. J. Med. 268: 80–82, 1963.
38. Meyer, M.W., Powell, H.C., Wagner, M., and Niwayama, G.: Thorotrast induced adhesive arachnoiditis associated with meningioma and schwannoma.
Hum. Pathol. 9: 366–370, 1978.
39. Dimant, I.N., Loktionov, G.M., and Sataev, M.M.: Induction of spinal cord meningeal tumor in rabbit with radioactive cobalt.
Vopr. Onkol. 11: 46–53, 1965.
40. Weiss, A.F., Portmann, R., Fischer, H., Simon, J., and Zang, K.D.: Simian virus 40-related antigens in three human meningiomas with defined chromosome loss.
Proc. Natl. Acad. Sci. USA 72: 609–613, 1975.
41. Weiss, A.F., Zang, K.D., Birkmayer, G.D., and Miller, F.: SV 40-related Papova-viruses in human meningiomas.
Acta. Neuropathol. (Berl.) 34: 171–174, 1976.
42. Zang, K.D., May, G., and Fischer, H.: Expression of SV 40-related T-antigen in cell cultures of human meningiomas.
Naturwissenschaften 66: 59, 1979.
43. Merletti, L., Panichi, G., Dall'Anese, A., and Ramundo, E.: Absence of SV 40-like T antigens in human meningiomas.
Bull. Soc. Ital. Biol. Sper. 52: 755–757, 1976.
44. Cuatico, W., Cho, J.R., and Spiegelman, S.: Particles with RNA of high molecular weight and RNA-directed DNA polymerase in human brain tumors.
Proc. Natl. Acad. Sci. USA 70: 2789–2793, 1973.
45. Bendheim, P.E., and Dinowitz, M.: Particles resembling oncorna-viruses. Spontaneous release from cultured meningioma cells.
Arch. Neurol. 34: 105–108, 1977.
46. Soo, A.Y.: Spinal epidural meningioma.
South. Med. J. 59: 141–144, 1966.
47. Ohry, A., and Rozin, R.: Late neoplasia after poliomyelitis. (Letter.)
Lancet 2: 823, 1975.

CHAPTER 7

The Possible Effect of Female Sex Hormones on Meningiomas

Mostly through the study of breast carcinomas, it was discovered that certain tumors respond to estrogens by accelerated growth. It also became known that whether a tumor cell will respond to estrogen stimulation depends on the presence of estrogen receptor proteins. When estradiol enters a cell it is bound to such proteins; then the complex migrates toward the nucleus and enters it. Shortly afterward there is a noticeable increase in the cell's RNA production. Mammary cells are not the only cells containing estrogen receptors; they have been found in the liver, pancreas, leiomyomas of the uterus, carcinoma of the endometrium, ovary, and colon, malignant melanoma, and other tissues.

TUMOR CHARACTERISTICS

That sex hormone receptors may be present in meningiomas is suggested by at least three interesting characteristics of these tumors: 1) the well-known preference for females (66% of intracranial and 80% of spinal canal meningiomas occur in females, and just about all the meningiomas en plaque occur in women); 2) increased clinical manifestations of meningiomas during pregnancy and menstruation; and 3) the more-than-chance association between breast carcinoma and meningioma in the same patient.

Preference for Females

The higher incidence of meningiomas in female patients is well recognized; for example, in our Vienna series of meningiomas, the ratio of females to males was 2.5:1 in the intracranial forms and 9:1 in the spinal cases. A closer examination of the statistics demonstrates, however, that this female preponderance applies primarily to middle-aged adults. At the extremes of life one does not find this feature. When it comes to meningiomas encountered as incidental findings at autopsies of the very old, the male/female ratio was found to be about 1:1.[1] Childhood meningiomas form another exception. Of the 313 meningiomas analyzed by Cushing and Eisenhardt,[2] five were in patients under the age of 20, three of whom were boys and two of whom were girls. Even more striking, of the 700 meningiomas included in the Vienna series of 1964–1974 that we reviewed, all seven patients under the age of 20 were male. It is quite possible, even likely, that if the higher estrogen levels in females do indeed have an effect on the growth of meningiomas, such influence would not exert itself over a very short time. Even in carcinomas of the breast and of the endometrium, in which estrogens are thought by many to play a role in the formation or growth rate of the tumor, such influence is believed to be slow and cumulative. Similarly, with meningiomas, this effect would not become evident shortly after puberty or even early in childbearing age, but rather in middle-aged persons. In very old women, several decades after the menopause, the role of estrogen stimulation may once again be limited or nonexistent. This would explain the high female/male ratio in middle-aged persons as well as the lack of female prevalence at the extremes of life.[3]

Changes in Meningiomas during Pregnancy

With regard to the rapid growth of meningiomas during pregnancy, this has been best recognized in meningiomas near the sella turcica (e.g., tuberculum sellae, parasellar, medial sphenoid ridge[4]), as in these instances the optic nerves are close and changes in visual acuity secondary to increased pressure from a neighboring mass are quickly noticeable by patients. Cushing and Eisenhardt[5] called attention to this phenomenon in 1929 (case 11 in their study). Their 52-year-old patient with a meningioma growing between the optic nerves experienced exacerbation of visual problems during her pregnancies. Similar instances were reported by Fischer,[6] Hagedoorn,[7] Walsh,[8] and Rucker and Kearns.[9] Weyand *et al.*[10] discussed the effects of pregnancies on intracranial meningiomas occurring above the optic chiasm in 10 patients. In those meningiomas surgically removed and histologically examined they could find no suggestion for increased rate of growth; that is, there was no increase in mitoses or anaplasia. They thought, however, that the tumor cells showed signs of hydropic swelling, as well as vacuolation, suggesting tissue edema.

It is difficult to estimate the relative importance of tumor enlargement versus the role of cerebral edema in hydremia of pregnancy, but at least it has been documented through serial angiograms by Michelsen and New[11] that a frontal mass caused by a meningioma in their patient decreased in size after her pregnancy terminated.

Correlation with Breast Carcinoma

As to the relationship between breast carcinoma and meningioma, numerous cases of patients suffering from both these tumors are on record. Fényes and Kepes[12] reported a patient with carcinoma of the breast, who died of a cerebellar metastasis. At autopsy, she was also found to have multiple convexity and falx meningiomas, one of which harbored a tumor embolus from the carcinoma. Buge *et al.*[13] tell of a 68-year-old woman with meningeal and cerebral metastases of breast carcinoma; she too had multiple meningiomas in addition, with "intrication of the two problems." Smith *et al.*[14] had two patients with breast carcinoma in whom meningiomas subsequently developed. This problem was discussed in great detail by Schoenberg *et al.*[15] In their analysis of a possible relationship between nervous system neoplasms and primary cancers of other sites, these authors found statistically significant connection between brain tumors and malignant tumors elsewhere only as it applied to meningiomas and breast carcinoma. Eight such cases were included in their study. In three patients a verified meningioma was followed by breast cancer; in the other five cases the breast carcinoma showed up first, followed by the discovery of meningioma (in two cases at autopsy). These investigators concluded that if a patient with known breast carcinoma develops symptoms and signs of an intracranial mass, these should be very carefully evaluated, as they may point to a curable lesion rather than to metastases. Failure to consider this possibility can lead to truly tragic consequences. Haar and Patterson[16] documented the case of a middle-aged women who, 2 years after mastectomy for breast cancer, developed an intracranial mass. Her physician husband was certain that it was a metastasis and refused to permit craniotomy. The patient died and was found to have a convexity meningioma and no residual cancer anywhere.

All these factors, that is, the higher incidence of meningiomas among women, the worsening of pressure signs during pregnancy in patients with meningiomas, and the cases in which breast carcinoma and meningioma develop in the same patient, point to the possibility that meningiomas respond to stimulation by female sex hormones.

SEX HORMONE RECEPTORS IN MENINGIOMAS

Donnell *et al.*[17] strongly considered the above implications when they examined six surgically removed meningiomas for the presence of estrogen receptors. Of the six cases that had frozen tumor tissue assayed, four were found to contain estrogen receptors, two at a high level. Of these four positive cases, one was a male. It is to be expected that this work will be followed by other, perhaps larger, series of meningiomas studied for the presence of estrogen receptors. In cases in which the size or location, or both, of the meningioma make complete surgical removal difficult, or in histologically malignant forms, the finding of estrogen receptors may even become an indication for some forms of hormone therapy.

Tilzer,[18] at Kansas University Medical Center, assayed six meningiomas for progesterone receptors. Four of the six tumors studied contained significant quantities of progesterone receptor (144–388 femtomoles/mg cytosol protein). Poisson *et al.*,[19] in their study of 22 meningiomas, found estrogen receptors to be present in 13 cases (59%), but receptors for progesterone were found in all 22 cases, further underlying the probable importance of these particular receptors in cells of meningiomas. The presence of these latter receptors may explain particularly well why meningiomas appear to grow more rapidly during pregnancy. This was also the conclusion of Schnegg *et al.*,[20] who recently examined meningiomas from 10 patients for sex hormone receptors. In this group of tumors *no* meningioma had estrogen receptors, while 4 had progesterone receptors. Interestingly, two meningiomas were found to have *androgen* receptors; the latter two patients were postmenopausal women.

References

1. Wood, M.W., White, R.J., and Kernohan, J.W.: One

hundred intracranial meningiomas found incidentally at necropsy.
J. Neuropathol. Exp. Neurol. 16: 337–340, 1957.

2. Cushing, H., and Eisenhardt, L.: *Meningiomas. Their Classification, Regional Behaviour, Life History and Surgical End Results.* Springfield, Ill., Charles C Thomas, 1938, pp. 57–68.
3. Quest, D.W.: Meningiomas: An update.
Neurosurgery 3: 219–225, 1978.
4. Bickerstaff, E.R., Small, J.M., and Guest, I.A.: The relapsing course of certain meningiomas in relation to pregnancy and menstruation.
J. Neurol. Neurosurg. Psychiatry 21: 89–91, 1958.
5. Cushing, H., and Eisenhardt, L.: Meningiomas arising from the tuberculum sellae with the syndrome of primary optic atrophy and bitemporal field defects combined with a normal sella turcica in a middle-aged person.
Arch. Ophthalmol. (Chic.) 1: 1–41, 166–205, 1929.
6. Fischer, F.: Über die Ursachen bitemporaler Hemianopsie bei Schwangerschaft.
Z. Augenheilkd. 85: 88–108, 1935.
7. Hagedoorn, A.: The chiasmal syndrome and retrobulbar neuritis in pregnancy.
Am. J. Ophthalmol. 20: 699, 1937.
8. Walsh, F.B.: *Clinical Neuro-Ophthalmology.* Baltimore, Williams & Wilkins, 1947, p. 416.
9. Rucker, C.W., and Kearns, T.P.: Mistaken diagnoses in some cases of meningioma.
Am. J. Ophthalmol. 51: 15–19, 1951.
10. Weyand, R.D., MacCarthy, C.S., and Wilson, R.B.: The effect of pregnancy on intracranial meningiomas occurring about the optic chiasm.
Surg. Clin. North Am. 31: 1225–1233, 1951.
11. Michelsen, J.J., and New, P.F.J.: Brain tumor and pregnancy.
J. Neurol. Neurosurg. Psychiatry 32: 305–307, 1969.
12. Fényes, G., and Kepes, J.: Über das gemeinsame Vorkommen von Meningeomen und Geschwülsten anderen Typs in Gehirn.
Zentralbl. Neurochir. 16: 251–260, 1956.
13. Buge, A., Escourolle, R., Martin, M., Poirier, J., and Devoise, L.: Metastases cerebro-méningées d'un epithelioma du sein. Méningiomatose multiple. Intrication des deux problèmes.
Rev. Neurol. (Paris) 114: 308–312, 1966.
14. Smith, F.P., Slavik, M., and MacDonald, J.S.: Association of breast cancer with meningioma: Report of two cases and review of the literature.
Cancer 42: 1992–1994, 1978.
15. Schoenberg, B.S., Christine, B.W., and Whisnant, J.P.: Nervous system neoplasms and primary malignancies of other sites.
Neurology (Minneapolis) 25: 705–712, 1975.
16. Haar, F., and Patterson, R.H., Jr.: Surgery for metastatic intracranial neoplasm.
Cancer 30: 1241–1245, 1972.
17. Donnell, M.W., Meyer, G.A., and Donegan, W.L.: Estrogen-receptor protein in intracranial meningiomas.
J. Neurosurg. 50: 499–502, 1979.
18. Tilzer, L.: Personal communication, 1980.
19. Poisson, M., Magdelenat, H., Foncini, J.F., Bleibel, J.M., Philippon, J., Pertuiset, B., and Buge, A.: Récepteurs d'oestrogènes et de progestérone dans les méningiomes. Étude de 22 cas.
Rev. Neurol. (Paris) 136: 193–203, 1980.
20. Schnegg, J. F., Gomez, F., LeMarchand-Beraud, T., and Tribolet, N.: Presence of sex steroid hormone receptors in meningioma tissue.
Surg. Neurol. 15: 415–418, 1981.

CHAPTER 8

Chemical Constitution and Enzyme Patterns of Meningiomas

Among the chemical constituents of meningiomas, lipids have been studied most extensively. Codegone *et al.*[1] found that lipids in meningiomas resembled those of schwannomas, but in the latter they were more alkaline resistant. Sunder-Plassmann and Bernheimer[2] compared the amount of gangliosides found in normal meninges and in meningiomas. Not surprisingly, of the three layers of meninges, the arachnoid had the greatest similarity to meningiomas with regard to its ganglioside composition. Gm_3, Gd_3, and $Gd_{1/a}$ were found to be the major ganglioside fractions. Kanazawa and Yamakawa[3] studied ceramides in human intracranial tumors. Ceramide monohexoside (CMH) and ceramide dihexoside (CDH) were found in all meningiomas as well as in gliomas. Meningiomas contained much more CDH than did normal meninges. The difference between meningiomas and benign gliomas was that the CMH in meningiomas contained glucosyl ceramide, the CMH in benign gliomas, exclusively a galactosyl ceramide. In malignant gliomas the two were mixed.

One noteworthy characteristic of meningiomas that Stewart *et al.*[4] detected was that in tissue cultures this tumor was found to have a very low uptake of glutamate, lower than either malignant glioma cultures or even fibroblast cultures. Mucous substances in meningiomas were extensively analyzed by Dahmen.[5]

With regard to enzymes, the phosphatases, particularly alkaline phosphatase, isoenzymes of lactic dehydrogenase, and the aldolases have attracted greatest interest.

PHOSPHATASES

As early as 1942, shortly after the introduction of Gomori's techniques for the histochemical detection of alkaline phosphatase, Landow *et al.*[6] examined the distribution of alkaline phosphatase in normal and noeplastic tissues of the nervous system. In all species studied, the leptomeninges gave a strong reaction for alkaline phosphatase, the greatest activity being localized in the cytoplasm of arachnoidal cells. This could be observed in every area, from the optic nerve sheath down to the cauda equina. As to meningiomas, 11 were studied by these authors, and seven gave a strongly positive reaction for alkaline phosphatase. Feigin and Wolf,[7] who examined 62 tumors for presence of this enzyme, found only a slight amount in gliomas, but a moderate to marked presence in meningiomas. With regard to subtypes of meningiomas, the literature contains some conflicting data. Büttger *et al.*[8] found alkaline phosphatase mostly in fibroblastic meningiomas and Gluszcz[9] in meningothelial forms. Kaufmann,[10] Nasu,[11] and Osske and Jänish[12] felt that the intensity of the reaction was not related to the histological type of mengingioma. As to distribution of the enzyme within a given mengingioma, Osske and Jänisch[12] separated meningiomas into three groups: those with alkaline phosphatase exclusively in the wall of blood vessels, those with predominance in the parenchyma, and those in which vessels and parenchyma alike contained the enzyme. By contrast, they found acid phosphatase only in the cytoplasm of tumors cells. Much acid phosphatase was found in intranuclear cytoplasmic inclusions and was considered a result of degeneration of trapped cytoplasm.[13] In a study of 28 surgically removed meningiomas Fabiani *et al.*[14] found alkaline phosphatase mostly in vessel walls and not in tumor parenchyma, except in whorls that have not yet calcified, particularly if the rest of the tumor was psammomatous. By contrast, Fischer and Müller[15] found more alkaline phosphatase in "cytoplasma active" than in "vessel active" (angioblastic?) meningiomas, whereas Lolova and Ivanova[16] observed a positive reaction in the parenchyma of meningiomas irrespective of their histological type.

Apparently a meningioma has to be very large or has to metastasize to other organs before elevation of serum alkaline phosphatase can be observed in a patient. This was documented in the case of Kepes *et al.*,[17] a peritorcular malignant meningioma, partly hemangiopericytic, partly papillary (see Chapter 25), in which alkaline phosphatase was histochemically demonstrated in the tumor as well as in its pulmonary metastases. Marked elevation of serum alkaline phosphatase was also found in the patient with malignant meningioma described by Mignot *et al.*[18] (see also Chapter 16).

A recent report on the subject of hydrolytic enzymes in meningiomas was a biochemical (not histochemical) study: Ramsey *et al.*[19] found alkaline phosphatase to be highest in the transitional type—higher than in either the meningothelial or the fibroblastic forms. This datum is hard to evaluate, because transitional meningiomas are a mixture of meningothelial and fibroblastic components. As to the physicochemical characteristics of alkaline phosphatase of meningiomas, Timperley and Warnes,[20] after extracting the enzyme, found that it could not be inhibited by C-phenylalanine, but that it was very heat sensitive.

LACTIC DEHYDROGENASE

Isoenzymes of lactic dehydrogenase (LDH) can be distinguished from one another by the speed with which they travel during electrophoresis. Customarily, five isoenzymes are identified. The fastest moving band, LDH-1, is characteristically found in tissues that use the aerobic process for their energy requirements. LDH-5 is the slowest-moving enzyme, characteristic of anaerobic activity, whereas LDH-2, -3, and -4 represent in-between types. It follows that in aerobically active tissues (heart, kidney, brain) the predominant activity is by the fastest-moving band, LDH-1, whereas tissues that use more anaerobic pathways of energy supply (liver, skeletal muscle) have more LDH-5. (Not surprisingly, in myocardial infarction LDH-1 is elevated in the serum, in acute hepatitis, LDH-5.)

Gerhardt *et al.*[21] found that most benign meningiomas are by far richest in LDH-2, -3, and -4; LDH-3 had the highest peak. Similar observations were made by Sherwin *et al.*[22] and McCormick and Allen.[23] All these workers pointed out that LDH-4 and LDH-5 were characteristic of malignant tumors, including malignant meningiomas. McCormick and Allen suggested that LDH analysis could be useful in the rapid diagnosis of a brain tumor, even to the point of replacing frozen sections. A case in point reported by Allen *et al.*[24] was that of a 14-year-old boy with a spinal meningioma. The tumor was found to be rich in LDH-4 and LDH-5, had very little LDH-2 and LDH-3, and no LDH-1 at all. This meningioma metastasized extensively to the lungs.

ALDOLASES AND OTHER ENZYMES

Isoenzymes of aldolase have been analyzed in various brain tumors. Gliomas were found to have a greater variety of this enzyme: aldolase A, C, and A + C hybrids were identified in them, whereas meningiomas contained only aldolase A.[25,26] Van Veelen *et al.*[27] studied the presence of pyruvate kinase in normal brain and brain tumors. He found mostly the muscle type (M) of this enzyme in the form of two subgroups: M_1, not inhibited in its action by alanin, and M_2, inhibited by alanin. The M_1 form was predominant in normal brain, the M_2 form in tumors, gliomas, and meningiomas alike.

Finally, Frattola *et al.*[28] discovered that soluble guanylate cyclase activity was much higher in meningiomas than either in normal brain or other primary brain tumors.

References

1. Codegone, M.L., Peres, B., and Schiffer, D.: Histochemical characterization of lipids in meningiomas and their comparison with neurinomas. *Acta Neurol. Napoli 25: 532–534, 1970.*
2. Sunder-Plassmann, M., and Bernheimer, H.: Ganglioside in Meningiomen und Hirnhäuten. *Acta Neuropathol. (Berl.) 27: 289–294, 1974.*
3. Kanazawa, I., and Yamakawa, I.: Presence of glucosyl ceramide and lactosyl ceramide in human intracranial tumors. *Jpn J. Exp. Med. 44: 379–387, 1974.*
4. Stewart, R.M., Martuza, R.L., Baldessarini, R.J., and Kornblith, P.L.: Glutamate accumulation by human gliomas and meningiomas in tissue culture. *Brain Res. 118: 441–452, 1976.*
5. Dahmen, H.G.: Studies on mucous substances in myxomatous meningiomas. *Acta Neuropathol. (Berl.) 48: 235–237, 1979.*
6. Landow, H., Kabat, E.A., and Newman, W.: Distribution of alkaline phosphatase in normal and neoplastic tissue of the nervous system. *Arch. Neurol. Psychol. 48: 518–530, 1942.*
7. Feigin, I., and Wolf, A.: The alkaline phosphomonoesterase activity of brain tumors. *J. Neuropathol. Exp. Neurol. 17: 522, 1958.*
8. Büttger, H.W., Scarlato, G., Müller, W., and Kemali, D.: Über das Vorkommen und die Verteilung der alkalischen und säuren Phosphatase in Meningeomen. *Dtsch. Z. Nervenheilkl. 176: 67–76, 1957.*

9. Glusczc, A.: A histochemical study of some hydrolytic enzymes in tumors of the nervous system. *Acta Neuropathol. (Berl.) 3: 184–201, 1963.*
10. Kaufmann, J.C.E.: Meningiomata and enzymes. *J. Lab. Clin. Med. 9: 112–118, 1963.*
11. Nasu, H.: Fermenthistochemische Untersuchungen an Meningeomen. *Acta Neuropathol. (Berl.) 3: 627–637, 1964.*
12. Osske, G., and Jänisch, W.: On the enzyme histochemistry of meningiomas. *Acta Neuropathol. (Berl.) 9: 290–297, 1967.*
13. Osske, G., and Jänisch, W.: Enzyme histochemical findings in nuclear excavations of meningiomas. *Acta Histochem. (Jena) 31: 159–165, 1968.*
14. Fabiani, A., Monticone, G.F., and Schiffer, D.: Rilievi istoenzimologici nei meningiomi. *Acta Neurol. Napoli 22: 193–195, 1967.*
15. Fischer, W., and Müller, E.: Untersuchungen über die alkalische Phosphatase in Meningeomen. *Enzymol. Biol. Clin. 11: 450–458, 1970.*
16. Lolova, I., and Ivanova, A.: A histochemical study of meningiomas. *Acta Neuropathol. (Berl.) 20: 110–121, 1972.*
17. Kepes, J.J., MacGee, E.E., Vergara, G., and Sil, R.: Malignant meningioma with extensive pulmonary metastases. *J. Kansas Med. Soc. 72: 312–316, 1971.*
18. Mignot, B., Hauw, J.J., Pasquier, P., DeSigalony, J.P.H., and Bricaire, F.: Perturbations biologiques reversibles evoluant parallelement à un méningiome recidivant et avec métastases. *Sem. Hop. Paris 54: 1231–1237, 1978.*
19. Ramsey, R.B., Fredericks, M., Crafts, D.C., Smith, K.R., and Chung, H.D.: Hydrolytic enzymes in meningioma subtypes. *Acta Neuropathol. (Berl.) 49: 63–65, 1980.*
20. Timperley, W.R., and Warnes, T.W.: Alkaline phosphatase in meningiomas. *Cancer 26: 100–103, 1970.*
21. Gerhardt, W., Clausen, J., Christensen, E., and Rüskede, J.: Changes of LDH-isoenzymes, esterases, acid phosphatases and proteins in malignant and benign human brain tumors. *Acta Neurol. Scand. 39: 85–111, 1963.*
22. Sherwin, A.C., Leblance, F.E., and McCann, W.P.: Altered LDH isoenzymes in brain tumors. *Arch. Neurol. 18: 311–315, 1968.*
23. McCormick, D., and Allen, I.V.: The value of LDH isoenzymes in the rapid diagnosis of brain tumors. *Neuropathol. Appl. Neurobiol. 2: 269–278, 1976.*
24. Allen, I.V., McClure, J., McCormick, D., and Gleadhill, C.A.: LDH isoenzyme pattern in a meningioma with pulmonary metastases. *J. Pathol. 123: 187–191, 1977.*
25. Sugimura, T., Sato, S., Kawabe, S., Suzuki, N., Chien, T.C., and Takakura, K.: Aldolase C in brain tumor. *Nature 222: 1070, 1969.*
26. Sato, S., Sugimura, T., Chien, T.C., and Takakura, K.: Aldolase isozyme patterns in human brain tumors. *Cancer 27: 223–227, 1971.*
27. Van Veelen, C.W., Staal, G.E., Verbiest, H., and Vlug, A.M.: Alanine inhibition of pyruvate kinase in gliomas and meningiomas. A diagnostic tool in surgery for gliomas? *Lancet 2: 384–385, 1977.*
28. Frattola, L., Carenzi, A., Cerri, C., Kumakura, K., and Trabucchi, M.: Regulation of the cyclic guanosine 3′-5′-monophosphate system in human brain tumors. *Acta Neurol. Scand. 54: 382–390, 1976.*

CHAPTER 9

The Search for Tissue-Specific Antigens in Meningiomas

With the worldwide interest in immunological aspects of neoplasms both for diagnostic and therapeutic purposes, meningiomas too have been examined for the presence of antigens specific for this particular tumor. The results so far are only tentative. For example, Catalano *et al.*[1] found that serum of patients with intracranial meningiomas reacted in immunofluorescent assays with cell cultures and imprints prepared from human meningiomas. This antibody, however, also showed some cross-reaction with neoplastic tissue of glial origin. The findings of Rich and Winters[2] were suggestive of more specificity: The sera of 14 out of 24 meningioma patients reacted positively with meningioma cells. Such sera could not be inactivated by anything except absorption with meningioma extract. In a related study Winters and Rich[3] found that antigens prepared from meningioma cells (meningioma-associated antigens or MSA) were not homogeneous. For example, sera from 53% of patients with *glial* tumors reacted with MSA. Winters and Rich concluded that there are at least three kinds of meningioma-associated antigens: MSA-A reacts specifically with sera from meningioma patients, MSA-B with sera of glioma patients, and MSA-C with sera of normal individuals or patients with nonneural tumors.

Kehayov *et al.*[4] produced antibodies in rabbit serum against human embryonic brain. Interestingly, this antiembryonic brain serum reacted with meningiomas, but not with gliomas or metastases. Kehayov *et al.* believe it to indicate the existence of a meningioma-associated antigen, having no crossreaction with either alpha-fetoprotein or carcinoembryonic antigen.

References

1. Catalano, V.W., Harter, D.H., and Hsu, K.J.: Common antigen in meningioma derived cell cultures. *Science 175: 180–183, 1972.*
2. Rich, J.R., and Winters, W.D.: Tumor associated antigen in human meningioma. *N. Engl. J. Med. 290: 164, 1974.*
3. Winters, W. D. and Rich, J. R.: Human meningioma antigens. *Int. J. Cancer 15: 815–827, 1975.*
4. Kehayov, I., Botev, B., Vulchanov, V., and Kyurkchiev, S.: Demonstration of a phase (stage)-specific embryonic brain antigen in human meningioma. *Int. J. Cancer 18: 587–592, 1976.*

CHAPTER 10

Incidence, Prevalence, and Mortality of Meningiomas

Statistical information on meningiomas, as indeed on other tumors as well, can be viewed in terms of incidence, prevalence, and mortality rate. A determining factor in the case of meningiomas is their often benign character. As is well known, many small meningiomas remain asymptomatic during life and are detected as incidental findings at autopsy. Also, thanks to advances in neurosurgery, many of the larger, clinically symptomatic, meningiomas will be cured by surgical intervention and therefore will fail to show up in mortality statistics. Thus, the literature actually provides us with three different sets of data:

1. The overall incidence and prevalence of meningiomas, including symptomatic cases as well as incidental findings in the general population.
2. The percentage of meningiomas among other primary brain tumors in large neurosurgical series—this is the most frequently tabulated datum.
3. The incidence of meningiomas leading to the patient's death—either because of lack of timely detection, inaccessibility for surgical removal, operative or postoperative complications, or biological malignancy of the tumor leading to recurrences or metastases.

Cases comprising group 3 are the meningiomas that show up in mortality statistics and will naturally be less numerous than those falling within group 1 or 2. An example of this difference can be found in the studies of Rausing *et al.*[1] In Malmö, Sweden (population 235,000), the autopsies performed during the 10-year period 1957–1966 were analyzed. (In that city, the autopsy rate for hospital patients is 99%, intracranial contents are examined in all autopsies.) Of a total of 11,793 autopsies over that 10-year period, 172 meningiomas were found: a prevalence of 1.44%. In only 11 of these 172 cases, however, were the meningiomas considered the chief cause of death.

In the United States the large neurosurgical series lists meningiomas as comprising, on the average, 14 to 15% of primary brain tumors. Yet, their relative benignity is reflected in the study of Choi *et al.*[2] on mortality from brain tumors, covering Minnesota for the years 1958–1962: During that period, 760 patients died of primary brain tumors, but among these, only 52 (6.8%) died of meningiomas.

GEOGRAPHIC PATHOLOGY

Over the last 20 years much information has accumulated from all over the world regarding the incidence and frequency of brain tumors, including meningiomas. In the United States meningiomas appear to make up about 15% of surgically treated brain tumors, as reflected in various large series: Cushing and Eisenhardt[3] had 13.4% in a series of 2,203 brain tumors; Grant[4] found a total of 17% meningiomas among 3,226 brain tumors of the University of Pennsylvania over a 30-year span. The incidence in European series is only slightly higher: 18% in Zülch's[5] material and 19.2% in the series of Hoessly and Olivecrona.[6] In India Dastur[7] and Balasubramaniam and Ramamurthi[8] encountered 13.1% and 13% meningiomas, respectively, in their series of brain tumors. In Japan, Katsura *et al.*[9] found meningiomas to form 15.9% in the brain tumor material from Japanese universities and major medical centers. In the People's Republic of China, meningiomas represent 12–13% of all primary brain tumors (Chai[10]).

Whereas these data suggest uniformity of incidence over much of the globe, reports and surveys from Africa indicate a much higher percentage of meningiomas among primary brain neoplasms on that continent. Thus, meningiomas were found to represent 23.5% of primary brain tumors on the Ivory Coast (Giordano and Lamouche[11]); 28.6% in a study covering Malawi, Rhodesia, and Zambia

(Levy[12]); 29.9% in the Nigerian African (Odeku and Adeloye[13]); and 30.3% in the Bantus of Transvaal (Froman and Lipshitz[14]). The highest incidence of all was found in a small series of 13 cases in Eritrea: 38% (Manfredonia[15]). Odeku and Adeloye,[13] reviewing the brain tumor material in the city of Ibadan in Nigeria, were able to state, "Meningiomas remain the single most common histologic type of all intracranial neoplasms in Ibadan." Their series differed from European and American findings in other important respects, as well. For example, males dominated their material, and a full 20% of their cases occurred during the second decade of life. This does not necessarily indicate an absolute increase in meningiomas on that continent, but it might reflect the low incidence of gliomas among Africans, accounting for the relatively high percentage of meningiomas encountered. Indeed, Froman and Lipschitz[14] estimate that the incidence of meningiomas among the Transvaal Bantus is only one-fifth that of a comparable population in Sweden; nevertheless, because gliomas among the Bantus number only one-tenth of gliomas in the Swedish population, the relative incidence of meningiomas among primary brain neoplasms appear therefore to be higher.

References

1. Rausing, A. Ybo, W., and Stenflo, J.: Intracranial meningioma—A population study of ten years. *Acta Neurol. Scand. 46: 102–110, 1970.*
2. Choi, N.W., Schuman, L.M., and Gullen, W.H.: Epidemiology of primary central nervous system neoplasms in Minnesota. *Am. J. Epidemiol. 91: 238–259, 1970.*
3. Cushing, H., and Eisenhardt, L.: Meningiomas. *Their Classification, Regional Behaviour, Life History and Surgical End Results.* Springfield, Ill., Charles C Thomas, 1938, p. 69.
4. Grant, F.G.: A study of the results of surgical treatment in 2,326 consecutive patients with brain tumor. *J. Neurosurg. 13: 479–488, 1956.*
5. Zülch, K.J.: *Brain tumors. Their Biology and Pathology.* New York, Springer-Verlag, 1957, p. 57.
6. Hoessly, G.F., and Olivecrona, H.: Report on 280 cases of verified parasagittal meningioma. *J. Neurosurg. 12: 614–626, 1955.*
7. Dastur, D.K., Lalitha, V.S., and Prabhakar, V.: Pathological analysis of intracranial space-occupying lesions in 1000 cases including children. Part I. Age, sex and pattern; and the tuberculomas. *J. Neurol. Sci. 6: 575–592, 1968.*
8. Balasubramaniam, V., and Ramamurthi, B.: Meningiomas. *Neurology India 18 (Suppl. 1): 81–88, 1970.*
9. Katsura, S., Suzuki, J., and Wada, T.: A statistical study of brain tumors in the neurosurgical clinics in Japan. *J. Neurosurg. 16: 570–580, 1959.*
10. Chai, W.: Personal communication, 1980.
11. Giordano, C., and Lamouche, M.: Méningiomes en Côte D'Ivoire. *Afr. J. Med. Sci. 4: 249–263, 1973.*
12. Levy, L.F.: Brain tumors in Malawi, Rhodesia and Zambia. *Afr. J. Med. Sci. 4: 393–397, 1973.*
13. Odeku, E.L., and Adeloye, A.: Cranial meningiomas in the Nigerian African. *Afr. J. Med. Sci. 4: 275–287, 1973.*
14. Froman, C., and Lipschitz, R.: Demography of tumors of the central nervous system among the Bantu (African) population of the Transvaal, South Africa.. *J. Neurosurg. 32: 660–664, 1970.*
15. Manfredonia, M.: Tumors of the nervous system in the African in Eritrea (Ethiopia). *Afr. J. Med. Sci. 4: 383–387, 1973.*

CHAPTER 11

Familial Occurrence

It has long been recognized that patients suffering from von Recklinghausen's neurofibromatosis, a familial disease inherited as an autosomal dominant trait, are susceptible to meningiomas, often multiple ones. This seems to be the most common setting in which familial meningiomas occur. Cushing and Eisenhardt[1] devoted an entire chapter of their classic text to "combined neurilemommas and meningiomas," reviewed the literature of such common occurrence in great detail, and added two cases of their own. Several other cases of this nature were described subsequently. A representative example was reported by Davidoff and Martin,[2] in which both a father and daughter were found to have multiple meningiomas in addition to bilateral cerebellopontine angle neurinomas.

However, there have been reports of multiple occurrence of meningiomas in families that did not have stigmata of von Recklinghausen's disease. For example, no evidence of neurofibromatosis was found in either a brother and sister with meningiomas, or their families, by Gaist and Piazza.[3] Nor was there evidence of neurofibromatosis in the families of other interrelated meningioma patients, for example, a 63-year-old mother and her 39-year-old daughter reported by Joynt and Perret,[4] the two brothers and one woman cousin described by Sahar,[5] or two brothers, seen by Grunert *et al.*[6] Of particular interest are the identical twin boys observed by Sedzimir *et al.*,[7] both of whom had cranial and spinal meningiomas that became symptomatic at ages 8 and 13 years, respectively. These boys and their family had no stigmata of neurofibromatosis.

There have been other patients, however, in whom only minor signs of von Recklinghausen's disease were present, some of which undoubtedly could easily have been overlooked. For example, Ectors and Van Bogaert[8] reported the case of a brother and sister, both of whom were operated on for meningiomas. Later the sister was found to harbor a bean-size schwannoma of the forearm, and the brother had a similar small mass in the thigh. Also, in the cases of Delleman *et al.*,[9] four members in two generations of the same family had meningiomas without any evidence of neurofibromatosis, but another family member had multiple meningiomas with bilateral acoustic neurilemommas, while still another relative had multiple café-au-lait spots. It is probably justified to assume in these latter cases that there was neurofibromatosis in the family with incomplete expression—clinical formes frustes cases—as should always be suspected in familial occurrence of meningiomas. But there appears to be no reason to surmise that meningiomas can never develop in several members of the same family without coexisting neurofibromatosis, as was demonstrated in some of the above-mentioned examples.

References

1. Cushing, H., and Eisenhardt, L.: *Meningiomas. Their Classification, Regional Behaviour, Life History and Surgical End Results.* Springfield Ill., Charles C Thomas, 1938, pp. 100–114.
2. Davidoff, L.M., and Martin, M.: Hereditary combined neurinomas and meningiomas. *J. Neurosurg. 12: 375–384, 1955.*
3. Gaist, G., and Piazza, G.: Meningiomas in two members of the same family (with no evidence of neurofibromatosis). *J. Neurosurg. 16: 110–113, 1959.*
4. Joynt, R.J., and Perret, G.E.: Meningiomas in a mother and daughter. Cases without evidence of neurofibromatosis. *Neurology (Minneapolis) 11: 164–165, 1961.*
5. Sahar, A.: Familial occurrence of neurofibromatosis. Case report. *J. Neurosurg. 23: 444–445, 1965.*
6. Grunert, V., Horcajada, J., and Sunder-Plassmann, M.: Familial occurrence of intracranial meningiomas. *Wien. Med. Wochenschr. 120: 807–808, 1970.*
7. Sedzimir, C.B., Frazer, A.K., and Roberts, J.R.: Cranial and spinal meningiomas in a pair of identical twin boys. *J. Neurol. Neurosurg. Psychiatry 36: 368–376, 1973.*
8. Ectors, L., and Van Bogaert, L.: Ablation d'un méningiome du trou occipital chez un frère et une soeur. *Acta Neurol. Belg. 53: 193–204, 1953.*
9. Delleman, J.W., De Jong, J.G., and Bleeker, G.M.: Meningiomas in five members of a family over two generations, in one member simultaneously with acoustic neurinomas. *Neurology (Minneapolis) 28: 567–570, 1978.*

CHAPTER 12

Multiple Meningiomas

The presence of more than one meningioma in a single patient is of interest to the pathologist. It can create serious problems in diagnosis and treatment for the clinician. Historically, Anfimow and Blumenau[1] were the first to report multiple meningiomas in one patient in 1889. (The article in which their findings were reported appeared in the journal *Vratsch* in Russian and was translated into German by Rosenbach for the *Neurologisches Centralblatt* that same year.) The patient was a 36-year-old man with multiple independent meningiomas in the left frontal lobe and one in the cerebellum. Altogether he had four large meningiomas and many small ones. Cushing and Eisenhardt[2] subdivided multiple meningiomas into three groups: 1) those occurring without the stigmata of von Recklinghausen's disease, 2) multiple meningiomas in patients with von Recklinghausen's disease, and 3) meningiomatosis. This latter term was used to describe the condition wherein innumerable tumors of varying sizes were found to stud the inside of the dura mater. No specific number, however, has been set to distinguish this last group form "ordinary" multiple meningiomas and, whereas some investigators accept this distinction, others fail to perceive a satisfactory cutoff between large numbers of multiple meningiomas and meningiomatosis. Thus Stöwsand[3] found 59 circumscribed meningiomas in a 40-year-old man and still believed this finding should be distinguished from meningiomatosis. Paillas *et al.*[4] found such distinction difficult, particularly in view of their patient, a 26-year-old man with three large meningiomas (parasagittal, intraventricular, and suprasellar) in addition to what looked like meningiomatosis of the falx at surgery. Scharrer and Brunngraber[5] also considered the distinction unclear, and more recently Bonnal *et al.*[6] stated, "Our observations show that all gradations between multiple meningiomas and meningiomatosis may be found."

Abtahi[7] proposed a classification somewhat different from that of Cushing and Eisenhardt[2]: 1) multiple meningiomas without von Recklinghausen's disease, 2) multiple meningiomas with von Recklinghausen's disease, and 3) multiple tumors found only at the second or third operation, suggesting (to him) postoperative implants from an original solitary tumor.

Multiple meningiomas may be present simultaneously, or they may occur in the same patient at different time intervals. More than one meningioma was found at surgery by several investigators,[8-10] whereas Ekong[11] had a woman patient who presented with a left convexity meningioma at age 47 only to return with a meningioma of the right sphenoidal ridge at age 63.

The overall incidence of multiple meningiomas is usually listed as between 1% and 2%.[12-15] A particularly high incidence was reported in the series of Horrax,[16] at 6.6%. It therefore appears that multiple meningiomas are uncommon, but not exceedingly rare, as attested by Russell's[17] seven cases and Levin and co-workers' [16] six cases. Other representative cases were contributed by Hosoi,[19] Echols,[20] Fényes and Kepes,[21] Zervas *et al.*,[22] Jimenez *et al.*,[23] and others.

Multiple meningiomas in the spinal canal are usually limited to two tumors.[24-27] In a case reported by Resnikoff *et al.*[27] two intraspinal meningiomas (at Th_8 and C_3 levels, respectively) occurred at a 7-year interval. Three spinal meningiomas in the same patient were reported by Patronas *et al.*[28] in a 32-year-old woman, who had a history of irradiation to the areas involved (C_7, Th_2, and Th_7 levels).

Scharrer and Brunngraber[5] raised the question whether multiple meningiomas could not possibly represent metastatic implants from each other, as was suggested by Abtahi for meningiomas occurring at different times in the same patient. These investigators felt, however, that this notion could be sustained only if the tumors in question showed histological signs of malignancy.

Multiple meningiomas in patients with known von Recklinghausen's disease have been described extensively in the literature. The case of Rodriguez and Berthrong[29] might serve as a typical example—a 24-year-old man with neurofibromatosis, who had numerous schwannomas and neurofibromas of the cranial nerves, including acoustic nerve tumors, and of spinal nerve roots, as well as multiple ependymomas and syringomyelia, in addition to multiple meningiomas.

References

1. Anfimow, J., and Blumenau, L.: Ein Fall Multipler Geschwülste in der Schädelhöhle. *Neurol. Centralbl. 8: 585, 1889.*
2. Cushing, H., and Eisenhardt, L.: *Meningiomas. Their Classification, Regional Behaviour, Life History and Surgical End Results.* Charles C Thomas, 1938, pp. 115–132.
3. Stöwsand, D.: Multiple meningiomas. *Acta Neurochir. 31: 279, 1975.*
4. Paillas, J.E., Bonnal, J., Legré, J., and Combalbert, A.: Des méningiomes multiples à la méningiomatose en plaques au cours de la maladie de Recklinghausen. *La Presse Med. 56: 2604–2606, 1961.*
5. Scharrer, E., and Brunngraber, C.V.: Über multiple Meningeome. *J. Neurol. 207: 227–246, 1974.*
6. Bonnal, J., Born, J.D., and Tremoulet, M.: Meningiomes multiples intracraniens. *Neurochirurgie 25: 78–83, 1979.*
7. Abtahi, H.: Multiple meningiomas. *Acta Neurochir. 31: 279, 1975.*
8. Wislawski, J., Bugusz, R., and Banack, S.: Mnogie oponiaki srodczaskowe. *Neur. Neurochir. Pol. 7: 435–442, 1973.*
9. Irger, I.M., Paramonow, L.V., and Stolypin, S.V.: Multiple meningiomas. *Vopr. Neurochir. 2(2): 11–17, 1974.*
10. Namba, S., Ishimitsu, H., and Tsuboi, M.: An operative case of multiple meningioma. *No Shinkei Geka 19: 571–575, 1978.*
11. Ekong, C.E., Paine, K.W., and Rozdilsky, B.: Multiple meningiomas. *Surg. Neurol. 9: 181–184, 1978.*
12. Elsberg, C.A.: The parasagittal meningeal fibroblastomas. *Bull. Neurol. Inst. NY 1: 389–418, 1931.*
13. Frazier, C.H., and Alpers, B.J.: Meningeal fibroblastomas of the cerebrum. A clinicopathologic analysis of 75 cases. *Arch. Neurol. Psychiatry 29: 935–989, 1933.*
14. Vestergaard, E. Multiple intracranial meningiomas. *Acta Psychiatr. Neurol. Kbh. 19: 389–411, 1944.*
15. Waga, S., Matsuda, M., Handa, H., Matshushima, M., and Ando, K.: Multiple meningiomas, report of four cases. *J. Neurosurg. 37: 348–351, 1972.*
16. Horrax, G.: Meningiomas of the brain. *Arch. Neurol. Psychiatry 41: 140–157, 1939.*
17. Russell, D.S.: Meningeal tumors: a review. *J. Clin. Pathol. 3: 191–211, 1950.*
18. Levin, P., Gross, S., Malis, L.I., Kirschenbaum, A.H., and Hollin, A.: Multiple intracranial meningiomas. *Surg. Gynecol. Obstet. 119: 1085–1092, 1964.*
19. Hosoi, K.: Meningiomas, with special reference to the multiple intracranial type. *Am. J. Pathol. 6: 245–260, 1930.*
20. Echols, D.H.: Multiple meningiomas. Removal of ten intracranial tumors from a patient. *Arch. Neurol. Psychiatry 46: 440–443, 1941.*
21. Fenyes, Gy., and Kepes, J.: Über das gemeinsame Vorkommen von Meningeomen und Geschwülsten anderen Typs im Gehirn. *Zentralbl. Neurochir. 16: 251–260, 1956.*
22. Zervas, N.T., Shintani, A., Kallar, B., and Berry, R.G.: Multiple meningiomas occupying separate neuraxial compartments, Case Report. *J. Neurosurg. 33: 216–220, 1970.*
23. Jimenez, J.P., Goree, J.A., and Parker, J.C., Jr.: An unusual association of multiple meningiomas, intracranial aneurysm and cerebrovascular atherosclerosis in two young women. *Am. J. Roentgenol. Rad. Ther. Nucl Med. 112: 281–288, 1971.*
24. Rand, R.W.: Multiple spinal cord meningiomas. *J. Neurosurg. 9: 310–314, 1952.*
25. Rath, J., Mathai, K.V., and Chandy, J.: Multiple meningiomas of the spinal cord. *J. Neurosurg. 26: 639–640, 1967.*
26. Devadiga, K.V., and Gass, H.: Multiple spinal cord meningiomas. *Neurol. India 20: 142–144, 1972.*
27. Resnikoff, S., Verdura, J.J., and Ardenas, J.: Multiple intraspinal meningiomas at different levels, operated on with a seven-year interval. A Case Report. *Ann. Surg. 176: 798–800, 1972.*
28. Patronas, N.J., Brown, F., and Duda, E.E.: Multiple meningiomas in the spinal cord. *Surg. Neurol. 13: 78–80, 1980.*
29. Rodriguez, H.A., and Berthrong, M.: Multiple primary intracranial tumors in von Recklinghausen's neurofibromatosis. *Arch. Neurol. 14: 467–475, 1966.*

CHAPTER 13

Meningiomas in Childhood

Meningiomas occur primarily in adults, particularly middle-aged people, and are distinctly rare in childhood. Taptas,[1] in a review of various reports totaling 1,760 meningiomas, found only 19 childhood examples (1.1%). Of the 313 meningiomas in Cushing and Eisenhardt's[2] series, there were six in the preadolescence age group (1.9%). Crouse and Berg,[3] defining childhood and adolescent meningiomas as occurring in patients less than 20 years of age, found 13 patients with meningiomas in that age group at the University of California, San Francisco, representing 2.3% of all pediatric intracranial tumors; these patients ranged in age from 2.5 months to 20 years.

It appears from the various series reviewed that 1) less than 2% of meningiomas occur in childhood, and 2) less than 2% of intracranial tumors in children are meningiomas—2.4% in Cuneo and Rand's[4] series, but only 0.5% in the Mayo Clinic series of 606 children with brain tumors.[5] Ingraham and Matson's[6] series of 313 brain tumors in childhood included only one meningioma, a parasagittal tumor in a 7-year-old boy. Odom *et al.*[7] also found only one meningioma among 164 brain tumors in children; there were, however, two meningeal sarcomas in the series.

Several cases of congenital meningiomas are on record.[8,9] An intracranial meningeal sarcoma in the newborn was described by Reigh and Decker,[10] and a spinal meningeal sarcoma in the same age group by Zwartverwer *et al.*[11] It appears, however, that the earliest occurrence of meningioma was reported by Solitare and Krigman[12] in a female fetus born at 32 weeks of gestation. The autopsy showed a meningioma with multinucleated giant cells in the middle cranial fossa.

Some investigators believe that childhood meningiomas have a few special characteristics, among them an apparent high incidence of malignant forms; for example, two out of seven childhood meningiomas reported by Cooper and Dohn[13] were histologically malignant. Crouse and Berg[3] found five sarcomas among 13 childhood and adolescent-age meningiomas (38%!). These investigators thought that because of the increased incidence of sarcomatous change, children with meningeal tumors had a significantly shorter survival time than did adults. Russell and Rubinstein[14] also suggest that there is a high percentage of malignant forms among childhood meningiomas. Nevertheless, there are quite a few cases of benign childhood meningiomas with good surgical results on record.[16–18] Meningiomas of children, like their adult counterparts, may develop in any of the usual intracranial sites and in the spinal canal, and even intraosseously in the cranial diploe."[20] Intraventricular meningiomas in children were described by Delandsheer,[21] Teng and Papatheodoru,[22] Sunder-Plassman *et al.*,[23] Vassilouthis and Ambrose,[24] Markwalder *et al.*,[25] and Lee *et al.*[26] reported an interesting meningioma of the third ventricle that clinically mimicked a colloid cyst. The unusually high incidence of intraventricular meningiomas in childhood was stressed by Kandel and Filatov.[27] In their own material, 6 of 22 patients with intraventricular meningiomas were under age 20 (27.2%). Childhood meningiomas also differ from adult forms with regard to sex ratio. The female predominance so characteristic of adults does not seem to apply to the childhood cases. For example, in the series of Cushing and Eisenhardt, five patients were under age 20, three of whom were males, two females. Our review of the Vienna series of 700 meningiomas found seven patients under age 20 (1%), all of whom were males. (See Chapter 7.) Paillas *et al.*[28] reviewed 110 cases of meningiomas in patients under age 20 and found 57 boys (51.8%) and 53 girls among them.

An unusually high percentage of spinal epidural meningiomas occurs in children. Five out of 35 such tumors (14.5%) collected from the literature by Calogero and Moossy[29] were in the pediatric age group. Male predominance was found in this group of tumors by Motomochi *et al.*[30]: of the seven cases reviewed by these investigators, five were males and only two were females. This is all the more striking when we consider that the female preponderance among intradural spinal meningiomas in adults is 90% in some series.

References

1. Taptas, J.N.: Intracranial meningioma in a four month old infant simulating subdural hematoma. *J. Neurosurg. 18: 120–121, 1961.*
2. Cushing, H., and Eisenhardt, L.: *Meningiomas. Their Classification, Regional Behaviour, Life History and Surgical End Results.* Springfield, Ill., Charles C Thomas, 1938, p. 69.
3. Crouse, S.K., and Berg, B.O.: Intracranial meningiomas in childhood and adolescence. *Neurology (Minneapolis) 22: 135–141, 1972.*
4. Cuneo, H.M., and Rand, C.W.: *Brain Tumors of Childhood.* Springfield, Ill., Charles C Thomas, 1952, pp. 116-125, 224.
5. Keith, H.M., Winchell, McK.C., and Kernohan, J.W.: Brain tumors in children. *Pediatrics 3: 839–844, 1949.*
6. Ingraham, F.D., and Matson, D.D.: Neurosurgery of infancy and childhood. Springfield, Ill., Charles C Thomas, 1954, p. 456.
7. Odom, G.L., Davis, C.H., and Woodhall, B.: Brain tumors in children. Clinical analysis of 164 cases. *Pediatrics 18: 856–870, 1956.*
8. Mendiratta, S.S., Rosenblum, J.A., and Strobos, R.J.: Congenital meningioma. *Neurology (Minneapolis) 17: 914–918, 1967.*
9. Gomez Bueno, J., Marquez Esteban, H., Botana Lopez, C., and Fernandez Puentes, M.L.: Congenital meningioma. *Child's Brain 3: 304–308, 1977.*
10. Reigh, E.E., and Decker, J.T.: Meningeal sarcoma in a two week-old infant simulating hydrocephalus. *J. Neurosurg. 19: 427–430, 1962.*
11. Zwartverwer, F.L., Kaplan, A.M., Hart, M.C., Hertel, G.A., and Spataro, J.: Meningeal sarcoma of the spinal cord in a newborn. *Arch. Neurol. 35: 844–946, 1978.*
12. Solitare, G.B., and Krigman, M.R.: Congenital intracranial neoplasm. A case report and review of the literature. *J. Neuropathol. Exp. Neurol. 23: 280–292, 1964.*
13. Cooper, M., and Dohn, D.F.: Intracranial meningiomas in childhood. *Cleveland Clin. Q. 41: 197–204, 1974.*
14. Russell, D.S., and Rubinstein, L.J.: *Pathology of Tumours of the Nervous System*, 4th ed. Baltimore, Williams & Wilkins, 1977, p. 66.
15. Garcia-Bengochea, F., Fusté, R., and Fernandez Carrera J.C.: Meningioma of the internal auditory meatus in a child 3 years old. *J. Neurosurg. 13: 215–218, 1956.*
16. Lecuire, J., Lapras, C., Tomasi, M., and Tusini, G.: Les méningiomes sus-tentorials de l'enfant. Considérations anatomo-cliniques et histopathologiques á propos de 6 observations. *Neurochirurgie 6: 147–155, 1960.*
17. Kosary, I. Z., Ouaknine, G. E., and Shacked, I. J.: Méningiomes frontaux et troubles psychiques chez l'enfant. *Neurochirurgie 15: 603–607, 1969.*
18. Klump, T. E., and McDonald J. V.: Successful removal of a large meningioma in a three-year-old boy. Case report. *J. Neurosurg. 34: 92–94, 1971.*
19. Lins, E.: Meningeome im Kindesalter. *Neurochirurgia (Stuttg.) 21: 28–31, 1978.*
20. Choux, R. Choux, M., Hassoun, J., Gomez, A., and Baurand, C.: Méningiome intra-osseux chez un enfant. *Neurochirurgie 21: 89–97, 1975.*
21. Delandsheer, J. M. Les méningiomes du ventricule latéral. *Neurochirurgie 11: 1–83, 1965.*
22. Teng, P., and Papatheodoru, Ch.: Suprachiasmal and intraventricular meningioma in a four year old child. *J. Neurosurg. 20: 174–176, 1963.*
23. Sunder-Plassmann, M., Jellinger, K., Kraus, H., and Regele, H.: Intraventriculäre Meningeome im Kindesalter. *Neurochirurgia (Stuttg.) 14: 54–63, 1971.*
24. Vassilouthis, J., and Ambrose, J. A.: Intraventricular meningioma in a child. *Surg. Neurol. 10: 105–107, 1978.*
25. Markwalder, T. M., Seiler, R. W., Markwalder, R. V., Huber, P., and Markwalder, H. M.: Meningioma of the anterior part of the third ventricle in a child. *Surg. Neurol. 12: 29–32, 1979.*
26. Lee, Y. Y., Lin, S. R., and Horner, F. A.: Third ventricle meningioma mimicking a colloid cyst in a child. *Am. J. Roentgenol. 132: 669–671, 1979.*
27. Kandel, E. I., and Filatov, Y. M.: Clinical picture and surgical treatment of meningiomas of the lateral ventricle. *In Proceedings of the Third International Congress of Neurological Surgery*, A. C. deVet (ed.). Copenhagen, 1965, pp. 719-723. Excerpta Medica Found., Amsterdam, 1966.
28. Paillas, J. E., Pellet, P., Guillermain, P., and Lavieille, J.: Les méningiomes intra-craniens de l'enfant et de l'adolescent. *Neurochirurgia (Stuttg.). 14: 41–53, 1971.*
29. Calogero, J. A., and Moossy, J.: Extradural spinal meningiomas. Report of four cases. *J. Neurosurg. 37: 442–447, 1972.*
30. Motomochi, M., Makita, Y., Nabeshima, S., and Aoyama, I.: Spinal epidural meningioma in childhood. *Surg. Neurol. 13: 5–7, 1980.*

CHAPTER 14

Meningiomas in the Elderly

Studies in large numbers of meningiomas occurring in very old people have shown that such patients share certain characteristics that set them apart from meningiomas in middle-aged persons. Many of them occur as incidental findings at autopsy. Wood et al.[1] reviewed 300 asymptomatic brain tumors detected at autopsy and found 100 (33.3%) to be meningiomas. These investigators noted that such incidental meningiomas tended to occur in elderly patients, with an average age of 69.8 years. Another unexpected finding was that the male/female ratio was 1:1.

Cooney and Solitare,[2] in reviewing the hospital records of Yale–New Haven Hospital for 1930–1967, found that out of 17,000 patients over 60 years of age, 497 had primary brain tumors, and of those 176 were meningiomas (35%). As many as 80% of the latter were incidental findings at autopsy. These authors distinguished in their series between *major meningiomas*, which were directly or indirectly related to the cause of the patient's death, and *subsidiary meningiomas*, that were not. Major meningiomas had their highest incidence in the sixth decade, subsidiary meningiomas in the eighth decade. Data from Japan also indicate that meningiomas become increasingly common autopsy findings in the older population compared with younger age groups. Otomo[3] found 10 primary intracranial tumors among 12,213 consecutive autopsy cases from a general hospital, with many geriatric patients. Of these 10 neoplasms, eight were meningiomas. A comparative series from the *Japanese Annual of Pathological Autopsy*, which comprises cases of mixed age groups, yielded only 18% meningiomas among primary intracranial tumors. Tsuyumu *et al.*,[4] also found meningiomas to comprise a high percentage among primary intracranial tumors in patients over sixty (44.5%). With regard to clinical problems in that age group, these workers warn against diagnostic pitfalls, one of them being that increased intracranial pressure is generally not found in elderly patients with meningiomas (perhaps because of atrophy of the brain?). Also, many of these cases are characterized by sudden onset, dementia, and intermittent course. Not too surprisingly, 12 of the cases were misdiagnosed as cerebrovascular disease.

Not all the meningiomas seen in old patients had their start after middle age. Probably the longest life-span for a meningioma was documented by Dudley *et al.*[5] in the remarkable case of an 81-year-old woman. This woman had migrainelike headaches in the region of the left eye since age 5. At age 50, a left sphenoid ridge meningioma was partly removed, but the tumor kept growing and killed her at the age of 81 in 1971. At the time of its first removal, this tumor was presented at the Annual Meeting in the American Association of Neuropathologists in 1940.

References

1. Wood, M.W., White, R.J., and Kernohan, J.W.: One hundred intracranial meningiomas found incidentally at necropsy.
   J. Neuropathol. Exp. Neurol. 16: 337–340, 1957.
2. Cooney, L.M., Jr., and Solitare, G.B.: Primary intracranial tumors in the elderly.
   Geriatrics 27: 94–104, 1972.
3. Otomo, E.: Brain tumor in the aged.
   Clin. Neurol. (Tokyo) 13: 120–127, 1973.
4. Tsuyumu, M., Suganuma, Y., Ohata, M., Hiratsuka, H., and Inada, Y.: Meningioma in the aged—on its differential diagnosis.
   No. Shinkei Geka (Tokyo) 4: 947–951, 1976.
5. Dudley, A.W., Jr., Erickson, T.C., Odom, G.L., Mathieson, G., and Penfield, W.: Fatal congenital meningioma in an 81 year old woman.
   J. Neuropathol. Exp. Neurol. 32: 178–179, 1973.

CHAPTER 15

Meningiomas and Intracranial Vascular Problems

Cerebrovascular diseases, or accidents, be they obstructive in nature (infarcts) or hemorrhages, may figure in the differential diagnosis of meningiomas, or they may be truly caused by or coexist with meningiomas. In the first group are patients with meningiomas who show the clinical features of cerebral vascular disease, sometimes leading to a mistaken diagnosis. This is usually the result of a sudden strokelike appearance of symptoms, entirely caused, however, by the tumor itself. This problem has been discussed in great detail by Moore[1] and more recently by Skultety[2] and Kalyanaraman *et al.*[3] Consideration of this set of problems rightfully belongs to the clinical differential diagnosis of meningiomas.

What concerns us here are those instances in which meningiomas truly cause or coexist with cerebral hemorrhages or infarcts. It seems that massive hemorrhage as a complication of meningiomas is altogether rather rare. For example, as Modesti[4] indicated, none was described in the series of Cushing and Eisenhardt[5] or the series compiled by Hoessly and Olivecrona.[6]

When a meningioma does cause hemorrhage, it may be *intracerebral*, *subdural*, or *subarachnoidal*, or the hemorrhage may remain mostly localized within the tumor itself but cause sudden enlargement of same. Goran *et al.*[7] observed four cases of *intracerebral* hemorrhage from meningiomas. In Modesti's[4] four cases of intracranial hemorrhage from meningiomas, one was intracerebral and subdural, the other three were subdural. All four of these meningiomas were found to be histologically very vascular. By contrast, in the two cases of intracerebral hemorrhages originating from a meningioma observed by Russell and Rubinstein,[8] the offending tumors were not particularly vascular. Walsh *et al.*[9] had a 77-year-old patient with a subfrontal meningioma who presented with a *subdural hematoma.* These investigators suggested that meningiomas may cause subdural hematomas in one of two ways: 1) by growth into the subdural space, and stretching the bridging veins until they rupture; and 2) through a hemorrhage from a meningioma that extends into the subdural space.

A meningioma and a subdural hematoma may coexist in the same patient without the tumor necessarily being responsible for the hemorrhage. In fact, even a reversed sequence is possible. In the case mentioned earlier, that of Cusick and Bailey,[10] a 47-year-old woman had bilateral ossified subdural hematomas since early childhood. Signs of a convexity meningioma developed at age 44. The possibility exists that long-lasting irritation by the chronic subdural hematomas may have had a role in the development of the meningioma. In still other cases, the patients with a subdural hematoma have actually suffered recent trauma that was blamed for the hemorrhage, and yet an underlying meningioma had been present that contributed to the hemorrhagic episode. Such a case was reported by Bingas and Meese.[11]

In most reported cases, hemorrhage was among the initial presenting signs of the tumor, but in Budny's[12] case, a 66-year-old women had a parasagittal meningioma removed without hemorrhagic complications, but 4 months later the recurrence of the same tumor caused a fatal hemorrhage.

Askenazy and Behmoaram[13] were the first to observe *subarachnoid hemorrhage*, as the presenting sign of meningiomas. In their two cases (a 34-year-old and a 28-year-old woman, respectively), the illness began abruptly with severe subarachnoid hemorrhage. The cause in both patients was the same: a meningioma involving the choroid plexus of the lateral ventricle. This may also occur in children, as in the 14-year-old female patient of Smith *et al.*,[14] who was in excellent health until the sudden onset of frontal headache, stiff neck, nausea, vomiting, and somnolence. A lumbar tap was grossly bloody. An aneurysm or arterial venous malformation was suspected, but instead, the angiogram showed a tumor in the trigone of the left lateral ventricle, which, at surgery, proved to be a meningioma. Meningiomas that produce massive subarachnoidal hemorrhage are not necessarily located, however, within the ventricles. Yasargil and So[15] reported two cases of subarachnoidal hemorrhage in patients who had meningiomas in the cerebellopontine angle, and Rosenberg *et al.*[16] have seen two cases of cavum Meckeli meningiomas with subarachnoid hemorrhage.

Hemorrhage, of course, can start *within the meningioma itself*, either because of the high degree of vascularity of some of these tumors, or as discussed in a Clinico-Pathologic Conference of the *New York State Journal of Medicine*,[17] as a result of hemorrhagic necrosis of the tumor. That patient had a thrombosis of the left internal carotid artery that was thought to have been responsible for infarction within the meningioma. Another hemorrhage within a meningioma that proved fatal within 24 hr was described by Bilodeau and Beraud.[18] Helle and Conley[18/a] provide an excellent review of all the reported cases of hemorrhages caused by meningiomas.

Venous occlusion caused by meningiomas happens most frequently when a meningioma near a major sinus will compress or invade the lumen of the sinus. If this develops slowly, as is usually the case, it will be tolerated, because the slow rate of occlusion permits the development of collaterals. A more rapid occlusion of a major sinus, whether or not related to surgery, may cause venous infarction in the draining area of the given vessel. Another complication of venous occlusion may be increased intracranial pressure. In two cases of Marr and Chambers,[19] the posterior portion of the superior sagittal sinus together with the torcula were occluded and both patients (a 65-year-old and a 26-year-old woman, respectively) had signs of increased cranial pressure with papilledema, suggesting to the clinicians the diagnosis of pseudotumor cerebri. The same year, Merli and Carteri[20] reported a case of a meningioma in the pineal region that obstructed the straight sinus with similar consequences. *Arterial occlusion* caused by meningioma is less common. We have seen a case where the right internal carotid was surrounded and smothered by a meningioma in the area of the foramen lacerum. The artery showed chronic fibrous obliteration, which was very likely secondary to the pressure from the meningioma. In the case of Bito and Sakaki[21] a middle fossa meningioma caused temporary occlusion of the right middle cerebral artery.

References

1. Moore, M.T.: The fate of clinically unrecognized intracranial meningiomas.
Neurology (Minneapolis) 4: 837–856, 1954.
2. Skultety, F.M.: Meningioma simulating ruptured aneurysm. Case report.
J. Neurosurg. 28: 380–382, 1968.
3. Kalyanaraman, K., Smith, B.H., and Alker, G.J., Jr.: Intracranial tumors of apoplectiform onset.
NY State J. Med. 73: 2133–2139, 1973.
4. Modesti, L.M., Binet, E.F., and Collins, G.H.: Meningiomas causing spontaneous intracranial hematomas.
J. Neurosurg. 45: 437–441, 1976.
5. Cushing, H., and Eisenhardt, L.: *Meningiomas. Their classification, Behaviour, Life History and Surgical End Results.* Springfield, ill., Charles C Thomas, 1938, p. 69.
6. Hoessly, G.F., and Olivecrona, H.: Report on 280 cases of verified parasagittal meningioma.
J. Neurosurg. 12: 614–626, 1955.
7. Goran, A., Ciminello, V.J., and Fischer, R.G.: Hemorrhage into meningiomas.
Arch. Neurol. 13: 65–69, 1965.
8. Russell, D.S., and Rubinstein, L.J.: Pathology of tumours of the nervous system, 4th ed. Baltimore, Williams & Wilkins, 1977, p. 72.
9. Walsh, J.W., Winston, K.R., and Smith, T.: Meningioma with subdural hematoma.
Surg. Neurol. 8: 293–295, 1977.
10. Cusick, J.F., and Bailey, O.T.: Association of ossified subdural hematomas and a meningioma. Case report.
J. Neurosurg. 37: 731–734, 1972.
11. Bingas, B., and Meese, M.: Subdurales Hämatom seltener Ätiologie. (Fallmitteilung).
Nervenarzt 37: 175–177, 1966.
12. Budny, J.L., Glassauer, F.E., and Sil, R.: Rapid recurrence of meningioma causing intracerebral hemorrhage.
Surg. Neurol. 5: 323–325, 1977.
13. Askenazy, H.M., and Behmoaram, A.D.: Subarachnoid hemorrhage in meningiomas of the lateral ventricle.
Neurology (Minneapolis) 10: 484–489, 1960.
14. Smith, V.R., Stein, P.S., and MacCarty, C.S.: Subarachnoid hemorrhage due to lateral ventricle meningiomas.
Surg. Neurol. 4: 241–243, 1975.
15. Yasargil, M.G., and So, S.C.: Cerebellopontine angle meningioma presenting as subarachnoid hemorrhage.
Surg. Neurol. 6: 3–6, 1976.
16. Rosenberg, G.A., Herz, D.A., Leeds, N., and Strully, K.: Meckel's cave meningiomas with subarachnoid hemorrhage.
Surg. Neurol. 3: 333–336, 1975.
17. Bruno, M.S., and Ober, W.B. (eds.): Clinico-Pathologic Conference. Intracranial lesion with hemorrhage.
NY State J. Med. 71: 1951–1959, 1971.
18. Bilodeau, B., and Beraud, R.: Hemorrhage in a meningioma.
Can. Med. Assoc. J. 95: 682–684, 1966.
18/a. Helle, T. L. and Conley, F. K. Haemorrhage associated with meningioma: A case report and review of the literature.
J. Neurol. Neurosurg. Psychiat. 43: 725–729, 1980.
19. Marr, W.G., and Chambers, J.W.: Occlusion of the cerebral dural sinuses by tumor simulating pseudotumor cerebri.
Am. J. Ophthalmol. 61: 45–49, 1966.
20. Merli, G.A., and Carteri, A.: Su un caso di meningioma della regione pineale svilsuppantesi nel seno retto con ostruzione competa di esso.
Sist. Nerv. 18: 62–67, 1966.
21. Bito, S., and Sakaki, S.: A case of a middle fossa meningioma with an infarction of the right middle cerebral artery.
(In Japanese) Brain-Nerve (Tokyo) 23: 953–957, 1972.

CHAPTER 16

Systemic Effects of Meningiomas

Most of the clinical symptoms and signs in patients with meningiomas are caused by local effects of the tumor mass. Except perhaps with meningiomas *en plaque*, there is always some pressure on the underlying tissues with resulting damage to cortex or other parts of the brain. The tumor may be large enough or grow rapidly enough to produce generalized increased intracranial pressure. It can be the cause of vascular occlusion, either venous or arterial. It may provoke hemorrhage, edema, or cyst formation in neighboring tissues. Meningiomas may also affect more distant portions of the brain not immediately adjacent to the tumor. For example, normal pressure hydrocephalus has been seen in a case of a tentorial meningioma by Kirschberg *et al.*[1]: the tumor obliterated the cerebrospinal fluid space next to the tentorium and thereby caused communicating hydrocephalus.

Some of the *indirect* effects of meningiomas are due to local pressure on the pituitary gland or hypothalamus. This is most often seen in cases of suprasellar meningiomas. Korsgaard *et al.*[2] analyzed endocrine functions in 35 patients who had suprasellar and hypothalamic nonpituitary tumors. Seven patients with meningioma were included in the group, and two of them had lowered urinary gonadotropin levels. Although impressive, such remote endocrine changes were more profound in patients with craniopharyngiomas and hypothalamic gliomas involving the same area.

In infants and young children hypothalamic tumors sometimes cause loss of appetite and massive weight loss—diencephalic syndrome of emaciation (Russell[3]). Such tumors are usually gliomas. An exceptional case was reported by Campiche and Oberson,[4] when the same syndrome was caused in a $3\frac{1}{2}$-year-old child by a tuberculum sellae meningioma.

Whereas the above hormonal changes are obviously caused by direct pressure on the hypothalamopituitary axis by meningiomas, there are also *distant* effects that are derived from the mere presence of the tumor or its chemical constituents.

During the last few decades, it has become increasingly evident that the presence of a neoplasm in the human body may significantly affect the immunological responses of the patient. That this should be so in tumors of the lymphoreticular system, the cells of which are primarily responsible for immunologic responses, should not be surprising. Other neoplasms, however, may also affect the patients' immunologic status, and meningiomas apparently are no exception. Mahaley *et al.*[5] studied patients with brain tumors with regard to their immunologic responses. Seventeen patients with meningiomas were included, and a degree of anergy was found in them. Cell-mediated immunity was tested with skin tests, using Streptokinase–Streptodornase (SK-SD), Trichophyton, and mumps test, all showing weakened response. Interestingly, skin reactions did not improve after removal of the tumor. Among the same group of patients, the authors also found lymphopenia and a decrease in humoral antibodies against influenza and tetanus after a booster shot. Thus, both cellular and humoral responses were to some extent decreased, as compared with normal subjects. Rather surprisingly, Tokumaru and Catalano[6] found an *increase* in IgM in the serum of patients with meningiomas, but Mahaley *et al.*[5] could not confirm this in their material, and Nakao *et al.*[7] found essentially normal plasma levels of the three major immune globulins in 18 patients with meningiomas. Some patients with meningiomas develop changes in the chemical constitution of the blood plasma. Mazzei *et al.*[8] found hypocalcemia and tetany in a patient with meningioma; these disappeared after removal of the tumor. By contrast, the patient of Liévre and Camus[9] had hypercalcemia. As to blood glucose levels, Jestico and Lantos[10] had a patient with a malignant meningioma of the right parasagittal area in whom hepatic metastases developed (the liver weighed 9 kg) as well as metastases in the kidneys, pancreas, and abdominal lymph nodes. This patient developed severe hypoglycemia with a blood glucose level down to 25 mg%; he suffered massive convulsive seizures as a result. It is known that some mesodermal tumors produce insulin or insulin-like substances, but in this patient radioimmunoassays (RIAs) of plasma insulin showed normal levels. It was therefore postulated that the low blood sugar was caused by massive liver destruction by tumor. The possibility that the huge total mass of tumor consumed too much glucose could not be ruled out.

Whereas no meningiomas have so far been implicated in causing hyperglycemia in a normal patient, Denton *et al.*[11] believed that the development of a meningioma aggravated their 54-year-old patient's existing diabetes mellitus. In this case, the brain tumor was responsible for a seizure that the authors believed to have precipitated hyperosmolar, hyperglycemic, nonketotic diabetic coma.

As to changes in circulating blood cells, in addition to the above-mentioned lymphopenia, a unique case of peripheral eosinophilia in a patient with meningioma was reported by Dietrich-Rap and Dziduszko.[12] One usually associates erythrocytosis in brain tumor patients with hemangioblastomas or occasionally metastatic renal cell carcinomas, both of which are known to elaborate erythropoietin. It is not a common feature with meningiomas, but Toyama *et al.*[13] found erythrocytosis in one of their patients with this tumor. The preoperative serum as well as the tumor tissue contained erythropoietin. Gabriel and Harrison[14] observed a patient whose meningioma apparently had systemic effects similar to those of a pheochromocytoma. There was a high urinary VMA level, which disappeared after the tumor was removed.

Whereas many meningiomas contain large amount of alkaline phosphatase within tumor cells (see pages 20–21) elevation of alkaline phosphatase levels in the serum is uncommon. It appears that such patients must have an unusually large tumor mass for this to affect the blood level of the enzyme. Such a case was reported by Kepes *et al.*,[15] a patient with a focally papillary hemangiopericytic meningioma of the peritorcular area, that metastasized extensively to both lungs. In this case, a large amount of alkaline phosphatase was found in the tumor cells histochemically, and it was thought that release of the enzyme from these cells was responsible for the high level of the enzyme in the serum. This case was also included in a report on metastatic meningiomas by Palacios and Azar-Kia[16] (Fig. 134). Mignot *et al.*[17] had a patient with a very similar problem, a posterior fossa meningioma that recurred twice locally; the patient eventually died with extensive pulmonary metastases. In that case, the blood levels of alkaline phosphatase seemed closely related to the tumor mass in the patient because after each removal of the tumor there was a precipitous drop in the serum level of this enzyme, but each time the tumor recurred the enzyme levels started rising again. (This was also true for the erythrocyte sedimentation rate, which rose to 142 mm/hr in the presence of the original tumor or its recurrences, but after surgeries it was as low as 3 mm/hr.) Mignot *et al.*[17] also believed the high serum levels of alkaline phosphatase to be caused by enzyme release from the tumor itself. It is possible that the elevated sedimentation rate was related to the malignant nature of the meningioma and its metastases.

References

1. Kirschberg, G.J., Epstein, I., Strasberg, Z., and White, N.F.: Normal-pressure hydrocephalus due to tentorial meningioma.
Can. Med. Assoc. J. 115: 154–155, 1976.
2. Korsgaard, O., Lindholm, J., and Rasmussen, P.: Endocrine function in patients with suprasellar and hypothalamic tumours.
Acta Endrocrinol. (Kbh) 83: 1–8, 1976.
3. Russell, A.: Diencephalic syndrome of emaciation in infancy and childhood.
Arch. Dis. Child. 26: 274–275, 1951.
4. Campiche, R., and Oberson, R.: Syndrome d'émaciation provoqué par un méningiome du tubercule sellaire.
Oto-Neuro-Ophthalmol. 44: 353–358, 1972.
5. Mahaley, M.S., Jr., Brooks, W.H., Roszman, T.L., Bigner, D.D., Dudka, L., and Richardson, S.: Immunobiology of primary intracranial tumors. Part I: Studies of the cellular and humoral general immune competence of brain tumor patients.
J. Neurosurg. 46: 467–476, 1977.
6. Tokumaro, T., and Catalano, L.W.: Elevation of serum immunoglobulin M (IgM) level in patients with brain tumor.
Surg. Neurol. 4: 17–21, 1975.
7. Nakao, S., Terano, M., Yamashita, J., and Handa, H.: Serum immunoglobulin (IgG, IgM, IgA) levels in patients with primary brain tumor.
No To Shinkei (Brain and Nerve) Tokyo 29: 1005–1009, 1977.
8. Mazzei, T.S., Mazzei, C.M., and Sanoner, A.: Hipocalcemia y tetania en el meningioma. Desaparicion despues de su extirpacion. Sindrome paraneoplasico.
Rev. Clin. (Espanol.) 141: 183–186, 1976.
9. Liévre, J.A., Camus, J.P., Joublin, M., and Schaeffer, A.: Hypercalcémie et méningiome. Le diagnostic différentiel des manifestations nerveuses de l'hypercalcémie.
Rev. Rhum. Malad. Resp. 37: 207–211, 1970.
10. Jestico, J.V., and Lantos, P.L.: Malignant meningioma with liver metastases and hypoglycemia. A case report.
Acta Neuropathol. (Berl.) 35: 357–361, 1976.
11. Denton, I.C., Jr., Kerlan, R.A., and McGraw, R., Jr.: Brain tumor with hyperosmolar hyperglycemic nonketotic diabetic coma.
JAMA 218: 256–257, 1971.

12. Dietrich-Rap, Z., and Dziduszko, J.: A case of brain tumor with raised eosinophil count (In Polish). *Neurol. Neurochir. Pol. 7: 749–751, 1973.*
13. Toyama, K., Fujiyama, N., Chen, T.P., Nakazawa, K., Suzuki, H., Hasegawa, M., and Toya, S. Erythrocytosis associated with various tumours; with a case report of meningioma associated with erythrocytosis *In Erythropoiesis*, K. Nakao, *et al.* (eds.), Baltimore University Park Press, 1975, pp. 435–446.
14. Gabriel, R., and Harrison, B.D.W.: Meningioma mimicking features of a phaeochromocytoma. *Br. Med. J. 2: 312, 1974.*
15. Kepes, J.J., MacGee, E.E., Vergara, G., and Sil, R.: Malignant meningioma with extensive pulmonary metastases. *J. Kansas Med. Soc. 72: 312–316, 1971.*
16. Palacios, E., and Azar-Kia, B.: Malignant metastasizing angioblastic meningioma. *J. Neurosurg. 42: 185–188, 1975.*
17. Mignot, B., Hauw, J.J., de Sigalony, J.P.H., and Bricaire, F.: Perturbations biologiques réversibles évoluant parallélement à un méningiome recidivant et avec métastases. *Sem. Hop. Paris 54: 1231–1237, 1978.*

CHAPTER 17

Meningiomas Combined with Non-Neoplastic Diseases

Meningiomas may coexist with other pathologic conditions that can affect the diagnosis or treatment of the brain tumor. Diagnostic problems are particularly likely to occur if the coexisting disease is one that also has central nervous system manifestations. Covey[1] described a 55-year-old woman who had suffered from essential hypertension for a long time; when signs of intracranial disease developed, they were thought to be caused by high blood pressure. Eventually, she was found to have a large right-sided parasagittal meningioma. The removal of the tumor relieved her intracranial symptoms. The reverse was true in the case of Hayreh *et al.*[2] Their patient, a 78-year-old woman, suffered from dementia with frontal lobe syndrome. Although she was found to have a 4 × 4 × 4 cm frontal meningioma, and the tumor was removed, her dementia did not improve after surgery; subsequent brain biopsy showed evidence of Creutzfeldt-Jakob disease.

The association of meningiomas with intracranial vascular disease in young people was reported by Jimenez *et al.*[3] in two women aged 28 and 44 years, respectively, both of whom had multiple meningiomas, intracranial aneurysms, and cerebrovascular atherosclerosis. The first patient had two meningiomas and a right internal carotid aneurysm. She died after surgery and was found to have atherosclerosis diffusely involving the cerebral vasculature. The second patient had three meningiomas plus an aneurysm of the left internal carotid artery. (See also Chapter 15.)

The presence of a symptomatic meningioma in an elderly male with multiple sclerosis was described by Spaar and Wikström.[4]

The occurrence of meningioma in a patient with progeria (Werner's syndrome) was first reported by Mogensen,[5] with a second case added by Hoppe and Koritsch.[6]

Blood dyscrasias may seriously interfere with the treatment of meningiomas by increasing the danger of hemorrhage during surgery. An interesting case of this type was reported by Gendelman *et al.*[7] whose patient had factor IX deficiency. One of the patient's brothers had already died of intracranial hemorrhage. This patient's meningioma, however, was successfully removed while he was receiving a large amount of factor IX during surgery.

References

1. Covey, A.H.: Meningioma coexisting with severe hypertension. Problems of diagnosis. *NY State J. Med. 72: 2561–2562, 1972.*
2. Hayreh, S.M., McDonnell, D.E., and Aschenbrenner, C.A.: Meningioma with Creutzfeldt-Jakob disease. (Letter.) *Arch. Neurol. 36: 179–180, 1979.*
3. Jiminez, J.P., Goree, J.A., and Parker, J.C., Jr.: An unusual association of multiple meningiomas, intracranial aneurysm and cerebrovascular atherosclerosis in two young women. *Am. J. Roentgenol. Rad. Ther. Nucl. Med. 112: 281–288, 1971.*
4. Spaar, F.W., and Wilkstrom, J.: Multiple sclerosis and malignant neoplasms in the central nervous system; a clinical anatomical report of three cases. *J. Neurol. 218: 23–33, 1978.*
5. Mogensen, E.F.: Konveksitetsmeningeom hos en patient med Werner's Syndrom. *Ugeskrift for Laeger 115: 18–21, 1953.*
6. Hoppe, W., and Koritsch, H-D.: Ein weiterer Fall von Meningeom bei einem Patienten mit Werner-Syndrome. *Psychiatr. Neurol. Med. Psychol. (Leipz.) 24: 611–617, 1972.*
7. Gendelman, S., Aledort, L., and Hollin, S.: Intracranial meningioma in Factor IX deficiency. *JAMA 239: 748–749, 1978.*

CHAPTER 18

Meningiomas Coexisting with Other Neoplasms

Numerous cases are on record that describe patients suffering from a meningioma as well as other intracranial or intraspinal tumor or tumors. This combination is frequently seen in von Recklinghausen's disease, in which meningiomas are usually accompanied by neurofibromas and neurilemmomas, as well as gliomas. Outside this group of patients, which will not be further discussed in this chapter, the most common combination is between meningiomas and tumors of the astrocytic series, particularly glioblastoma multiforme. Cushing and Eisenhardt[1] described the prototype of such a patient, a man who had both a peritorcular meningioma and a glioblastoma of the corpus callosum. Other reports included those of Barla-Szabo,[2] Myerson[3] (with four meningiomas and two gliomas in one patient), Arieti[4] (astrocytoma and meningioma), Kirschbaum,[5] Feiring and Davidoff[6] (two meningiomas and a glioblastoma), Alexander,[7] Russell,[8] Gass and van Wagenen[9] (an oligodendroglioma combined with meningioma), Brihaye *et al.*[10] Hoffman,[11] and Fényes and Kepes[12] (one patient with meningioma and glioblastoma, the other with an olfactory groove meningioma and an ependymoma of the fourth ventricle), King and Botton,[13] Shapiro *et al.*,[14] Madonick *et al.*,[15] Nagashima *et al.*,[16] Bingas and Brunngraber,[17] Sahar and Streifler,[18] Cooper,[19] Sackett *et al.*,[20] Wilson and Ashley,[21] Tanaka *et al.*,[22] Strong *et al.*,[23] Mikhael,[24] Marra *et al.*,[25] Antunes *et al.*,[26] and Karapowsky and Chernashov.[27] Manuelidis and Solitare,[28] reviewing combined tumors in a study dealing primarily with glioblastomas, tabulated these cases, including an additional 10 reports of glioblastomas occurring together with meningiomas.

Russell and Rubinstein,[29] who observed five cases of meningiomas coexistent with gliomas (all glioblastomas), considered such concurrence to be most likely coincidental, as both meningiomas and gliomas are relatively common. If, however, the meningioma and glioma develop in close juxtaposition, it was felt that a relationship between the two may exist, particularly if the meningioma is malignant. Not all meningiomas closely juxtaposed to gliomas are malignant; however, of the abovementioned cases, those reported in refs. 9, 16, 19, and 22–25 fulfilled this criterion. In the cases of Gass and van Wagenen,[9] the meningioma and the underlying oligodendroglioma was removed in one sitting; Nagashima *et al.*[16] were also able to report successful removal of a meningioma and contiguous glioma, whereas Cooper[19] first thought that a layer of gliosis was underlying the meningioma of his patient, only to return subsequently after the biopsy from the tumor bed proved to represent a glioma. In the case of Tanaka *et al.*,[22] the meningioma developed 24 years after the removal of an oligodendroglioma of the same location. The tumors were later found in combined form.

After gliomas, adenomas of the pituitary gland appear to be the most common second intracranial tumor associated with meningiomas (again, not counting the combination of meningiomas and neurilemmomas in von Recklinghausen's disease). In the case of Bankl *et al.*,[30] the patient had a meningioma as well as an eosinophilic adenoma of the pituitary and acromegaly, as did the patients described by Stock *et al.*,[31] Bunick *et al.*,[32] and Hainer *et al.*[33] The patient of Bankl *et al.*[30] also had a carcinoid of the small intestine, whereas Gaffney and Coyle[34] had a patient with a posterior fossa meningioma and a carcinoid tumor of the gallbladder. A parathyroid adenoma accompanied the intracranial meningioma in the patient described by Grinblat *et al.*[35] As to nonfunctioning endocrine tumors, Brennan *et al.*[36] described a large chromophobe adenoma with a middle fossa meningioma, the two tumors together forming a dumbbell-shaped lesion. Finally, the interesting combination of a meningioma and a melanoma of the choroid plexus described by Aron-Rosa *et al.*[37] deserves special mention. The coexistence of breast carcinoma and meningioma in the same patient and its implications were alluded to earlier (Chapter 7).

References

1. Cushing, H.J., and Eisenhardt, L.: *Meningiomas. Their Classification, Regional Behaviour, Life History and Surgical End Results.* Springfield Ill., Charles C Thomas, 1938, p. 507.
2. Barla-Szabó, L.: Ueber multiple Hirngeschwülste. *Zentralbl. Allg. Pathol. 74: 397, 1940.*
3. Myerson, P.G.: Multiple tumors of the brain of diverse origin. *J. Neuropathol. Exp. Neurol. 1: 406–415, 1942.*
4. Arieti, S.: Multiple meningioma and meningiomas associated with other brain tumors. *J. Neuropathol. Exp. Neurol. 3: 255–270, 1944.*
5. Kirschbaum, W.R.: Intrasellar meningioma and multiple cerebral glioblastoma. *J. Neuropathol. Exp. Neurol. 4: 370–378, 1945.*
6. Feiring, E.H., and Davidoff, L.M.: Two tumors, meningioma and glioblastoma multiforme in the same patient. *J. Neurosurg. 4: 282–289, 1947.*
7. Alexander, W.S.: Multiple primary intracranial tumor. Meningioma associated with a glioma. Report of a case. *J. Neuropathol. Exp. Neurol. 7: 81–88, 1948.*
8. Russell, D.S.: Meningeal tumours: A review. *J. Clin. Pathol. 3: 191–211, 1950.*
9. Gass, H., and van Wagenen, W.P.: Meningioma and oligodendroglioma adjacent in the brain. Case report. *J. Neurosurg. 7: 440–443, 1950.*
10. Brihaye, J., Danis, P., and Drochmaus, P.: Tumeur cérébrale multiple avec syndrome de Foster Kennedy: Gliomes du corpus calleux et du lobe temporal, méningiome du nerf optique. *Acta Neurol. Belg. 51: 28–55, 1951.*
11. Hoffmann, G.R.: Astrocytome et méningiome associés chez même sujet. *Acta Neurol. Belg. 52: 57–60, 1952.*
12. Fényes, Gy., and Kepes, J.: Über das gemeinsame Vorkommen von Meningomen und Geschwülsten anderen Typs im Gehirn. *Zentralbl. Neurochir. 16: 251–260, 1956.*
13. King, A.B., and Botton, J.E.: Multiple tumors of the central nervous system. *Guthrie Clin. Bull. 27: 49–56, 1957.*
14. Shapiro, S.K., Segal, M., and Horwitz, C.A.: Two primary intracranial tumors of different histological type. Report of a case with both a glioblastoma and a meningioma. *Minn. Med. 59: 84–87, 1976.*
15. Madonick, M.J., Shapiro, J.H., and Torack, R.M.: Multiple diverse primary brain tumors. Report of a case with review of the literature. *Neurology (Minneapolis) 11: 430–436, 1961.*
16. Nagashima, C., Nakashio, K., and Fujino, T.: Meningioma and astrocytoma adjacent in the brain. *J. Neurosurg. 20: 995–999, 1963.*
17. Bingas, B., and Brunngraber, C.V.: Das gleichzeitige Vorkommen von Meningeom und Glioblastom. *Zentralbl. Neurochir. 24: 271–280, 1964.*
18. Sahar, H., and Streifler, M.: Multiple intracranial tumors of diverse origin. *Neurochirurgia (Stuttg.) 9: 18–27, 1966.*
19. Cooper, D.R.: Contiguous meningioma and astrocytoma in brain. *NY State J. Med. 69: 969–972, 1969.*
20. Sackett, J.F., Stenwig, J.T., and Songsinjul, P.: Meningeal and glial tumors in combination. *Neuroradiology 7: 153–160, 1974.*
21. Wilson, P.J.E., and Ashley, D.J.B.: Meningioma after contralateral hemispherectomy for malignant glioma, case report. *J. Neurol. Neurosurg. Psychiatry 38: 493–499, 1975.*
22. Tanaka, J., Garcia, J.H., Netsky, M.G., and Williams, J.P.: Late appearance of meningioma at the site of partially removed oligodendroglioma. Case report. *J. Neurosurg. 43: 80–85, 1975.*
23. Strong, A.J., Symon, L., MacGregor, B.J.L., and O'Neill, B.P.: Coincidental meningioma and glioma. Report of two cases. *J. Neurosurg. 45: 455–458, 1976.*
24. Mikhael, M.A.: Case report: Diminished density surrounding a meningioma verified to be an overlying cystic astrocytoma. *J. Comput. Assist. Tomogr. 1: 349–351, 1977.*
25. Marra, A., Ramponi, G., and Grimaldi, G.: Simultaneous occurrence of right supratentorial meningioma and glioblastoma multiforme. Case report. *Acta Neurochir. 36: 83–91, 1977.*
26. Antunes, A.C.M., Coutinho, M.F., and Coutinho, L.M.B.: Meningeoma e glioblastoma concomitantes. Registro de un caso. *Arq. Neuropsiquiatr. 36: 265–269, 1978.*
27. Karapowsky, M.I., and Chernashov, I.M.: On primary multiple tumors of the brain. (In Russian.) *Vopr. Neurokhir. 1: 52–55, 1979.*
28. Manuelidis, E.E., and Solitare, G.: Glioblastoma multiforme. *In Pathology of the Nervous System*, J. Minckler (ed.), Vol. 2. New York, McGraw-Hill, 1971, pp. 2026–2071.
29. Russell, D.S., and Rubinstein, L.J.: *Pathology of Tumours of the Nervous System*, 4th ed. Baltimore, Williams & Wilkins, 1977, p. 89.
30. Bankl, H., Grunert, V., and Sunder-Plassmann, M.: Endokrine Polyadenomatose kombiniert mit einem Tentoriummeningeom. *Wien. Klin. Wochenschr. 82: 257–259, 1970.*
31. Stock, J.M., Ghatak, N.R., and Oppenheimer, J.H.: Unsuspected meningioma in a patient with pituitary gigantism. Case report with autopsy findings. *Metabolism 24: 767–775, 1975.*
32. Bunick, E.M., Mills, L.C., and Rose, L.I. Association of acromegaly and meningiomas. *JAMA 240: 1267–1268, 1978.*
33. Hainer, V., Krejcik, L., Pelikan, J., Tvarok, F., and Urbanek, J.: Meningiom nasadajici na eosinofilni adenom u pacienta s akromegalii. *Cas. Lek. Cesk. 117: 829–831, 1978.*
34. Gaffney, P.R., and Coyle, L.J.: Carcinoid tumor of the gallbladder associated with a meningioma. *Ir. J. Med. Sci. 147: 318–321, 1978.*
35. Grinblat, J., Seidenstein, B., Lerman, P., and Lewitus, Z.: Meningiomas associated with parathyroid adenoma. *Am. J. Med. Sci. 272: 327–330, 1976.*
36. Brennan, T.G., Jr., Rao, C.V., Robinson, W., and Itani, A.: Case report. Tandem lesions: Chromophobe adenoma and meningioma. *J. Comput. Assist. Tomogr. 1: 349–351, 1977.*
37. Aron-Rosa, D., Laloi, M., Man, H.X., Dhermy, P., and Girard, G.: Tumeur double méningiome et melanome malin de la choroide associés (á propos d'un cas). *Bull. Soc. Ophtalmol. Fr. 77: 895–897, 1977.*

CHAPTER 19

Epidural Meningiomas

By far most cranial and spinal meningiomas develop inside, that is, deep to, the dura mater, and they may or may not be attached to that membrane. Some meningiomas, of course, not only attach themselves to the dura, but grow right through it. Much less commonly, one finds meningiomas with their main bulk situated on the outer surface of the dura mater. Such tumors are called epidural meningiomas, and they occur both intracranially and within the spinal canal. Of course, in the head, where the dura is lying tightly against the bone, an extradural meningioma is by definition intraosseus, or may grow through and beyond the bone into the soft tissues of the scalp. Although, as stated before, the greatest bulk of these tumors is extradural, many of them nevertheless do have an intradural component, while others involve the substance of the dura, but not the intradural space. Still others—epidural meningiomas in the purest sense—are found only on the outer surface of the dura.

SPINAL EPIDURAL MENINGIOMAS

The first such tumor was described by Tissier in 1898.[1] Subsequent examples are found in many series. For example, Ellsberg[2] saw two patients with such tumors: a 9-year-old boy and a 44-year-old woman. Frazier and Alpers[3] described one in a 10-year-old girl, as did Ingraham,[4] who found an epidural meningioma in another 10-year-old girl. (That latter patient, however, also suffered from neurofibromatosis.) Other well-documented reports are by Haft and Shenkin[5] (one case), Soo[6] (two cases), Singh *et al.*[7] (two cases), Fortuna *et al.*[8] (four cases), and Rao *et al.*[9] (three cases). An excellent summary of the literature prior to 1972 was given by Calogero and Moossy,[10] who collected 35 cases and added four of their own. Some interesting findings emerged from their study: among the 35 reviewed cases, the sexes were about equally divided. This is all the more striking because, in general, among spinal meningiomas the ratio of females versus males has been recorded as high as 20:1 in some series. Also, the number of children in the series was unusually high—five children among the 35 cases (14.2%). Many of the reviewed cases had some minor intradural component. Calogero and Moossy[10] believe that epidural meningiomas make up about 15% of all spinal meningiomas. Cases reported since this review article were by Borovich *et al.*,[11] Gandolfi and Bertolino,[12] Krishnan *et al.*,[13] Ohaegbulam,[14] and Motomochi *et al.*[15] Of these, Ohaegbulam's case was particularly noteworthy, because it was found at the level of the cauda equina, a region in which meningiomas occur with utmost rarity.

EXTRADURAL MENINGIOMAS OF THE CRANIUM

As in the spinal extradural forms, such meningiomas may have involvement of the dura, but the greatest bulk is on the outer surface of this membrane. As stated before, such tumors frequently invade through the bone and may also cause hyperostosis. The bony mass thus produced or the tumor itself may be palpable in such patients. One such case, often quoted, was reported by Zachariae[16]: a 58-year-old woman whose extradural meningioma caused marked swelling in the left temporal area. Hyperostosis was also present in the case of Siegel and Anderson.[17] Excess bone formation, however, does not have to be present in such cases. No bone was reported to be present in a giant epidural childhood meningioma of the occipital area,[18] and in the patient of McWhorter *et al.*,[19] an extradural meningioma presented as a lytic skull lesion: the tumor replaced the outer table and greatly thinned the inner table of the skull. Other extracalvarial meningiomas in the recent literature were reported by Ito *et al.*[20] and Hamada *et al.*[21]

PRIMARY INTRAOSSEOUS MENINGIOMAS

Since, as stated above, the dura mater forms the endosteum for cranial bones, any meningioma growing into extradural tissue will involve bone. The dural component may be represented by no more than an area of diffuse thickening underlying the involved bone. In such cases, it is not always clear whether the dura was the source of the tumor or might have been secondarily invaded by a meningioma that originated in the bone. Many cases in the literature are listed as intraosseous meningiomas, that, on closer examination, showed dural involvement.[22,23] It is probably best to consider as truly primary intraosseous meningiomas those cases wherein the tumor was entirely within the bone and the dura was found intact on careful examination. Such were the first two cases of Azar-Kia *et al.*,[23] the childhood case of Choux *et al.*,[24] and the intradiploic meningioma of the orbital roof reported by Reale *et al.*[25] Case 1 of Waga *et al.*[26] may also be listed in this category; although the authors considered the tumor an extracalvarial meningioma arising from the outer table of the skull, as it was still covered by periosteum, it was, strictly speaking, an intraosseous, although not intradiploic, meningioma.

References

1. Tissier, H.: Compression lente de la moelle. *Bull. Soc. Anat. Fr. 73: 304–308, 1898.*
2. Ellsberg, C.A.: Concerning the clinical features and the diagnosis of extramedullary meningeal and perineurial fibroblastomas of the spinal cord. *Bull. Neurol. Inst. NY 3: 124–137, 1933.*
3. Frazier, C.H., and Alpers, B.J.: Meningeal fibroblastomas of the cerebrum. A clinicopathologic analysis of 75 cases. *Arch. Neurol. Psych. 29: 935–989, 1933.*
4. Ingraham, F.D.: Intraspinal tumors in infancy and childhood. *Am. J. Surg. 39: 342–376, 1938.*
5. Haft, H., and Shenkin, H.A.: Spinal epidural meningioma. Case report. *J. Neurosurg. 20: 801–804, 1963.*
6. Soo, L.Y.: Spinal epidural meningioma. *South. Med. J. 59: 141–144, 1966.*
7. Singh, R., Coerkamp, G., and Luyendijk, W.: Spinal epidural meningiomas. *Acta Neurochir.* (*Wien*) *18: 237–245, 1968.*
8. Fortuna, A., Gamacorta, D., and Occhipinti, E.M.: Spinal extradural meningiomas. *Neurochirurgia* (*Stuttg.*) *12: 166–180, 1969.*
9. Rao, S.B., Dinakar, I., and Rao, K.S.: Spinal epidural meningiomas. *Neurol. India 18: 126–128, 1970.*
10. Calogero, J.A., and Moossy, J.: Extradural spinal meningiomas. Report of four cases. *J. Neurosurg. 37: 442–447, 1972.*
11. Borovich, B., Wilson, E., and Palomo, J.: Extradural spinal meningioma. *Acta Neurol. Lat. Am. 16: 231–236, 1970.*
12. Gandolfi, A., and Bertolino, G.: Simultaneous cervical cord compression from herniated disk and extradural meningioma. Report of a case. *Acta Neurol.* [*Quad.*] *33: 273–278, 1978.*
13. Krishnan, K.L.M., Narayanan, R., Kalyanaraman, G., and Ramamurthi, B.: Spinal epidural meningioma. *Int. Surg. 63: 42–43, 1978.*
14. Ohaegbulam, S.C. Cauda equina epidural meningioma. *Acta Neurochir.* (*Wien*) *46: 287–291, 1979.*
15. Motomochi, M., Makita, Y., Nabeshima, S., and Aoyama, I.: Spinal epidural meningioma in childhood. *Surg. Neurol. 13: 57–66, 1980.*
16. Zachariae, L.: A case of extracranial primary meningioma. *Acta Pathol. Microbiol. Scand.* [*B*] *31: 57–66, 1952.*
17. Siegel, G.J., and Anderson, P.J.: Extracalvarial meningioma. Case report. *J. Neurosurg. 25: 83–86, 1966.*
18. Rao, S.B., Dinakar, I., and Rao, K.S.: Giant intracranial epidural meningioma. Case report. *J. Neurosurg. 35: 748–750, 1971.*
19. McWhorter, J.M., Ghatak, N.R., and Kelly, D.L.: Extracranial meningioma presenting as lytic skull lesion. *Surg. Neurol. 5: 223–224, 1976.*
20. Ito, M., Tomizawa, M., Takagi, S., and Ishii, S.: Extracalvarial meningioma. Report of a case. *No Shinkei Geka 5: 465–471, 1977.*
21. Hamada, H., Kadota, K., Uetsukara, K., Asakura, T., and Igakura, T.: Extracalvarial meningioma. A case report. (In Japanese.) *No Shinkei Geka 5: 633–639, 1977.*
22. Wagman, A.D., Weiss, E.K., and Riggs, H.E.: Hyperplasia of the skull associated with intra-osseous meningioma in the absence of gross tumor. *J. Neuropathol. Exp. Neurol. 19: 111–115, 1965.*
23. Azar-Kia, B., Sarwar, M., Marc, J.A., and Schechter, M.M.: Intra-osseous meningioma. *Neuroradiology 6: 246–253, 1974.*
24. Choux, R., Choux, M., Hassoun, J., Gomez, A., and Baurand, C.: Meningiome intra-osseux chez un enfant. *Neurochirurgie 21: 89–97, 1975.*
25. Reale, F., Delfini, R., and Cintorino, M.: An intradiploic meningioma of the orbital roof: Case report. *Ophthalmologica 177: 82–87, 1978.*
26. Waga, S., Nishikawa, M., Ohtsubo, K., Kamijyo, Y., and Handa, H.: Extracalvarial meningiomas. *Neurology* (*Minneapolis*) *20: 369–372, 1970.*

CHAPTER 20

Meningiomas of the Orbit

Meningiomas form an important part of intraorbital tumors. According to Craig and Gogelo,[1] the first intraorbital meningioma was described in 1816 by Scarpa. Since that first report, it has become a well-known entity for ophthalmologists and neurosurgeons alike. It should not be surprising that meningeal tumors sometimes involve the orbit. After all, the orbit is part of the skull and is connected to the middle cranial fossa through the optic foramen and the superior orbital fissure. It is therefore fairly easy for intracranial meningiomas to grow by extension into the orbit. In addition, the orbit houses the optic nerve with its full complement of meningeal sheaths: dura, arachnoid, and pia mater, tissues that themselves may give rise to meningiomas. Rarely, meningiomas apparently unconnected to either the optic nerve or intracranial masses are believed to originate from ectopic nests of arachnoidal tissue within the orbit or its walls.

As to incidence, Reese,[2] in an analysis of 504 consecutive cases of expanding lesions in the orbit, found 17 meningiomas to account for 3% of the total. Many of these people are young.[3] In their series of 25 primary orbital meningiomas, Karp *et al.*[4] found their patients to be mostly young white females. Ten of the 25 were less than 20 years old and six were under the age of 10. Of these 10 children, eight were girls and four suffered from von Recklinghausen's disease.

With regard to relative incidence of the sources of orbital meningiomas, those invading the orbit secondarily as an extension from an intracranial tumor form the majority. Meningiomas arising from the optic nerve sheath are less common. In the series of Craig and Gogelo,[1] 17 tumors originated from the optic sheath as contrasted to 35 patients whose orbital tumor was an extension of an intracranial meningioma. Of the latter, tumors of the sphenoid ridge are the most common, although other sites may also play the role of a primary source. Some of these tumors are bilateral. The medially located sphenoid ridge meningiomas may extend into, and impinge on, the contents of the optic canal, causing visual impairment, but obstruction of the superior orbital fissure may also result in problems for the contents of the orbit. Similarly, the *en plaque* meningiomas of the pterion often cause exophthalmus through tumor growth as well as through hyperostosis, thereby endangering vision.

As to meningiomas of the optic nerve sheath, they may start their development in the area of the optic foramen, sometimes forming a dumbbell tumor with a small intracranial extension,[5] but most are located farther anteriorly, involving the optic nerve behind the globe. Like meningiomas elsewhere, they are believed to originate from the arachnoid sheath, but as a rule they do not remain intradural; instead, they penetrate the dura mater and involve to a varying extent the soft tissues of the orbit. Their presence and growth usually leads to severe atrophy of the optic nerve (22 of the 25 patients in the Karp *et al.*[4] series), as the nerve is caught in the center of this tumor mass (Fig. 125). An additional circulatory problem for the eye may be caused by the shunting effect of ectatic opticociliary veins that develop in patients with orbital meningiomas.[6]

Rarely, the tumor will penetrate the globe and invade the choroid and the retina, usually through the area of the optic disc. Henderson and Campbell,[7] who reported a case of this type, reviewed the pertinent literature covering this complication of orbital meningiomas. A case of this type is shown in our Fig. 124.

Once an intraorbital tumor attains a large size, its precise place of origin may become difficult to determine. As stated, truly ectopic meningiomas of the orbit are rare. A representative case, involving the superior orbital ridge, was found by Wolter and Benz[8]; their patient had neither an intracranial nor an optic sheath meningioma.

References

1. Craig, W., McK., and Gogelo, L.J.: Intraorbital meningiomas. A clinico-pathologic study. *Am. J. Ophthalmol. 32: 1663–1680, 1949.*

2. Reese, A.B.: *Tumors of the eye*, 3rd ed. Hagerstown, Md., Harper & Row, 1976, pp. 148–153.
3. Walsh, F.B.: Meningiomas primary within the orbit and optic canal. *In* Neuro-Ophthalmology, J. S. Glaser and J. Lawton Smith (eds.). London, Henry Kimpton, 1975, Vol. 8, p. 166.
4. Karp, L.A., Zimmerman, L.E., Borit, A., and Spencer, W.: Primary intraorbital meningiomas. *Arch. Ophthalmol. 91: 24–28, 1974.*
5. Russell, D.S., and Rubinstein, L.J.: *Pathology of Tumours of the Nervous System*, 4th ed. Baltimore, Williams & Wilkins, 1977, pp. 308–309.
6. Zakka, K.A., Summerer, R.W., Yee, R.D., Foos, R.Y., and Kim, J.: Optociliary veins in a primary optic nerve sheath meningioma. *Am. J. Ophthalmol. 87: 91–95, 1979.*
7. Henderson, J.W., and Campbell, R.J.: Primary intraorbital meningioma with intraocular extension. *Mayo Clin. Proc. 52: 504–508, 1977.*
8. Wolter, J.R., and Benz, S.C.: Ectopic meningioma of the superior orbital rim. *Arch. Ophthalmol. 94: 1920–1922, 1976*

CHAPTER 21

Meningiomas in Other Unusual Sites

It might appear somewhat arbitrary to separate tumors in this chapter from the previously discussed spinal and cranial extradural meningiomas; it is done mostly for clinical considerations. The cranial and spinal meningiomas, even when extradural, or intraosseous, are still in the domain of the neurosurgeon for diagnosis and operative removal. The ophthalmologist is very likely first to encounter a meningioma involving the optic nerve, orbit, or eyeball. But those meningiomas that occur elsewhere "belong to" other specialists. Tumors of the paranasal sinuses or the middle ear are usually discovered and treated by an otolaryngologist. Meningiomas of the skin will probably be the responsibility of a plastic surgeon or a dermatologist, not to mention the still more distant areas, such as neck, mediastinum, or other locations, which may be handled by general surgeons, thoracic surgeons, and so on.

GENERAL ASPECTS

Hoye *et al.*[1] provided a very useful classification for ectopic meningiomas. The categories suggested by these authors are as follows:

1. Meningiomas that originate intracranially or intraspinally, but later extend into neighboring structures (e.g., paranasal sinuses, orbit, ear). Any of these may initially present as a truly ectopic tumor, and in every case one must rule out the existence of an underlying intracranial or intraspinal meningioma that may have only a tenuous connection with the ectopic portion of the tumor. Most extracranial and extraspinal meningiomas really belong to this category.
2. Meningiomas that originate from extracranial and extraspinal arachnoidal cell nests in or near foramina that serve as exit points for cranial nerves. In these instances, the arachnoidal cell nests are often supposed to have formed part of the covering for the nerve exiting through that given foramen, although an alternate theory for the origin, namely, metaplasia from nerve sheath cells, has been proposed by Smith *et al.*[2] and Shuangshoti and Panathanya.[3]
3. Extracranial and extraspinal meningiomas with no obvious connections to foramina or nerves, ocurring at remote sites, such as skin or thoracic cavity.
4. Metastases of malignant meningiomas.

Perhaps the most detailed and all-inclusive series of ectopic meningiomas was compiled by Farr *et al.*[4] from New York Hospital and Memorial Hospital. Their 405 cases of meningioma included 30 in the orbit, 25 involving the outer table of the skull and scalp, 10 from the nasal or paranasal area, five in the parotid and parapharyngeal region, and two in the neck as deep parotid tumors.

NASAL CAVITY AND PARANASAL SINUSES

One of the early important papers on meningiomas in these areas was by New and Devine.[5] They described four meningiomas, three of them in the frontal sinus, and one in the midline attached to the roof of the nose. Secondary invaders from intracranial sites above were not included. Other reports represent a mixture of secondary invaders and truly primary tumors. Olfactory meningiomas growing into the nose from above were described by Belal *et al.*,[6] Rosalki *et al.*,[7] and Caruel *et al.*[8] Tumors attached to lower surface of the cribriform plate and filling the nasal cavity have been seen by Pathak,[9] So *et al.*,[10] and others, whereas an another apparently "true" primary intranasal meningioma was found by McGavran *et al.*[11] Vakil,[12] from India, also reported what appeared to be a primary meningioma of the nose and ethmoid as well as sphenoid sinus in a 10-year-old girl. In the two cases of Kjeldsberg and Minckler,[13] the meningiomas presented as nasal polyps. On the other hand, the oft-quoted "ectopic meningioma in infant" of Khanna *et al.*[14] turns out to be a nasal glioma on closer examination of the published picture.

The meningioma observed by Majoros[15] and the two cases of Rao *et al.*[16] were located within a frontal sinus with no apparent tumor elsewhere, as in the cases of New and Devine.

Shaheen[17] described a case of a 12-year-old boy with a maxillary sinus meningioma that extended into the ethmoidal sinus, but had no connection to the dura. Other similar cases were reported by Shuangshoti and Panyathanya[3] and Stanisavljevic *et al.*[18]

ORAL CAVITY

Suzuki *et al.*[19] have seen a meningioma of the pterygopalatine fossa that bulged into the oral cavity, causing swelling of the right cheek. Brown *et al.*[20] reported a meningioma, part of which presented as an intraoral mass, the main bulk of the tumor, however, was in the maxillary sinus. The second patient of So *et al.*[10] had a retromandibular meningioma; inspection of the oral cavity showed medial displacement of the tonsil.

PAROTID

The parotid gland may be involved by the extracranial portion of an intracranial meningioma. Grundy *et al.*[21] described such a case, in which a right sphenoid ridge meningioma has extended into this gland. By contrast, the patient of Wolff and Rankow[22] had a meningioma that apparently originated within the parotid. The authors speculated about the role of displaced arachnoid cells that may have followed the facial nerve into this salivary gland.

EAR

Woltman and Love[23] had a patient with multiple intracranial meningiomas, one of them growing through the petrous bone presented as a warty mass in the right external auditory canal. A very similar case was described by Risch.[24] By 1964, Nager[25] was able to compile a monograph on meningiomas involving the temporal bone; to the 30 cases found in the literature he added seven of his own. In a later work,[26] he and Masica provided beautiful illustrations of intrapetrous extension of the tumor. Singh *et al.*[27] have seen a meningioma confined to the internal auditory meatus in a 14-year-old boy; the tumor did not extend medially beyond the porus acousticus. Russell and Rubinstein[28] have also observed two cases of petrous bone meningiomas, one involving the facial nerve. We have seen a patient who presented with otitis media with granulation tissue protruding through the perforated eardrum. This was curetted and microscopically showed an underlying meningioma. Many new cases have been added to the list; Buchheit *et al.*[29] summarized the literature of the last few years.

NECK

Meningiomas of the base of the skull may extend into the neck or they may originate within the cervical structures. Important reported cases include the ones by Hoye *et al.*[1]: a 22-year-old man with a retromandibular meningioma, and Hallgrimson *et al.*,[36] a 15-year-old boy with the tumor found behind the sternomastoid muscle. Shuangshoti *et al.*[31] found a parapharyngeal meningioma in a 36-year-old man, whereas the ectopic meningioma described by Russell and Rubinstein[28] was found at the carotid bifurcation. We have seen three histologically typical deep cervical meningiomas in the Kansas University material and examined one in consultation from the Mayo Clinic (Figs. 137 and 138).

MEDIASTINUM

Located even farther away from the CNS was the meningioma described by Wilson *et al.*[32] Their patient was a 63-year-old physician, who had an asymptomatic lesion in the apex of the right lung, discovered on routine x-ray film of the chest. This tumor was removed and found to be a meningothelial meningioma. The investigators postulated that the cells of origin were possibly related to the stellate ganglion.

SKIN

Winckler[33] was the first to describe ectopic meningiomas in the skin. His patient was a 10-year-old girl with raised dermal and subcutaneous nodules of the back. In the area of the lowermost lesion there was also hypertrichosis of the skin. Bain and Shnitka[34] reported on a 38-year-old man who had a painless lump 2 inches in diameter within the skin posterior to the frontal hairline. The patient later died of uremia and heart failure and autopsy showed no residual meningioma in the scalp and brain. (There was no sign of neurofibromatosis, either, but a pheochromocytoma was found in the right adrenal.)[35] The 31-year-old woman patient of Brown and Cherry[36] had a left frontoparietal subcutaneous nodule that appeared first as a sebaceous cyst, but later turned out to be a meningioma. Nothing was found intracranially. Junaid *et al.*[37] reported a 3-year-old girl from Ibadan, Nigeria, who had an ovarian fibroma and multiple skin swellings in the neck (just as Winckler's first patient did), which proved to be cutaneous meningiomas. A useful classification of meningiomas in the skin was offered by Lopez *et al.*,[38] who reviewed 25 cases at the Armed Forces Institute of Pathology (AFIP) and divided cutaneous meningiomas into three types, Types I, II, and III.

Type I. Tumors of the scalp, face, and paravertebral skin, occurring mostly in children. These tumors probably originate from congenitally displaced arachnoidal cells that create hamartoma-like growths. Such tumors usually have a benign course.

Type II. Meningiomas in the skin near the sensory organs (eye and ear).

Type III. Meningiomas originating intracranially or intraspinally, and reaching the skin by growing through the bone or through a bone defect.

The prognosis is best for type I.

PERIPHERAL NERVE

Some meningiomas of the soft tissues of head and neck are believed to develop from arachnoidal cell clusters accompanying the sheaths of cranial nerves (*vide supra*). A much more distant meningioma was described in the brachial plexus of a 26-year-old woman by Harkin and Reed.[39] There was no clinical evidence that the tumor involved the vertebral canal.

References

1. Hoye, S.J., Hoar, C.S., Jr., and Murray, J.I.: Extracranial meningioma presented as tumor of the neck. *Am. J. Surg. 100: 486–389, 1960.*
2. Smith, A.T., Selecki, B.R., and Stening, W.A.: Ectopic meningioma. *Med. J. Aust. 1: 1100–1104, 1973.*
3. Shuangshoti, S., and Panyathanya, R.: Ectopic meningiomas. *Arch. Otolaryngol. 98: 192–105, 1973.*
4. Farr, H.W., Gray, G.F., Vrana, M., and Panio, M.: Extracranial meningioma. *J. Surg. Oncol. 5: 411–420, 1973.*
5. New, G.B., and Devine, K.D.: Neurogenic tumor of nose and throat. *Arch. Otolaryngol. 46: 163–179, 1947.*
6. Belal, A.: Meningiomas infiltrating the nasal cavity, nasal sinuses and the orbit. *J. Laryngol. Otol. 69: 59–69, 1959.*
7. Rosalki, S.B., and McGee, L. I.: Meningioma presenting as nasopharyngeal tumour. Report of two cases. *J. Laryngol. Otol. 76: 133–139, 1962.*
8. Caruel, N., Houtteville, J.P., and Pertuiset, B.: Le prolongement nasal des méningiomes olfactifs. *Neurochirurgie 17: 160–162, 1971.*
9. Pathak, P.N.: Ectopic meningioma of the nose. *J. Laryngol. Otol. 83: 1115–1118, 1969.*
10. So, N.C., Ngan, H., and Ong, G. B.: Ectopic meningiomas. Report of two cases and review of literature. *Surg. Neurol. 9: 231–237, 1978.*
11. McGavran, M.H. Biller, H.F., and Ogura, J.H.: Primary intranasal meningioma. *Arch. Otolaryngol. 93: 95–97, 1971.*
12. Vakil, R.E.: Meningioma of the nose and paranasal sinuses. *Neurology (India) 22: 95–96, 1974.*
13. Kjeldsberg, C.R., and Minckler, J.: Meningiomas presenting as nasal polyps. *Cancer 29: 153–156, 1972.*
14. Khanna, S.D., Singh, G., and Saigal, R.K.: Ectopic meningioma in an infant. *Arch. Surg. 89: 752–754, 1964.*
15. Majoros, M.: Meningioma of the paranasal sinuses. *Laryngoscope 80: 640–645, 1970.*
16. Rao, S.B., Dinakar, I., and Reddy, C.R.: Meningioma of the frontal sinus; report of two cases. *J. Neurosurg. 36: 363–365, 1972.*
17. Shaheen, H.B.: Psammoma in the maxillary antrum. *J. Laryngol. Otol. 46: 117, 1931.*
18. Stanisavljevic, B., Stefanovic, P., Pejcic M., and Djordjevic, M.: Cas d'un rare méningiome ectopique primaire du nez et du sinus maxillaire chez l'enfant. *Rev. Otol. Rhinol (Bord.) 96: 85–84, 1975.*
19. Suzuki, H., Gilbert, E.F., and Zimmermann, B.: Primary extracranial meningioma. *Arch. Pathol. 84: 202–206, 1967.*
20. Brown, A.M., Fordham, K.C., and Lally, E.T.: Meningioma presenting as an intraoral mass. *Oral Surg. 41: 771–776, 1976.*
21. Grundy, D.J., Hobsley, M., and Ranger, D.: Recurrent meningioma presenting as a parotid swelling. *Proc. R. Soc. Med. 64: 1002, 1971.*
22. Wolff, M., and Rankow, R.M.: Meningioma of the parotid gland: An insight into the pathogenesis of extracranial meningiomas. *Hum. Pathol. 2: 453–459, 1971.*
23. Woltman, H.W., and Love, J.G.: Multiple intracranial meningiomas with extension to the external auditory canal: Successful removal. Presentation of case. *Mayo Clin. Proc. 10: 497–501, 1935.*
24. Risch, O.C.: Meningioma with unusual involvement of the temporal sphenoid and occipital bone. *Laryngoscope 52: 732–744, 1942.*
25. Nager, G.T.: *Meningioma Involving the Temporal Bone. Clinical and Pathological Aspects.* Springfield, Ill., Charles C Thomas, 1964.

26. Nager, G.T., and Masica, D.N.: Meningiomas of the cerebello-pontine angle and their relation to the temporal bone.
Laryngoscope 80: 863–895, 1970.
27. Singh, K.P., Smyth, G.D., and Allen, I.V.: Intracanalicular meningioma.
J. Laryngol. Otol. 89: 549–552, 1975.
28. Russell, D.S., and Rubinstein, L.J.: *Pathology of Tumours of the Nervous system*, 4th ed. Baltimore, Williams & Wilkins, 1977, p. 68.
29. Buchheit, F., Greiner, D., Maitrot, D., and Braun, J.J.: Meningiome intrapetreux primitif.
Oto-Neuro-Ophthalmol. 49: 25–32, 1977.
30. Hallgrimsson, J., Ornsson, A., and Gudmundsson, G.: Meningioma of the neck. Case report.
J. Neurosurg. 32: 695–699, 1970.
31. Shuangshoti, S., Netsky, M.G., and Fitz-Hugh, G.S.: Parapharyngeal meningioma with special reference to cell of origin.
Ann. Otol. Rhinol. Laryngol. 80: 463–473, 1971.
32. Wilson, A.I., Ratliff, J.L., Lagios, M.D., and Aguilar, M.J.: Mediastinal meningioma.
Am. J. Surg. Pathol. 3: 557–562, 1979.
33. Winckler, M.: Über Psammome der Haut und des Unterhautgewebes.
Virchows Arch. [*Pathol. Anat.*] *178: 323–350, 1904.*
34. Bain, G.O., and Shnitka, T.K.: Cutaneous meningioma (psammoma).
Arch. Dermatol. Syphil. 74: 590–594, 1956.
35. Shnitka, T.K., and Bain, G.O.: Cutaneous meningioma (psammoma). Autopsy findings in a previously reported case.
Arch. Dermatol. Syphil. 80: 410–412, 1959.
36. Brown, J.M., and Cherry, A.P.: Subcutaneous meningioma.
Med. J. Aust. 2: 1972–1973, 1971.
37. Junaid, T.A., Nkoposong, E.O., and Kolawole, T.M.: Cutaneous meningiomas and an ovarian fibroma in a three year old girl.
J. Pathol. 108: 165–167, 1972.
38. Lopez, D.A., Silvers, D.N., and Hellwig, E.B.: Cutaneous meningiomas—A clinicopathologic study.
Cancer 34:728–744, 1974.
39. Harkin, J.C., and Reed, R.J.: Tumors of the peripheral nervous system. *In Atlas of Tumor Pathology*, 2nd series. Washington, D.C., Armed Forces Institute of Pathology, 1969, fasc. 3, p. 18.

CHAPTER 22

Chromosomal Patterns in Meningiomas

The relationship between chromosomal abnormalities and neoplasia has interested many investigators, and a huge body of scientific literature has evolved from the studies related to this matter. Very broadly speaking, there have been two main lines of studies of abnormal chromosomal patterns as they relate to neoplasms: 1) abnormalities in the karyotype of the host who develops tumors. An example of this would be the patients with Down's syndrome, who have a known higher incidence of developing malignancies, particularly myeloid leukemia. 2) The other avenue of study is that of chromosomes and chromosomal patterns of the tumors themselves. With regard to meningiomas, a similar division can be made: There have been studies of karyotype of somatic cells in patients who harbor meningiomas, and the karyotypes of meningioma cells themselves have also been investigated. It is in the latter area that some very striking developments have taken place in the last decade:

Chromosomal abnormalities in human and experimental neoplasms have been known for quite some time to exist. However, departure from the normal diploic chromosomal pattern was always more likely to be associated with malignant tumors rather than benign neoplasms. In fact, according to Robbins and Cotran,[1] most human cancers are aneuploid. Such cytogenic changes as are present may in part be secondary phenomena acquired during active replication of the tumor cells, but at least some are supposed to be present from the very beginning of tumor development. As a rule, such chromosomal changes do not constitute markers of a specific neoplastic process. (A notable exception is chronic myelocytic leukemia with its specific marker, the Philadelphia chromosome.) It was therefore of significant interest when Zang and Singer[2] first reported in a letter to *Nature* that in eight out of eight meningiomas they cultured from 4 to 9 days, the karyotype showed loss of a chromosome of the G group (monosomy G). The missing chromosome was identified as one belonging to the number 22 pair, by fluorescent banding[3,4] and also by Giemsa banding.[5]

These findings created so much interest among geneticists that Mark[6] could point out, "Cytogenetically the meningioma is currently the most thoroughly studied tumor type of all human solid neoplasms." By 1977, more than 200 meningiomas had been studied and other reports have been added since. In general, consistent with Zang and Singer's original report, hypoploidia is predominating among chromosomal changes—75% according to Robbins and Cotran[1]—and among these karyotypes those with 45 chromosomes outnumber the others. This means that there is a pronounced tendency in meningiomas to lose chromosomes during their karyotypic evolution.

A similar stemline pattern has not been observed in any other tumor type studied in detail. Interestingly, in the cultures examined, not every tumor cell was involved in the loss of chromosomes. There seemed to be a sideline of variant cells that have a normal karyotype. Apparently, when meningiomas develop in the body they start with a normal karyotype and then deviate from it. Mark[6] believed that the loss of one G chromosome might be advantageous for the tumor under *in vivo* conditions. Because *in vitro* the normal karyotype will slowly overgrow the monosomy G cells, it appears that cells with a normal karyotype thrive better in culture.

As to the nature of the chromosome loss, Zankl *et al.*[7] showed that the missing chromosome was not lost to translocation, as neither partial nor total translocation was observed in the karyotypes. In addition to the typical loss of chromosome 22 (Fig. 1), the absence of other chromosomes was detected in some tumors. Most notably, in six out of 24 meningiomas of male patients, the Y chromosome was also missing (Fig. 2).[8] Whereas the absence of one chromosome did not have an apparent effect on the general cytology of the cells, if two or more

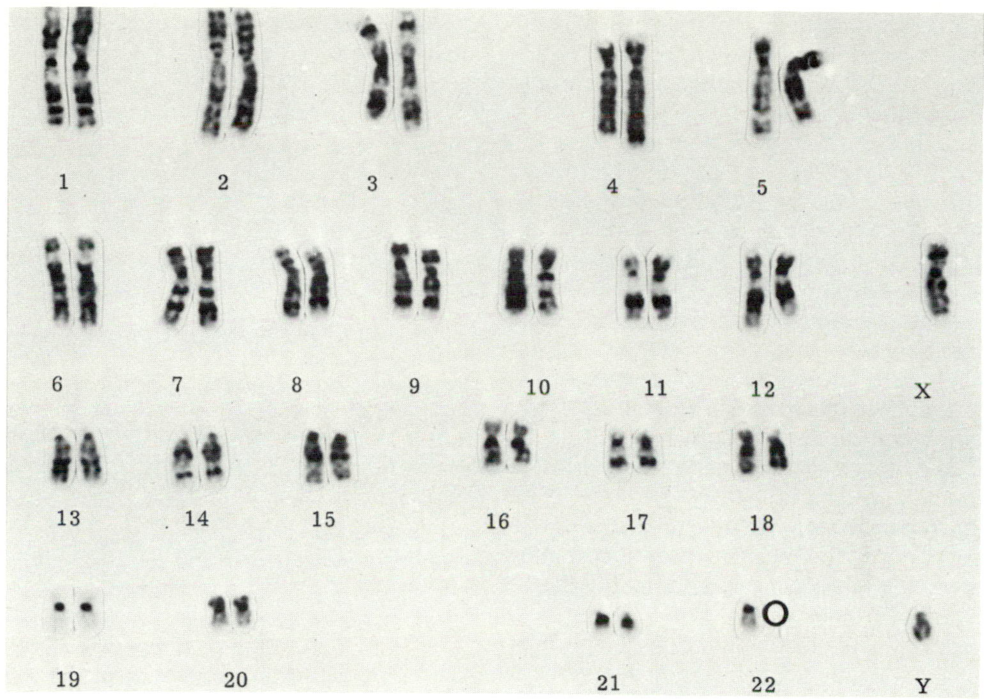

FIGURE 1
Karyotype of a meningioma in cell culture. There are only 45 chromosomes: one No. 22 chromosome is missing. This is the most common chromosomal abnormality seen in cultured meningiomas. (Courtesy Prof. Dr. H. Zankl.)

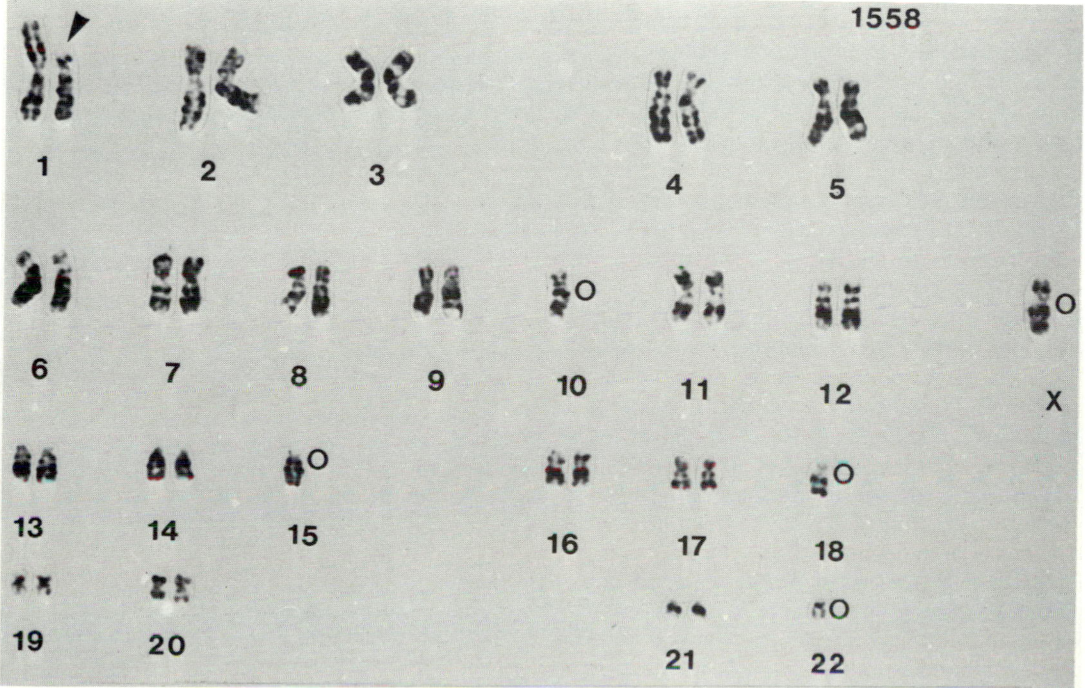

FIGURE 2
Karyotype of another meningioma. Here, in addition to the missing No. 22 chromosome, No. 10, No. 15, No. 18, and an X chromosome are absent as well. (Courtesy Prof. Dr. H. Zankl.)

acrocentric chromosomes were lost, there was a decrease in nucleoli in the tumor cells.[3] It will be of interest to follow the relationship of chromosomal changes to specific histologic variants of meningiomas. In this regard, one interesting fact has already emerged: A 47/48 hyperdiploid stemline was found by Mark[9] in a benign-appearing angioblastic meningioma. Mark[10] also reported a histologically benign meningioma having a ring chromosome. According to this author, ring chromosomes have been seen in many malignant tumors, such as carcinomas and malignant gliomas, but this meningioma was the first benign neoplasm to show such anomaly.

In summary, if one disregards for the time the much less common other chromosomal aberrations in meningiomas, one can state with Mark *et al.*[4] that a large number of meningiomas—better than 70%, according to Yunis[11]—have nonrandom chromosomal evolution involving primarily the loss of one G-22 chromosome.

Compared with the rich literature on chromosomal anomalies in meningiomas themselves, very few data exist about abnormal karyotypes of the patients who have meningiomas. One such patient was reported by Ayraud,[12] a 60-year-old woman with a right frontal meningioma. This patient had a short neck, small, poorly developed breasts, and, although her external genitalia appeared normal, she was never regular in her menstrual periods. She also had coxa vara and polycystic kidneys. Buccal smears showed Barr bodies in only 3% of the cells examined. Her karyotype was 45X-46XX and 47XXX in equal proportions. The karyotype of her meningioma was not examined, and whether the fact that she had a meningioma was related to her general chromosomal makeup is not known.

The traditional method of determining chromosomal patterns in tumor cells is through culturing the cells and establishing a karyotype by arresting mitosis and counting chromosomes. There are now newer techniques available, in particular flow through cytometry, making it possible to compare the DNA content, size, and viability of meningioma cells obtained directly from surgical specimens with the same cells after a period of culture. Such techniques have been applied to meningiomas by Fredericksen *et al.*[13,14] Kajikawa *et al.*[15] as well as Lehmann and Krug.[16] Whereas polyploidia characterizes cells of malignant tumors, in meningiomas the cell populations were found essentially to be diploid, with only a small proportion of tetraploid cells by Kajikawa *et al.*[15] and Lehmann and Krug.[16] When discussing diploidia, these studies did not take into consideration the monosomy so commonly seen in meningiomas (*vide supra*).

References

1. Robbins, S.L., and Cotran, R.S.: *Pathologic Basis of Disease*, 2nd ed. Philadelphia, W.B. Saunders, 1979, p. 165.
2. Zang, K.D., and Singer, H.: Chromosomal constitution of meningiomas. *Nature 216: 84–85, 1967.*
3. Zankl, H., and Zang, K.D.: The role for acrocentric chromosomes in nucleolar organization I. Correlation between the loss of acrocentric chromosomes and a decrease in number of nucleoli in meningioma cell cultures. *Virchows Arch. [Cell Pathol.] 11: 251–256, 1972.*
4. Mark, J., Levan, G., and Mitelman, F.: Identification by fluorescence of the G chromosome lost in human meningiomas. *Hereditas 71: 163–172, 1972.*
5. Paul, B., and Porter, I.H.: Giemsa banding in an established line of human malignant meningioma. *Humangenetik 18: 185–187, 1973.*
6. Mark, J.: Chromosomal abnormalities and thier specificity in human neoplasms: An assessment of recent observations by banding techniques. *Adv. Cancer Res. 24: 165–222, 1977.*
7. Zankl, H., Weiss, A.F., and Zang, K.D.: Cytological and cytogenetical studies on brain tumors VI. No evidence for a translocation in 22-monosomic meningiomas. *Humangenetik 30: 343–348, 1975.*
8. Zankl, H., Seidel, H., and Zang, K.D.: Cytological and cytogenetical studies on brain tumors V. Preferential loss of sex chromosomes in huamn meningiomas. *Humangenetik 27: 119–128, 1972.*
9. Mark, J.: Two benign intracranial human tumors with an abnormal chromosomal pattern. *Acta Neuropathol. (Berl.) 14: 174–184, 1969.*
10. Mark, J.: Chromosomal aberration and their relation to malignancy in meningiomas. *Acta Pathol. Microbiol. Scand. [A] 79: 193–200, 1971.*
11. Yunis, J.J., and Chandler, M.E.: The chromosomes of clinical and biologic significances. *Am. J. Pathol. 88: 466–496, 1977.*
12. Ayraud, N., Duplay, J., Grellier, P. Bezon, A., and Martinon, J.: Caryotype 45, X/ 46, XX/47, XXX et tumeur du systéme nerveux. *Nouv. Presse Med. 1: 2902, 1972.*
13. Fredericksen, P., Reske-Nielsen, E., and Bichel, P.: Flow cytometry in tumours of the brain. *Acta Neuropathol. (Berl.) 41: 179–183, 1978.*
14. Fredericksen, P., Reske-Nielsen, E., and Bichel, P.: DNA content of meningiomas. *Acta Neuropathol. (Berl.) 46: 65–68, 1979.*
15. Kajikawa, H., Kawamoto, K., Herz, F., Wolley, R.C., Hirano, A., and Koss, L.G.: Flow-through cytometry of meningiomas and cultured meningioma cells. *Acta Neuropathol. (Berl.) 44: 183–187, 1979.*
16. Lehmann, J., and Krug, H.: Flow-through fluorocytometry of different brain tumours. *Acta Neuropathol. (Berl.) 49: 123–132, 1980.*

CHAPTER 23

Topography and Gross Characteristics of Meningiomas

COMMON LOCALIZATION OF MENINGIOMAS

Meningiomas may occur in any area where there are meninges or at least cell clusters of meningeal derivation, but it has long been recognized that they have a distinct predilection for certain intracranial and intraspinal locations. For one thing, there appears to be a close relationship between the distribution of arachnoidal granulations and favored sites of meningiomas. The arachnoidal granulations of Pacchioni serve to redirect the cerebrospinal fluid into the major venous sinuses of the dura mater. Their relationship to the great sinuses is best observed when viewed from the inside of an opened dural sinus (Fig. 3).

The sites of predilection for meningiomas have important implications for neurosurgeons, as localization of these tumors will, to a great extent, determine the clinical symptomatology and possible operative approaches. It has become customary since the Cushing and Eisenhardt monograph to classify meningiomas according to their site of origin.

Meningiomas of the cerebral convexity may involve any one of the major lobes. They are usually globular in shape but they may have a somewhat bumpy nodular surface, particularly on their deep surface facing the brain. In benign meningiomas, such nodular extensions of the tumor may press into the underlying brain but as a rule no true infiltration occurs. By contrast, the outer surface of the tumor often has a broad-based attachment to the overlying dura (Fig. 4). On coronal sections of autopsy specimens, pressure atrophy of the underlying cortex may be well appreciated (Fig. 5). Not infrequently, the tumor penetrates the dura, in some cases continuing its growth through the bones of the skull, and even into muscle and soft tissues of the scalp. The fact that the tumor usually has a broad-based attachment to the dura has some surgical implications (Fig. 6).

Meningiomas of the anterior cranial fossa may be of the convexity type, but they also occur in the subfrontal region, in the region of the tuberculum sellae (Fig. 7), the olfactory groove (Fig. 8), and other locations. Parasagittal meningiomas develop near the midline, often with attachment to the wall of the superior sagittal sinus, the falx cerebri or both. They may involve the frontal, parietal or occipital medial cortex (the temporal lobe is not represented in the parasagittal area). Meningiomas of the falx may be unilateral (Fig. 9) or dumbbell-shaped, sometimes with equal-size masses on both sides of this dural partitioning membrane. The sphenoid ridge (formed medially by the free edge of the lesser wing, laterally by the greater wing of the sphenoid bone) is a common site of origin for meningiomas. Because of the location of this structure (separating the anterior and middle cranial fossae), meningiomas of the sphenoid ridge may in time involve the contents of both of these cranial compartments. Tumors of the medial third often impinge on the optic nerve canal and its contents, thus causing visual disturbances. These are usually globular in shape (Fig. 10) as are the meningiomas of the middle third. In the lateral third, the tumors may be globular or they may form a flat, granular, carpetlike growth (Fig. 11). Such *en plaque* meningiomas have a marked predilection for women, even more than the run-of-the-mill meningiomas. They usually provoke hyperostosis of neighboring bony structures. These tumors of the pterion many times present clinically with exophthalmus.

Other favored sites for meningiomas include the cavum of Meckel, the peritorcular area (near the confluens sinuum or torcular Herophili), edge and the lower surface of the tentorium cerebelli, the cerebellar convexity, the pontocerebellar angle (Fig. 12) (originating from the petrous dura), the clivus, and the edge of the foramen magnum (Fig. 13). Meningiomas may also occur without dural attachment (pial forms) sometimes in the depth of

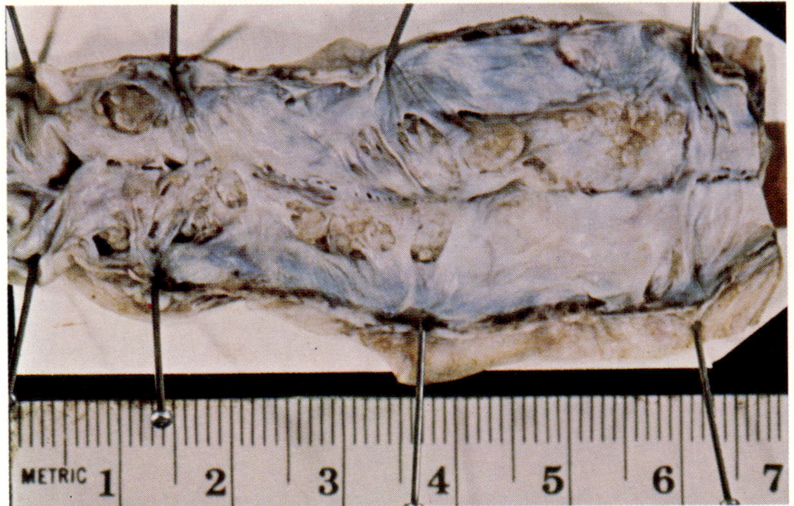

FIGURE 3.
Segment of the superior sagittal sinus in a middle-aged man. The sinus has been opened to show arachnoidal granulations (here yellow nodular masses) protruding into its lumen.

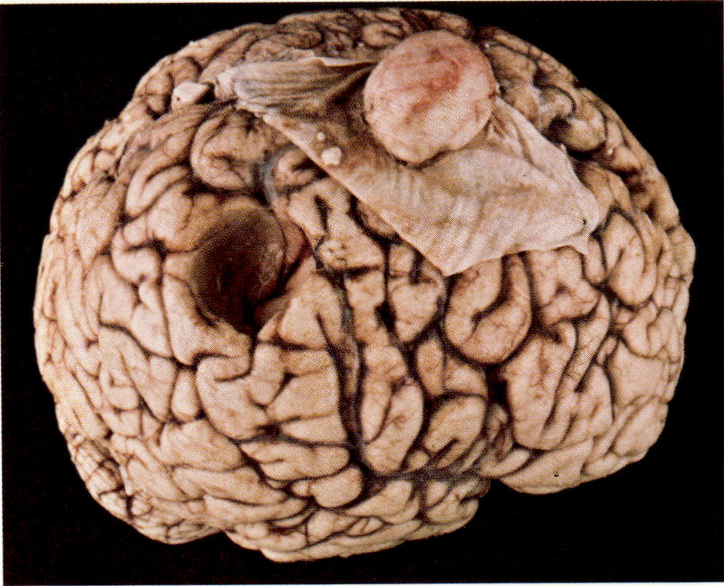

FIGURE 4.
Convexity meningioma at the junction of the right parietal and occipital lobes. (Courtesy Dr. H. Okazaki.)

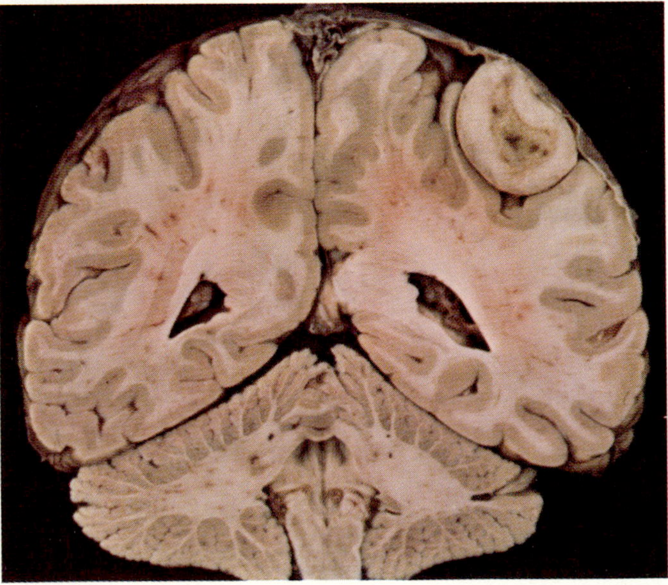

FIGURE 5
The same tumor shown in Figure 4 replaced into its original position and sectioned in the coronal plane. The brain is compressed and the cortex underlying the tumor is thinned. (Courtesy Dr. H. Okazaki.)

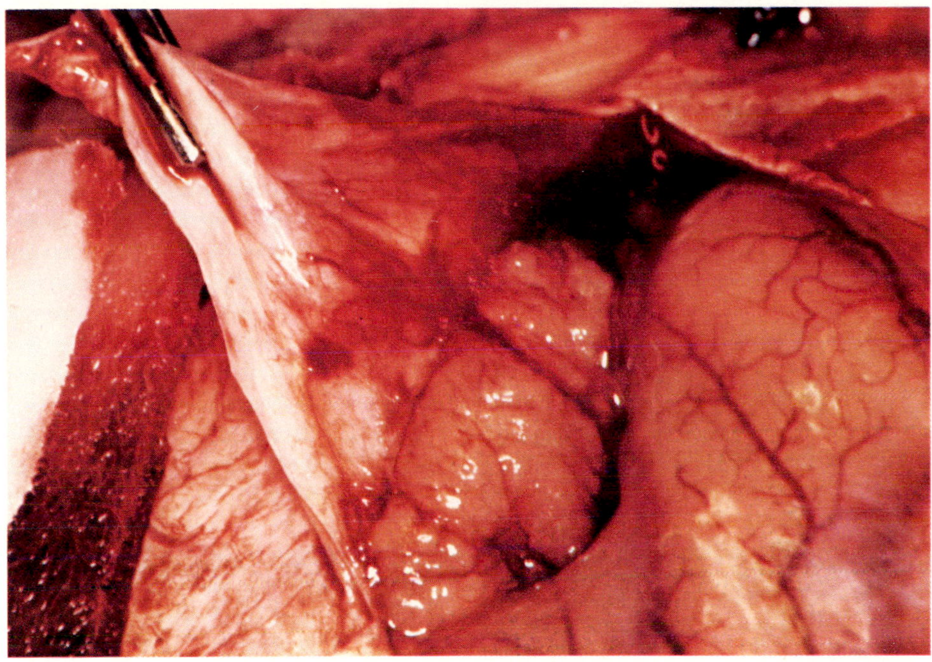

FIGURE 6
Attachment of convexity meningioma to dura mater facilitates surgical removal through gentle tugging on dura. (S. Rengachary, Kansas City VA Hospital.)

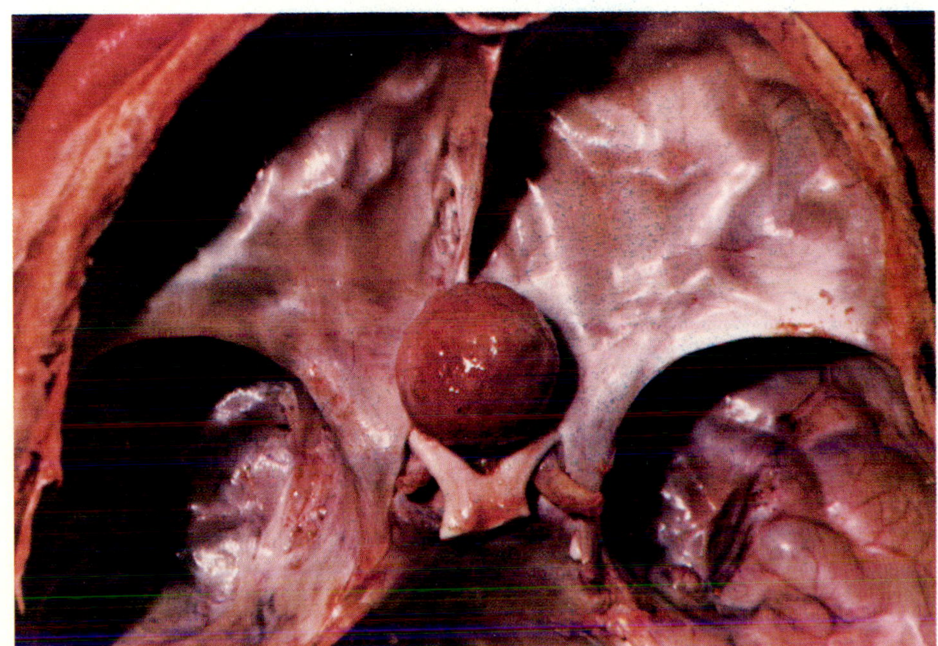

FIGURE 7
Meningioma arising from the tuberculum sellae. (Courtesy Dr. H. Okazaki.)

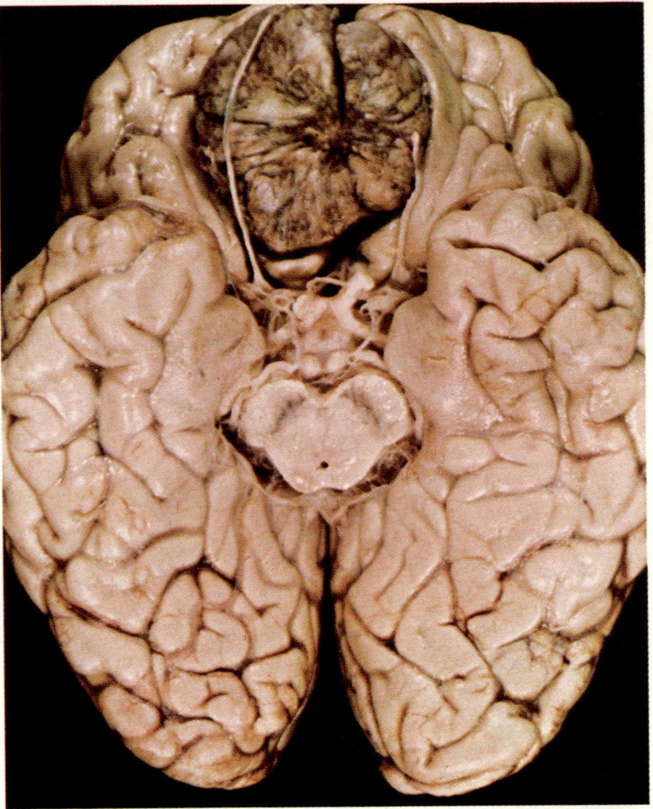

FIGURE 8
Right olfactory groove meningioma. The olfactory tract is intact and stretched over the tumor. (Courtesy Dr. H. Okazaki.)

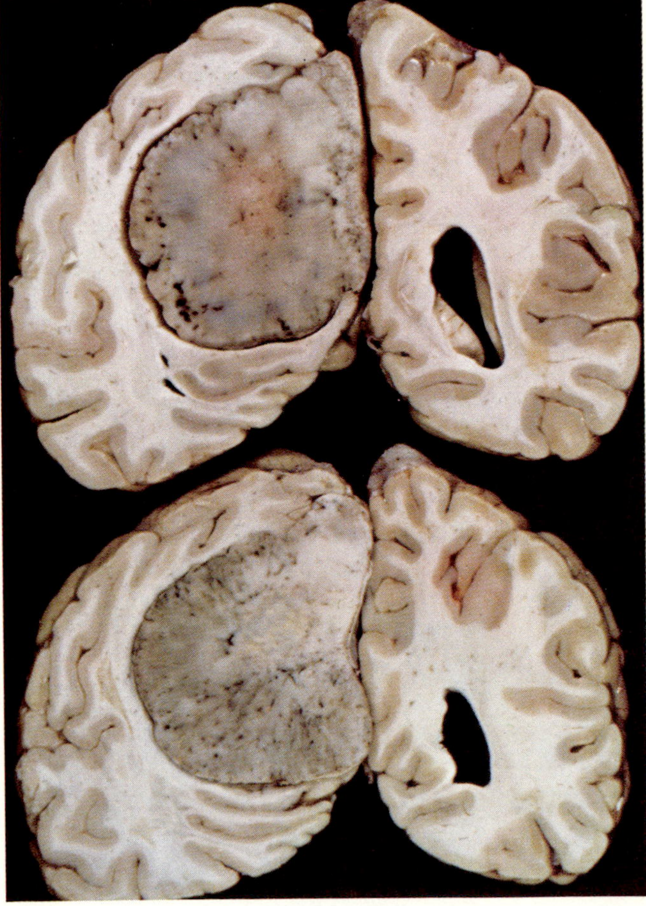

FIGURE 9
Falx meningioma of left occipital lobe. (Courtesy Dr. H. Okazaki.)

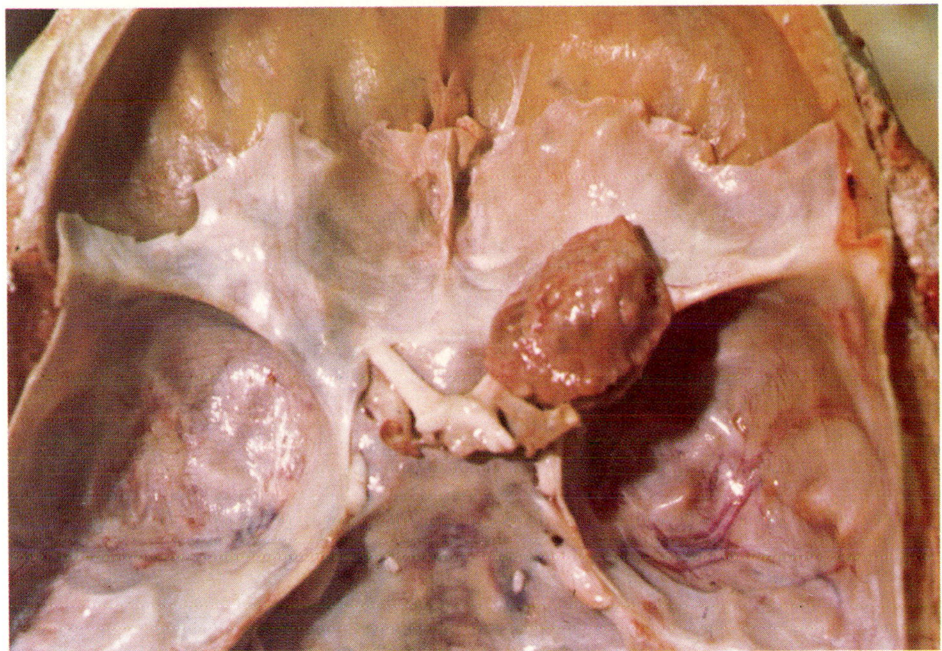

FIGURE 10
Meningioma of the medial third of the right sphenoid ridge. (Courtesy Dr. H. Okazaki.)

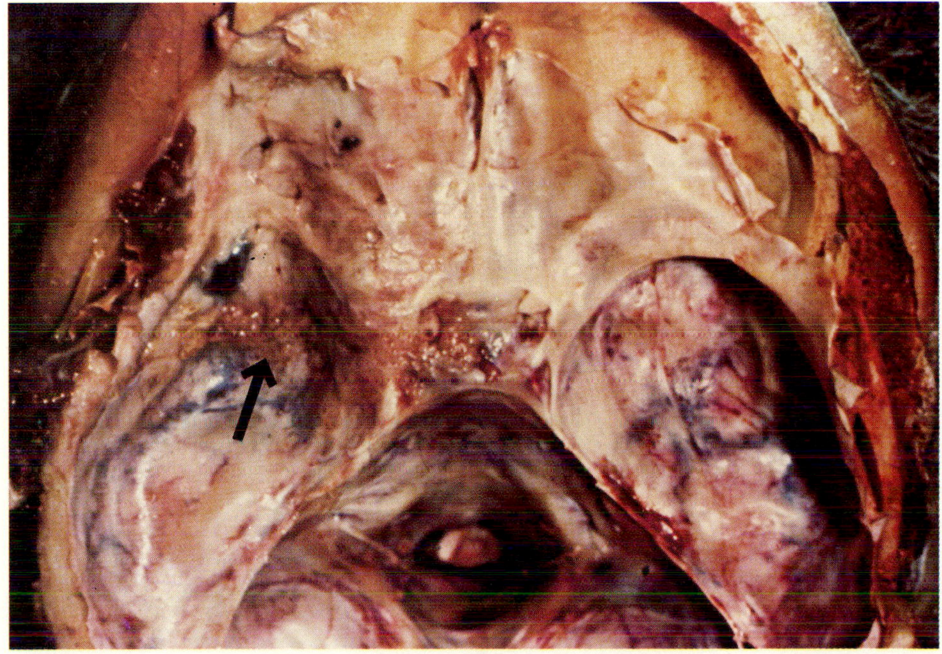

FIGURE 11
Meningioma enplaque involving area of left pterion (lateral third of sphenoid ridge). The tumor appears as a flat granular carpetlike growth (*arrow*) at the base of the skull. (Courtesy Dr. H. Okazaki.)

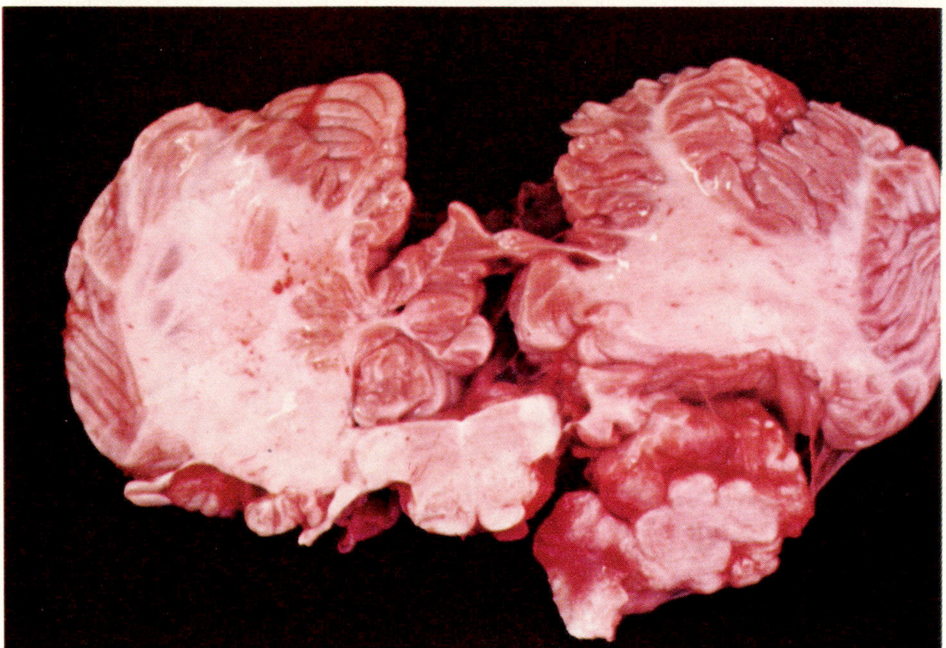

FIGURE 12
Meningioma of the right pontocerebellar angle (here lying against medulla oblongata). (Courtesy Dr. H. Okazaki.)

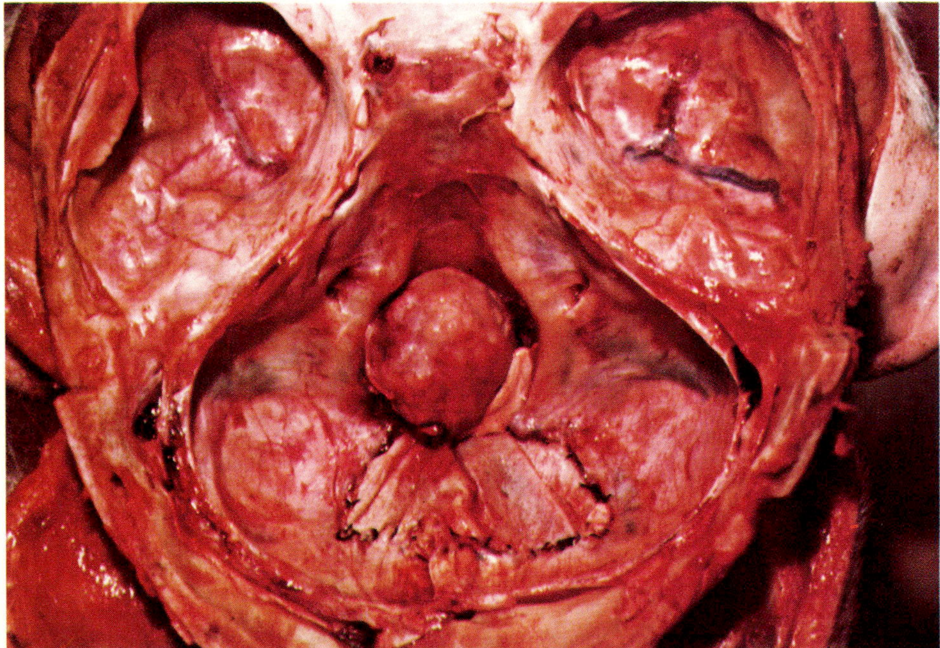

FIGURE 13
Meningioma arising from posterior margin of foramen magnum (a recurrence—suture of dura marks previous craniectomy). (Courtesy Dr. H. Okazaki.)

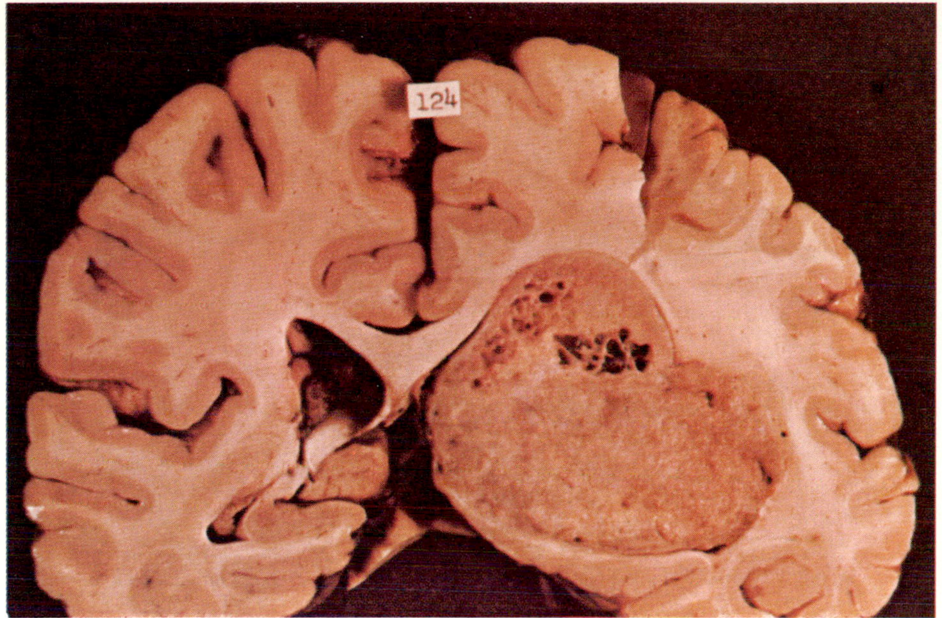

FIGURE 14
Meningioma of the right lateral ventricle. The tumor is somewhat spongy and has multilocular cysts.

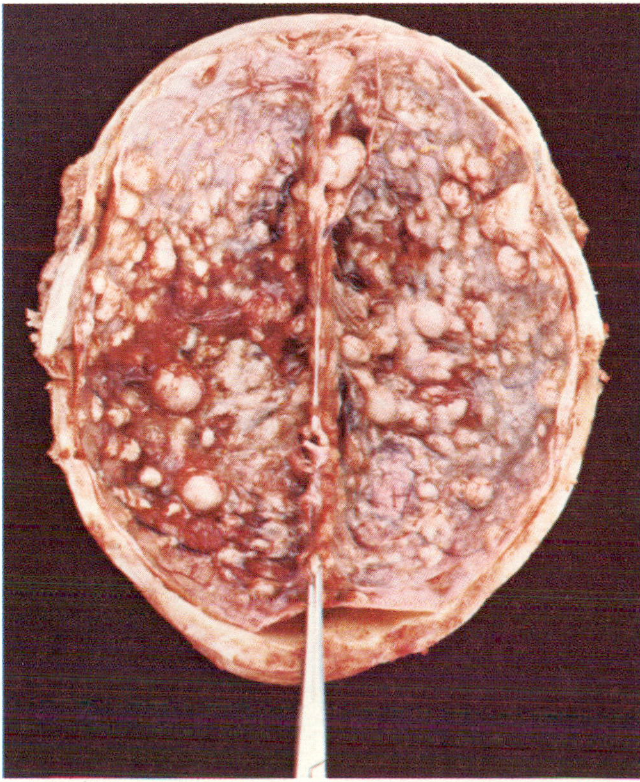

FIGURE 15
Inside of the calvaria is studded by large numbers of meningiomas (meningiomatosis). (Courtesy Dr. H. Okazaki.)

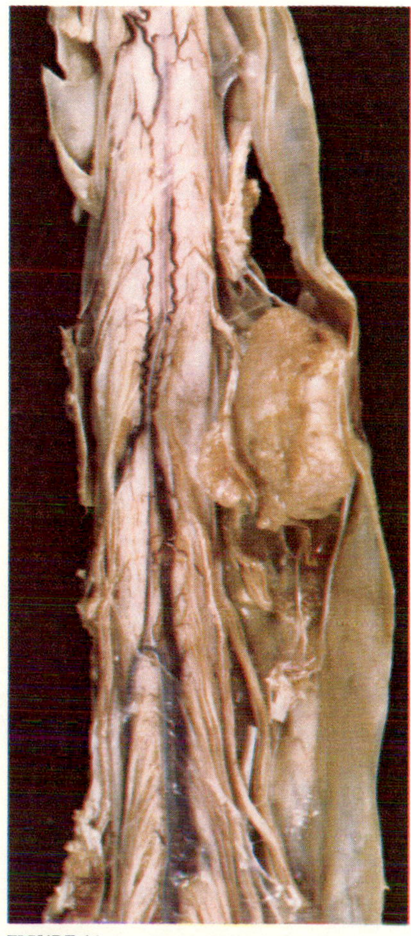

FIGURE 16
Meningioma of the thoracic spinal cord. Note depression on surface of cord. (Courtesy Dr. H. Okazaki.)

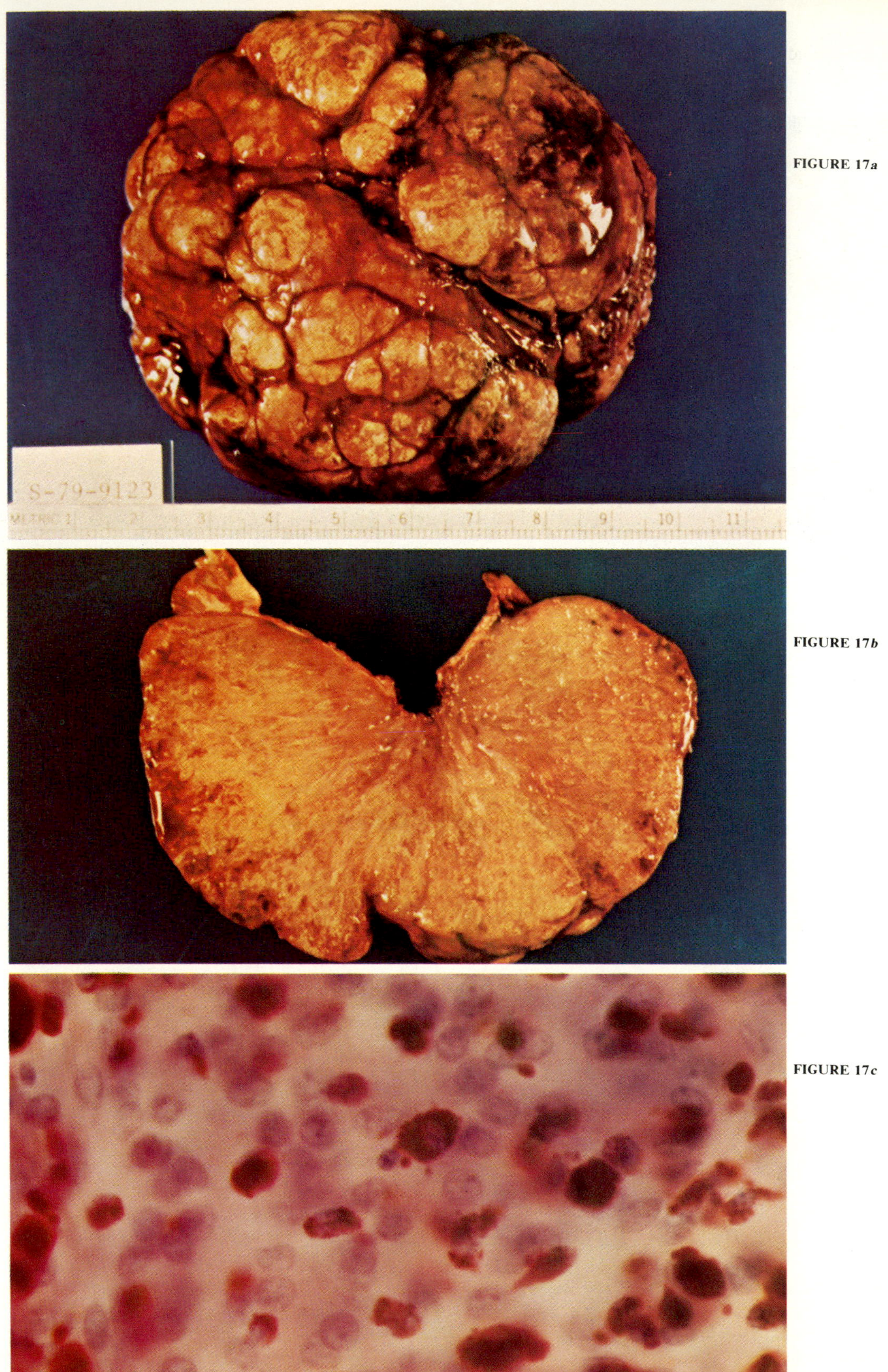

FIGURE 17*a*

FIGURE 17*b*

FIGURE 17*c*

FIGURE 17
Meningioma with xanthomatous changes causing yellow discoloration of the tumor. (*a*) Outer surface of surgically removed specimen. (*b*) Cut surface of tumor. (*c*) Frozen section with Oil-red-O stain shows lipid-filled cells in tumor.

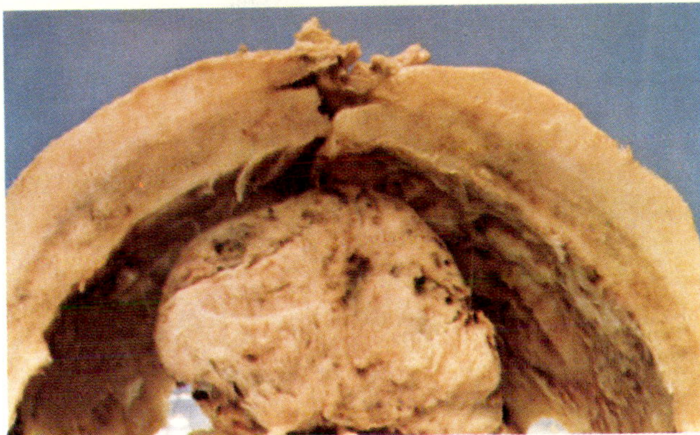

FIGURE 18
Hyperostosis of frontal bone caused by meningioma. Note that hyperostotic changes involve the midline as well.

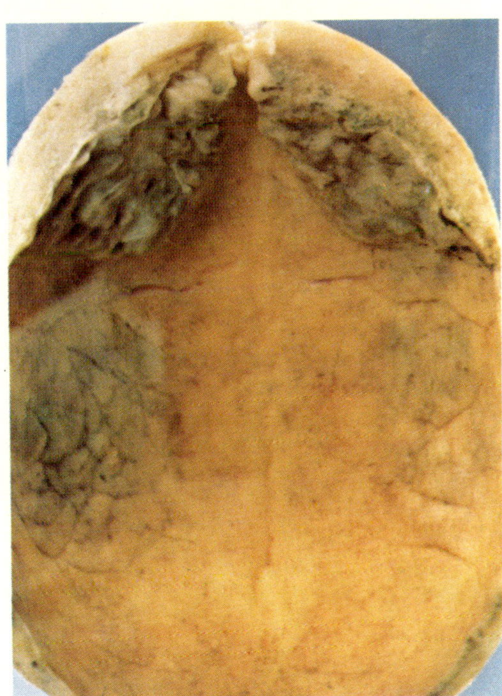

FIGURE 19
Hyperostosis frontalis interna in a patient without meningioma. Despite bilateral marked bony thickening, the midline sturctures are spared.

major fissures, such as the Sylvian fissure. Intraventricular meningiomas may occur in any of the ventricles, but are most common in one of the lateral ventricles (Fig. 14). These are considered to originate from arachnoidal cell nests located within the stroma of the choroid plexus and the tela chorioidea. Multiple intracranial meningiomas may range in number from just a few to a multitude of tumors, literally studding the dura mater (Fig. 15).

In the spinal canal, meningiomas are usually (but not always) attached to the dura and after attaining sufficient size will compress the spinal cord (Fig. 16). They are more common in the upper half of the spinal canal, particularly the thoracic segments, whereas meningiomas of the lumbosacral region and of the cauda equina are distinctly rare.

Meningiomas that are primarily extradural, occurring in the orbit or in other ectopic locations, have been discussed in Chapters 19–21.

GROSS CHARACTERISTICS OF MENINGIOMAS

Meningiomas range in size from tiny tumorlets, barely visible to the naked eye, to huge tumor masses. The clinical disturbances caused by these tumors obviously will bear a relationship to their size, but in this respect the localization is also of great importance. A relatively small meningioma of the spinal canal may cause cord compression with irreversible paraplegia, and as to meningiomas developing in the bony optic canal, a very small tumor can go a long way in creating serious visual disturbance.

The color of meningiomas is usually pink-gray in the fresh state, changing to gray-white after formol fixation. Recent and old hemorrhages within the tumor will cause red and brown discoloration, respectively, whereas the presence of numerous lipid-filled cells in the meningioma will produce a yellow color of both the external and the cut surface of the tumor (Figs. 17a–c). The consistency of meningiomas is usually rather firm and rubbery. The presence of numerous psammoma bodies (as often found in spinal meningiomas) or of bone and cartilage lends special hardness to the tumor. Cut surfaces of psammomatous meningiomas have a characteristic gritty feel to them. By contrast, advanced mucoid or fatty degeneration, edema, and spongy changes as well as recent necrosis are likely to produce a softer consistency. The occasional cystic meningioma may feel quite fluctuant on palpation. Highly vascularized meningiomas may ooze much blood from fresh-cut surfaces.

GROSS CHANGES IN THE IMMEDIATE NEIGHBORHOOD OF MENINGIOMAS

In addition to pressure atrophy of the underlying brain, one occasionally sees the formation of one or several cysts in the nervous parenchyma next to a meningioma. Unlike cysts that develop within the meningioma itself, these adjacent cysts are lined by glial tissue, sometimes showing some proliferative tendencies of the astrocytes. A meningioma growing through a cranial bone may cause lytic changes, but more often the bone responds to the presence of a nearby meningioma by the formation of increased numbers of bony spicules: hyperostosis. (This reactive hyperostosis must not be confused with osseous changes within a meningioma, where the process is the result of metaplasia of the tumor tissue or its stroma.) Cranial hyperostosis caused by a meningioma is often a diffuse process, which, should it develop near the sagittal plane, does not spare the midline structures (Fig. 18). By contrast, excess bone formation in the condition known as hyperostosis frontalis interna does not involve the midline (Fig. 19).

(*Comment:* Localization of meningiomas is of great importance for neurosurgeons, since it plays an important role in planning and executing the surgical removal of these neoplasms. In some instances the localization alone will determine whether the tumor is operable or not. Surgical texts dealing with meningiomas strongly emphasize data relating to localization and relative frequency of meningiomas in certain anatomic sites. These data, together with suggested surgical approaches to meningiomas of the three cranial fossae and the spinal canal, will be the subject of a future section of this work, representing the views of a neurosurgeon on clinical diagnosis and surgical treatment of meningiomas.)

CHAPTER 24

Histology of Non-Neoplastic Arachnoidal Cells

When viewed with the light microscope, the outer surface of the arachnoid membrane is covered by flat, elongated cells that form a single layer in most areas, but not uncommonly are six to 10 layers thick. Such accumulations of arachnoidal cells may occur haphazardly, but are more regularly seen on the surface of arachnoidal villi or granulations. By light microscopy the bottom layer of arachnoidal cap cells does not seem to be sharply demarcated from the underlying connective tissue (Fig. 20). Sometimes, particularly in arachnoidal granulations, the delineation from the stroma is so indistinct that some of the cap cells actually appear to have migrated into deeper zones of the arachnoid (Fig. 21). Arachnoidal cell clusters covering villi may also be seen within the lumen of venous sinuses of the dura (Fig. 22).

The familiar basic histologic features of meningiomas may often be recognized in non-neoplastic clusters of meningothelial cells of the normal leptomeninges. Such features include the tendency of cells to form whorls, often with secondary hyalinization, and even calcification (Fig. 23).

The fact that meningiomas may originate within cerebral ventricles may seem puzzling until one examines the stroma of the choroid plexus. There, particularly in the heavy tufts of the glomus portion in the trigonal area of the lateral ventricles (but to a lesser extent also elsewhere), one can

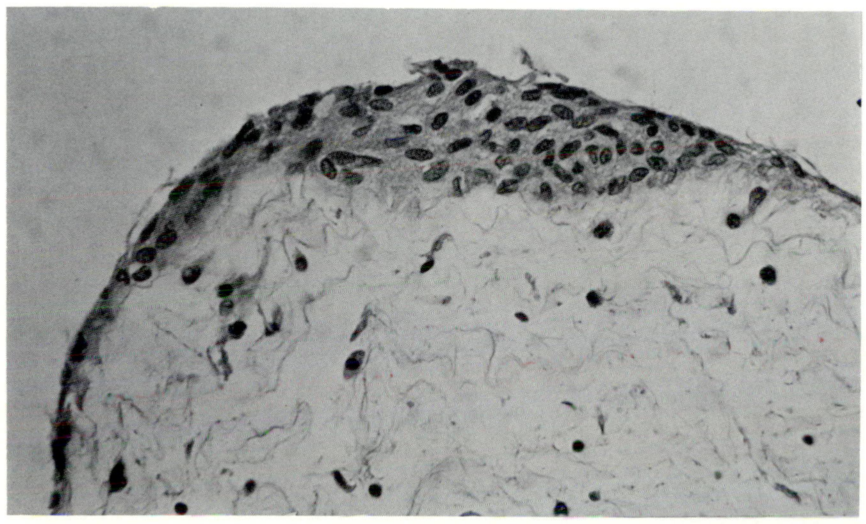

FIGURE 20
Normal leptomeninges from convexity of brain. The outer aspect of the arachnoid is formed by so-called cap cells. They form a single layer in some areas; in the center of this figure they are 6 to 8 layers thick. Light microscopy shows no sharp demarcation between cap cells and underlying loose stroma.

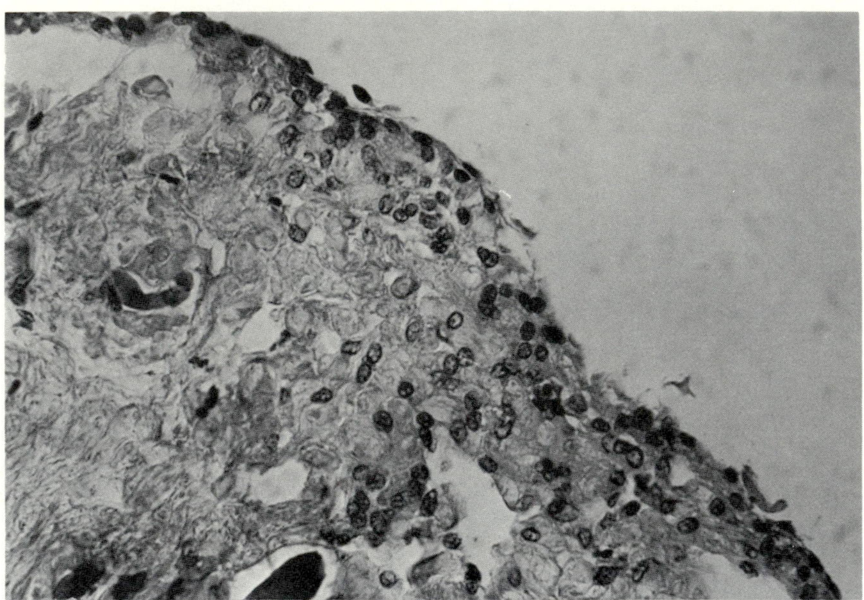

FIGURE 21
Surface of an arachnoidal (Pacchionian) granulation. The demarcation between cap cells and stroma appears quite indistinct.

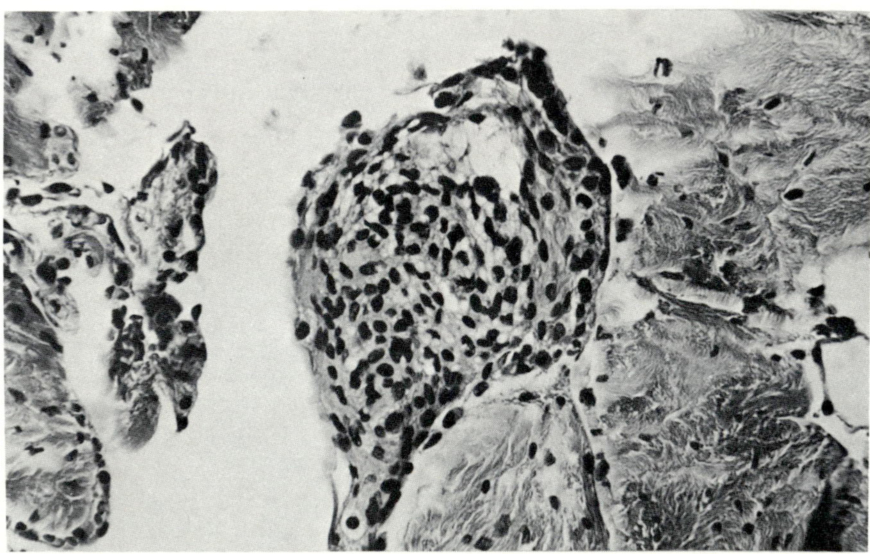

FIGURE 22
Arachnoidal granulation protruding into lumen of superior sagittal sinus. The outermost cells covering the granulation are an extension of the endothelial lining of the sinus.

easily find nests and clusters of arachnoidal cells. Such cells are not exposed to the ventricular lumen; they are separated from the latter by choroid plexus epithelium (Fig. 24). The presence of arachnoidal cell clusters in that location can be explained by the invagination of the leptomeninges to form part of the tela chorioidea. Much of this takes place in the area of the transverse cerebral

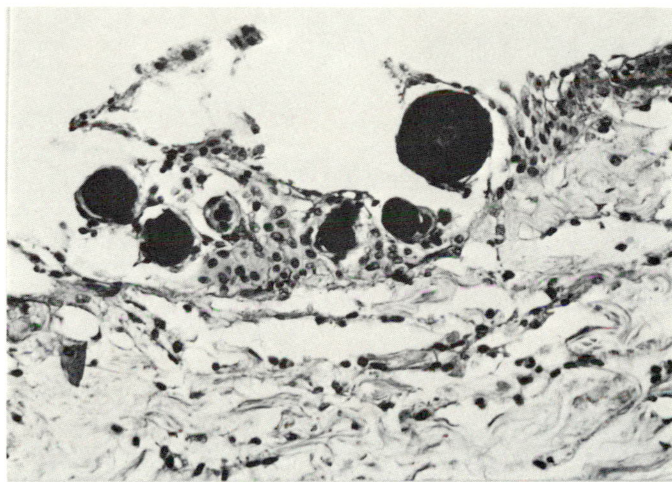

FIGURE 23
Formation of cellular whorls with psammoma bodies may be found in non-neoplastic arachnoidal cells of the normal brain.

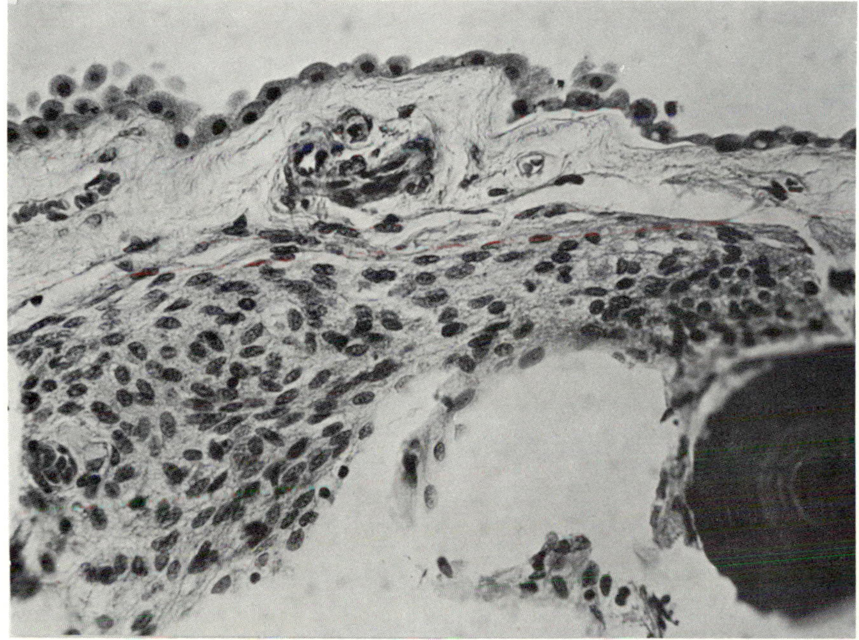

FIGURE 24
Arachnoidal cell clusters in the stroma of the choroid plexus (lateral ventricle). Such cell clusters are believed to be the source of intraventricular meningiomas.

fissure, where the invaginating membranes will form the floor of the lateral ventricles and the roof of the third ventricle. A similar arrangement takes place in the choroid plexus of the fourth ventricle. As a result, meningiomas may occur in any of the cerebral ventricles, although they are most commonly found in one of the lateral ventricles (Fig. 14).

CHAPTER 25

Light-Microscopic Features of Meningiomas

Many cellular characteristics of normal arachnoidal cap cells are recapitulated in meningiomas (*vide supra*). Probably as a reflection of the epithelioid arrangement of the most superficial cells of the normal arachnoid, many meningiomas consist of closely packed cells, suggesting an almost epithelial arrangement. Whorling tendency is often noted. Although not invariably present, intranuclear vacuoles are regarded by many as a helpful hint in identifying meningothelial cells—not that such vacuoles may never occur in other types of tumors, but in meningiomas they do so with great frequency and regularity (Fig. 25). As will be shown later, in Chapter 26, these intranuclear vacuoles may represent cytoplasmic invaginations, dissolution of nuclear material, or both.

The term syncytial is used to describe some meningiomas, because the cell boundaries between neighboring tumor cells cannot always be discerned under the light microscope. Electron microscopy has shown that we are not dealing with a real syncytium, that is, the tumor cells do possess cell membranes individually, but these membranes are so intertwined and dovetailing that often the light microscope cannot resolve their zig-zagging, meandering course; thus, with no cell walls seen between neighboring cells, the appearance of a syncytium suggests itself very strongly. In such areas, the nuclei of the tumor cells are seen against a seemingly continuous eosinophilic, sometimes slightly fibrillary background. If the cells in these areas are more spindly than polyhedral the tumor may resemble connective tissue more than an epithelial growth (Fig. 26).

The tendency of meningothelial cells to form whorls is a well-known basic phenomenon, manifested in the non-neoplastic arachnoidal cells as well and seen also in tissue cultures of meningiomas. Some meningiomas may show only an occasional whorl (Fig. 27). In others they may dominate the histologic picture throughout (Fig. 28). Whorls owe their existence to the peculiar tendency of meningothelial cells to wrap themselves in a concentric fashion around structures they encounter during their proliferation. Within meningiomas the central element of the whorl is most often another meningothelial cell, but whorls may form around collagen fibers, blood vessels and still other structures. For example, when a meningioma infiltrates striated muscle (most often the temporalis muscle) the tumor cells may wrap themselves around muscle fibers (Fig. 29). In the rare instance of a collision between a metastatic carcinoma and meningioma, meningothelial cells may envelop clusters of metastatic tumor cells (Fig. 30). Meningothelial whorls may consist exclusively of cells without intervening extracellular substances. Very often, however, precollagen and collagen fibers are found deposited in the center of the whorl and also between neighboring layers of concentrical cells. Some fibers may be shown by silver impregnation as reticulin fibers (Fig. 31). More mature collagen can be visualized by one of the modifications of Masson trichrome stain (Fig. 32a,b) or by the Van Gieson's solution (Fig. 33). Often, an amorphous substance appears to impregnate the whorls, having tinctorial characteristics of glycoproteins staining positively with periodic acid-Schiff (PAS) stain (Fig. 34) and appearing deep red on Masson trichrome stain (Fig. 32a,b). The internal structure of some whorls may become less discernible, more homogenized, that is, hyalinized. Some meningiomas abound in such hyalinized whorls. In still others, the whorls become calcified, that is, calcium apatite crystals appear between the meningothelial cells. With appropriate histochemical methods, both the phosphate component and the calcium ions can be demonstrated in these deposits (Figs. 35 and 36). Whereas the presence of calcium in the whorls is well known, a more detailed examination will frequently indicate the presence of iron as forming part of the mineral deposits (Fig. 37). Very rarely, one may find amyloid, or at least a substance with

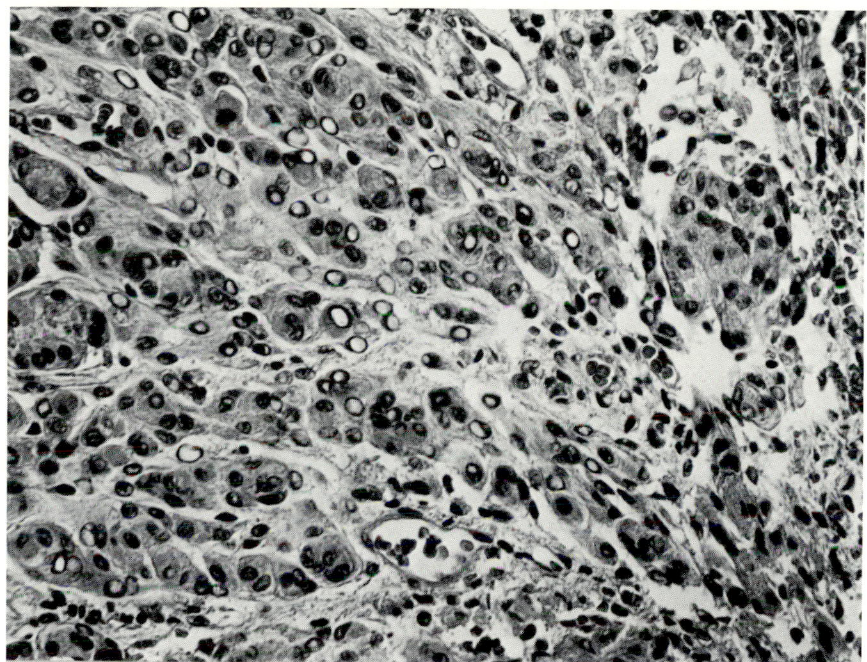

FIGURE 25
Meningothelial meningioma. Tumor cells are closely packed much as epithelial cells, yet they lack sharp demarcation from each other. Many nuclei are vacuolated. Left from center, early whorl formation is noted.

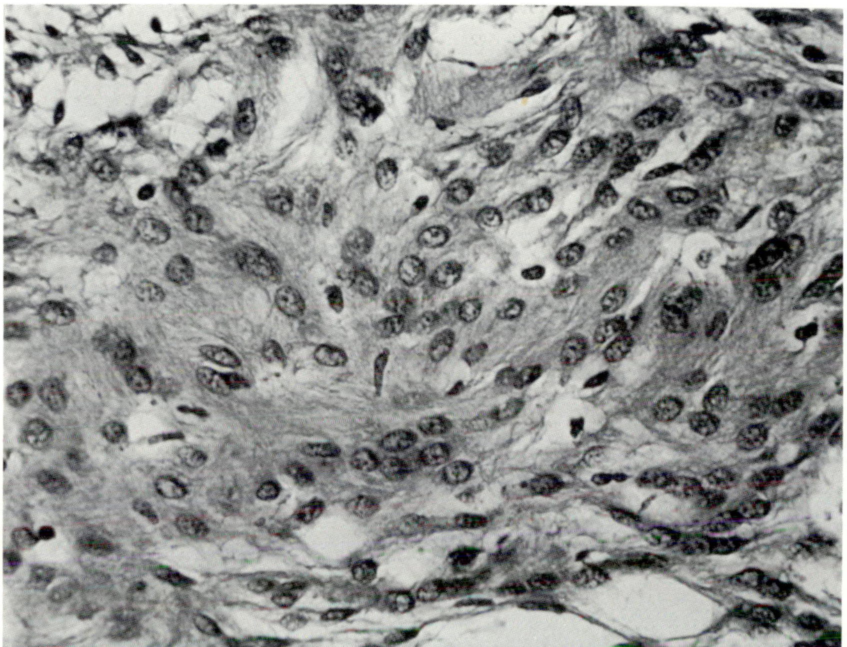

FIGURE 26
Lack of discernible cell margins leads to a syncytial appearance in this tumor. In reality, the cell bodies of neighboring cells are not continuous, but light microscopy fails to resolve the intricate interdigitation of cell membranes. Instead, the nuclei are seen against a continuum of a fine fibrillary background.

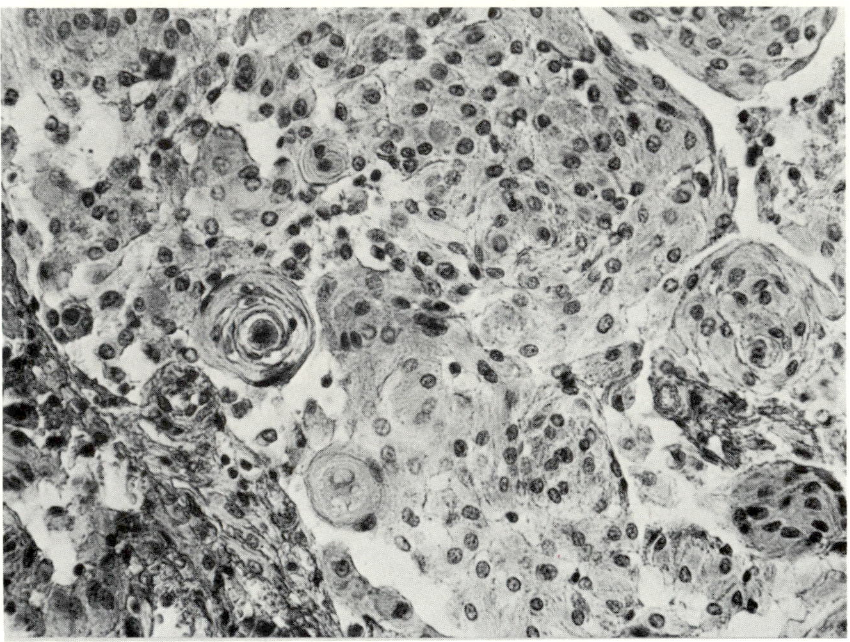

FIGURE 27
This meningioma shows epithelioid and syncytial patterns together. A few whorls have formed.

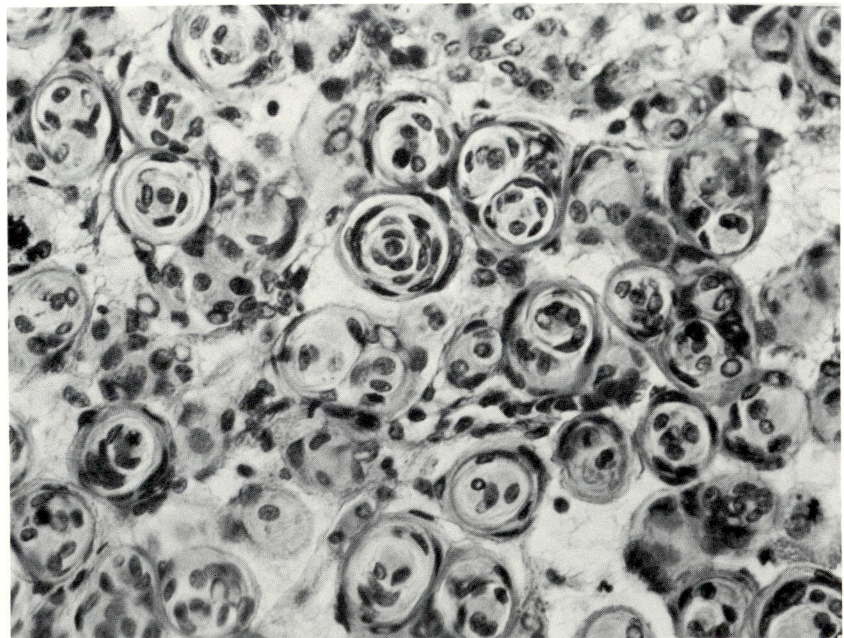

FIGURE 28
Meningioma composed almost entirely of cellular whorls. None was calcified in this case.

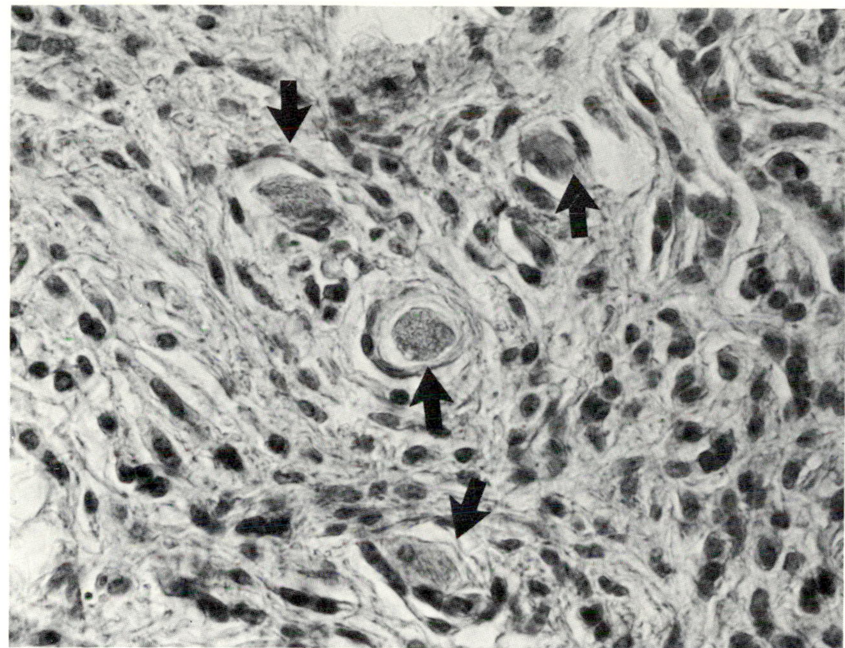

FIGURE 29
Meningioma infiltrating the temporalis muscle. Striated muscle fibers (*arrows*) form the center of the meningothelial whorls in this instance.

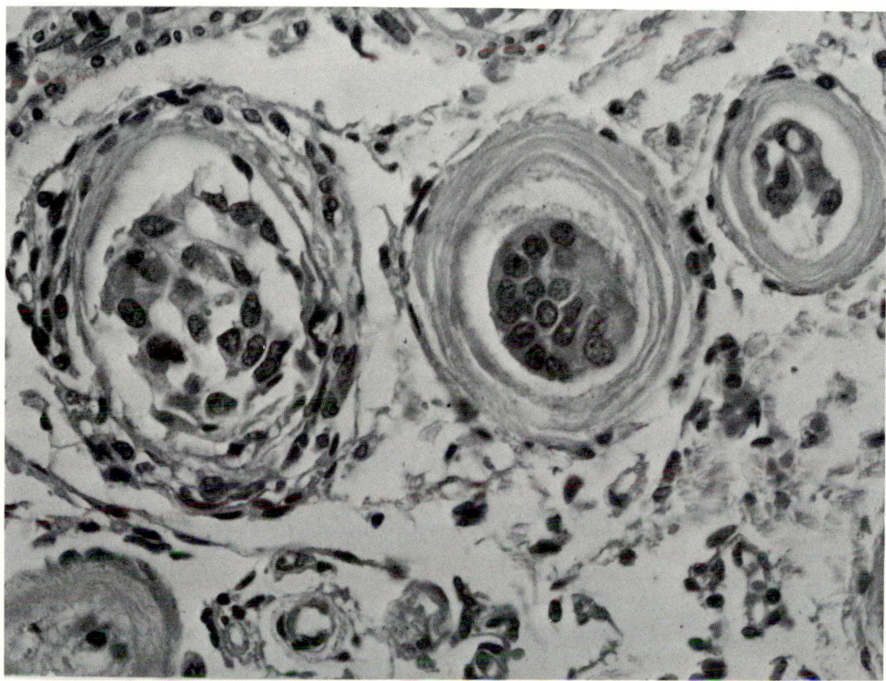

FIGURE 30
Interface between a meningioma and a dural metastasis of a breast carcinoma. Meningothelial cells have wrapped themselves around clusters of carcinoma cells.

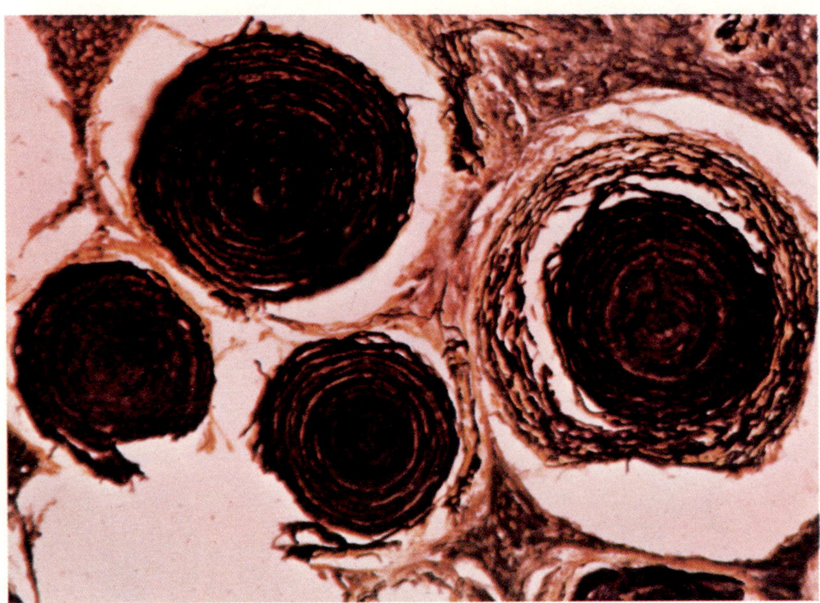

FIGURE 31
Reticulin fibers (pre- or protocollagen) are demonstrated within hyalinized cellular whorls. Wilder's reticulin stain.

the staining characteristics of amyloid, deposited in hyalinized whorls (Figs. 38–40). It has become customary to refer to mineralized concentric bodies in meningiomas as psammoma bodies, from the Greek word *psammos* (sand). Meningiomas that are predominantly composed of such structures are sometimes referred to as psammomatous meningiomas. They may occur anywhere but they reach highest proportion in spinal canal meningiomas (Fig. 41). Perhaps this is related to the slow growth of meningiomas in this location—they seldom become malignant—or perhaps to pressure on the tumor in the tightly confined space of the spinal canal. The orderly arrangement of calcium apatite crystals and the underlying concentric collagenous fibers are the source of striking birefringency of many psammoma bodies when examined under the polarizing microscope. The Maltese cross pattern seen under these circumstances can be quite striking (Fig. 42).

Whereas some meningiomas are composed entirely of epithelioid elements with or without whorl formation, the tendency of the tumor cells to become increasingly spindly is observed in many others. When epithelioid or meningothelial and spindly areas coexist in the same tumor, the term *transitional meningioma* has been applied. The term is certainly justified because these meningiomas do not have a truly dual cell population, and one can easily observe a transition from plump to more elongated cells (Figs. 43–45).

There are some differences of interpretation when one encounters a meningioma that is predominantly composed of long, slender, slightly wavy, bipolar cells. Such tumors are sometimes referred to as fibroblastic meningiomas, even though the tumor cells do not show a tendency for collagen formation. It is only their elongated, bipolar shape that makes them appear fibroblastic. Purists may want to refer to such forms as meningothelial tumors with greatly elongated cell forms, and restrict the term fibroblastic to variants in which the formation of precollagen or mature collagen, or both, can be observed between tumor cells. But such clear distinction is not always possible. When one observes the reticulin network in a given meningioma (Fig. 46a,b), in some areas (Fig. 46a) the reticulin fibers are entirely confined to connective tissue septa and vessel walls, whereas the tumor "parenchyma" is entirely free of such fibers. Elsewhere, however, in the same tumor (Fig. 46), a dense reticulin network can be observed between and around individual tumor cells, strongly suggesting that the latter had a role in the formation of reticulin fibers. Parallel and almost identical cellular patterns may be observed in different meningiomas with spindly tumor cells forming wavy bundles, the only difference being that collagen fibers have been deposited between the tumor cells in one tumor, but not the other

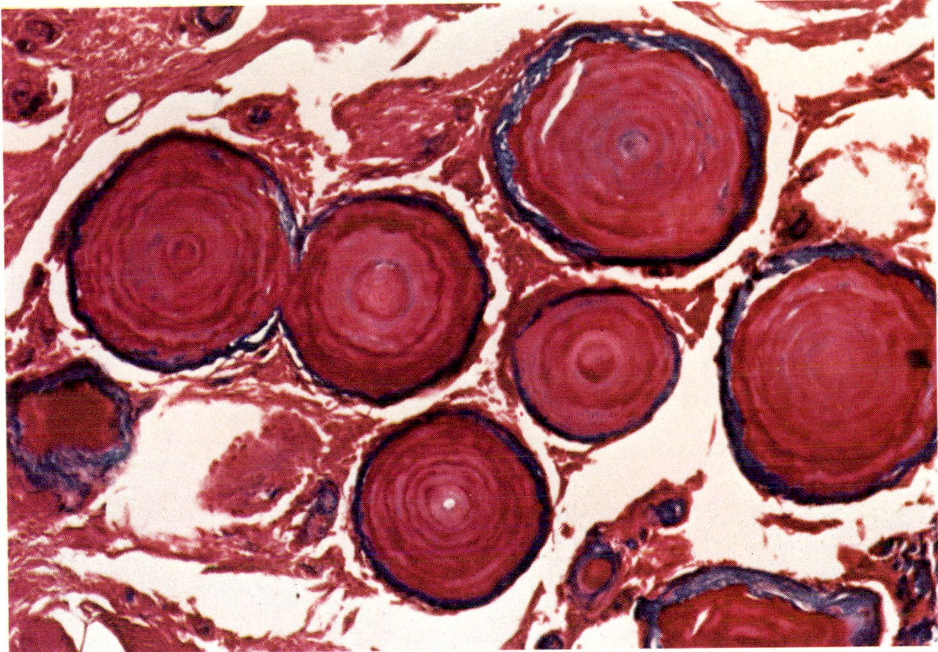

FIGURE 32*a*.
On trichrome stain of hyalinized whorl, blue-staining collagen fibers are seen to form part of whorls. Masson's trichrome stain, ×120.

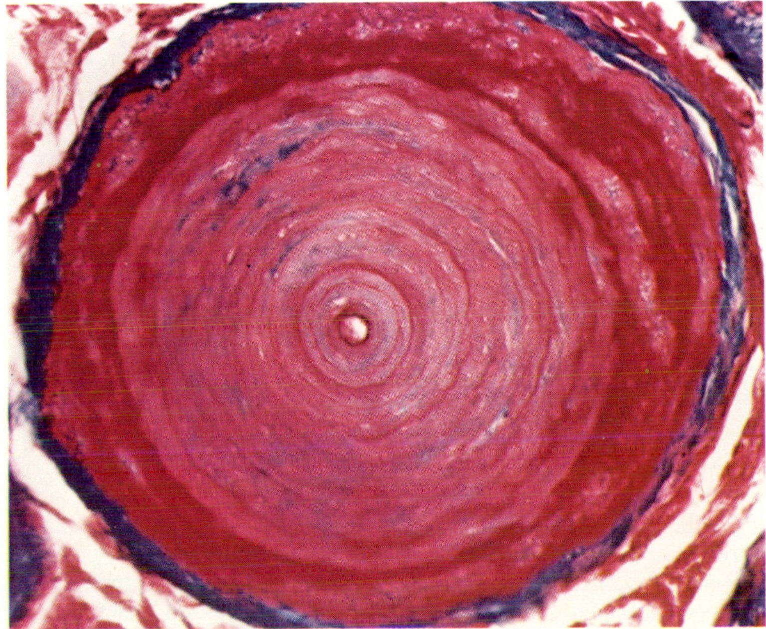

FIGURE 32*b*.
Higher-power magnification shows alternating layers of blue-staining collagen and amorphous red staining proteinaceous matrix. Masson's trichrome stain ×360.

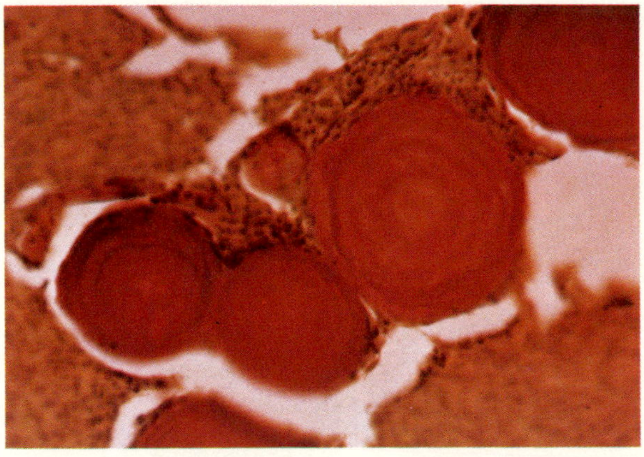

FIGURE 33

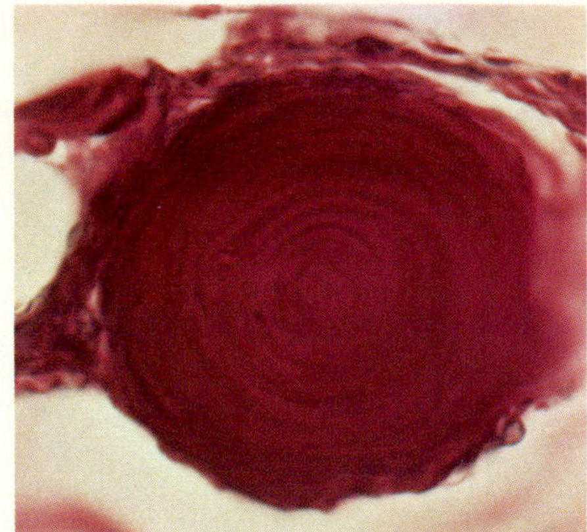

FIGURE 34

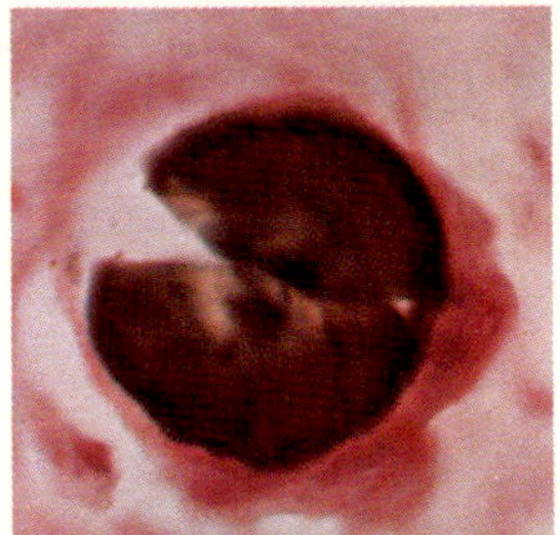

FIGURE 35

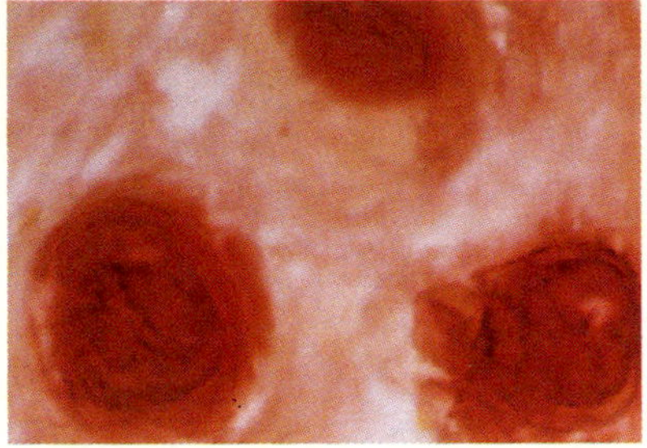

FIGURE 36

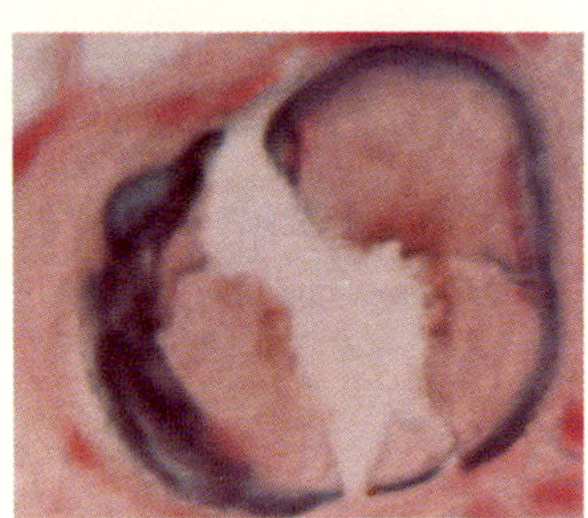

FIGURE 37

FIGURE 33
Presence of collagen in whorls shown here through positive staining with acid fuchsin. Van Gieson stain.

FIGURE 34
Glycoproteins within hyalinized whorl stain positively on periodic acid-Schiff (PAS) stain.

FIGURE 35
Whorl with central calcification. The phosphate component of calcium phosphate stains black with silver nitrate. Van Kossa's phosphate stain.

FIGURE 36
The calcium ion component in the psammoma bodies may be selectively stained red. (Alizarin-S stain.)

FIGURE 37
In some psammoma bodies in addition to calcium, iron may be found as part of the process of mineralization. Perl's iron stain.

(Fig. 47a,b). The term fibrous or fibroblastic meningioma is applied by most pathologists to those tumors where collagen can be demonstrated between the spindly tumor cells, but the identical shape and arrangement of cells in other meningiomas without collagen deposition strongly suggest that one is dealing with a similar tumor, but one having a lesser tendency actually to lay down collagen fibers. It is for this reason that some pathologists refer to meningiomas with a predominantly spindle cell population as fibroblastic, even without demonstrable reticulin or collagen between tumor cells.

Figure 48a,b also introduces another cellular pattern commonly seen in meningiomas, one that in other neoplasms is often referred to as a storiform or pinwheel pattern. This consists of elongated spindly cells arranged in such fashion that

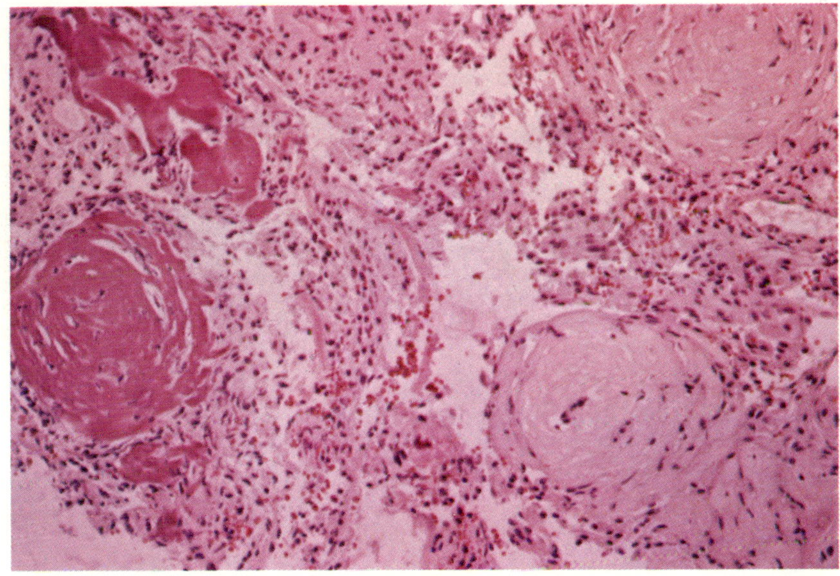

FIGURE 38
Some of the hyalinized whorls and portions of connective tissue septa (*left*) stain positively for amyloid. Sirius-red amyloid stain. (Case for Figs. 38–40 was submitted by Dr. G. Froio.)

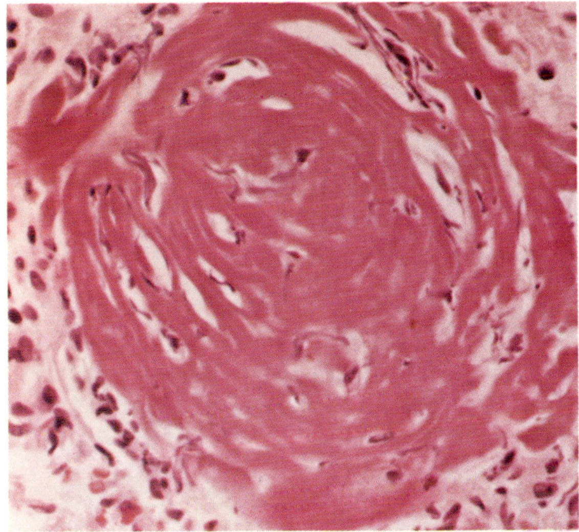

FIGURE 39
Higher-power view of sclerosed whorl with positive staining for amyloid. Sirius red stain.

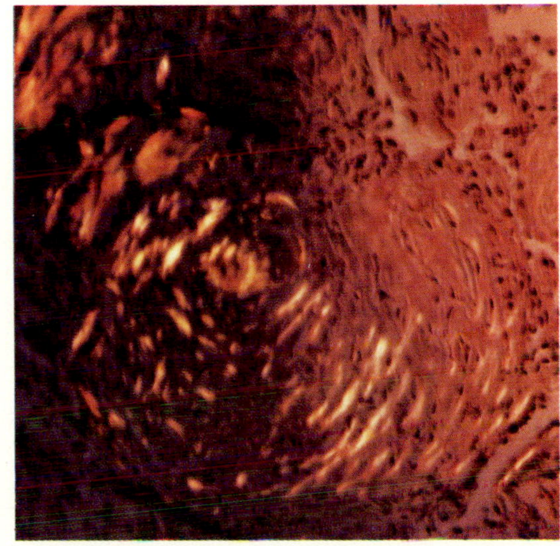

FIGURE 40
Same whorl shown in Figure 39, as it appears when viewed with polarized light. Apple-green birefringence is consistent with presence of amyloid.

a central area contains only cytoplasmic material without nuclei; from this area, the cells stream forth in different directions and in a slightly wavy pattern, imitating the blades of a toy pinwheel. In general, pathology this pattern is most commonly associated with fibrous histiocytomas and their variants, but thecomas of the ovary, certain primary bone tumors, as well as the so-called storiform neurofibromas of Bednar, also display this arrangement of their cells. As shown in Figure 48a,b, this pattern may be quite frequently seen in meningiomas as well. Whether the presence of a

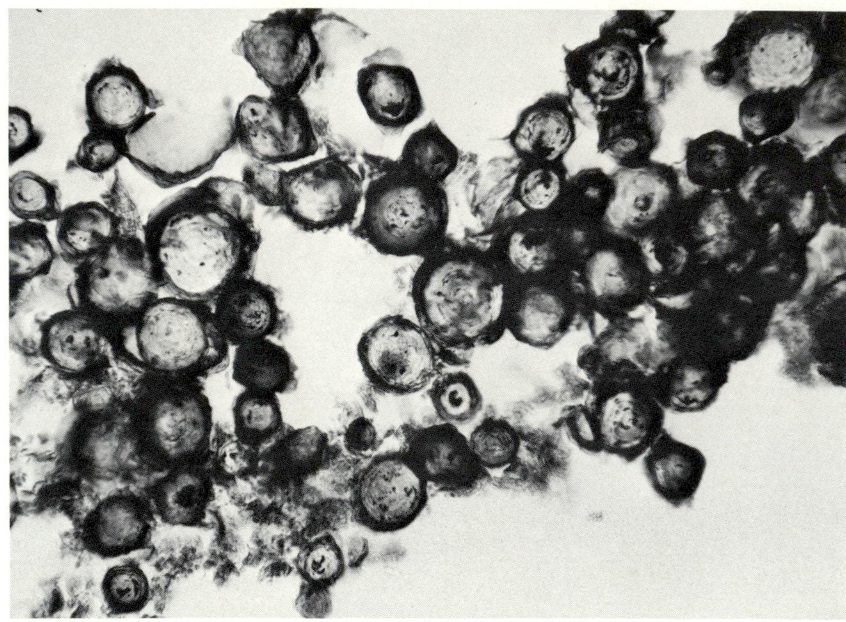

FIGURE 41
Some meningiomas, particularly those in the spinal canal, contain very large numbers of calcified whorls (psammomatous meningiomas).

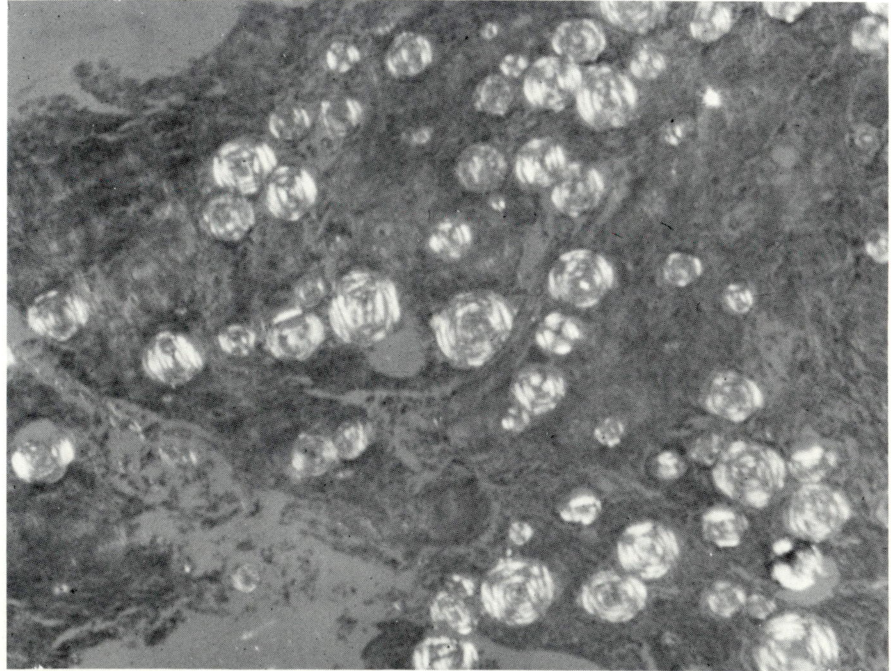

FIGURE 42
Psammoma bodies examined under polarized light. Marked birefringence is noted, resulting from concentric arrangement of collagen fibers underlying calcification.

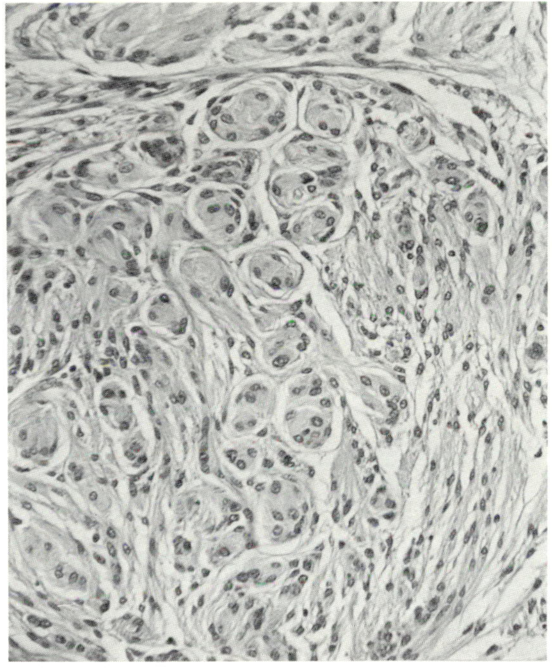

FIGURE 43
Transitional meningioma composed of plump cells forming cellular whorls and elongated, bipolar cells with transitions between the two cell types. In this area, the whorls predominate.

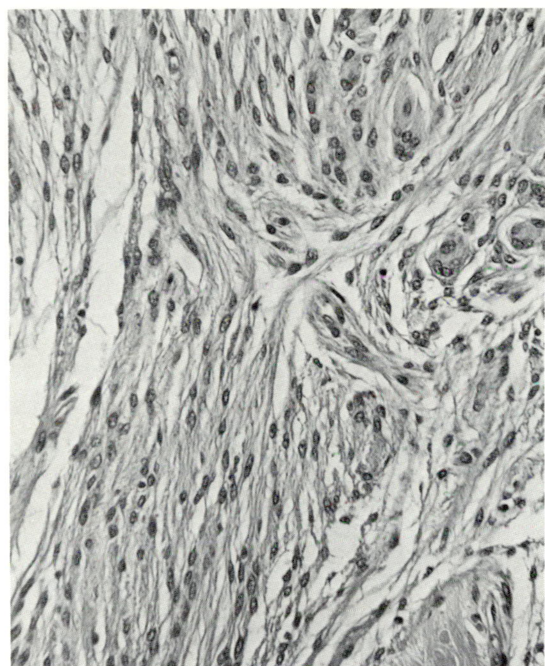

FIGURE 44
Another area of the tumor shown in Figure 43. Here, most cells are elongated.

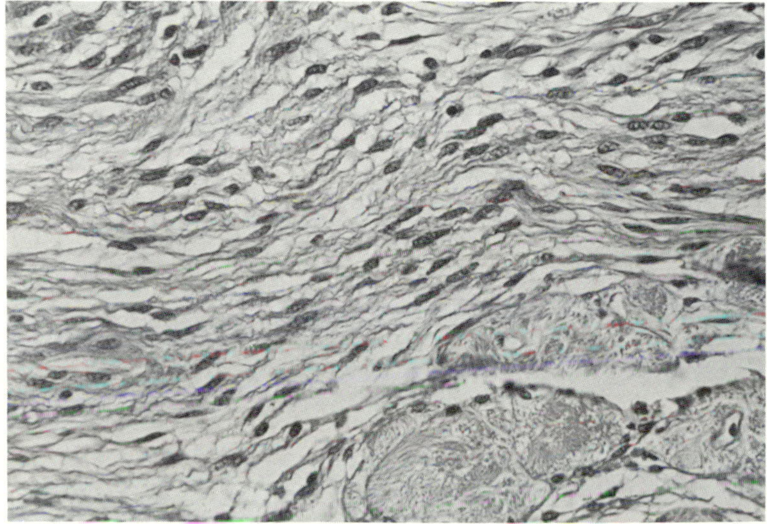

FIGURE 45
This area of the same tumor is entirely made up of very long, wavy fibroblastlike cells, that, however, do not form collagen. An unrelated feature is the marked fibrous thickening of the blood vessel walls (*right lower corner*).

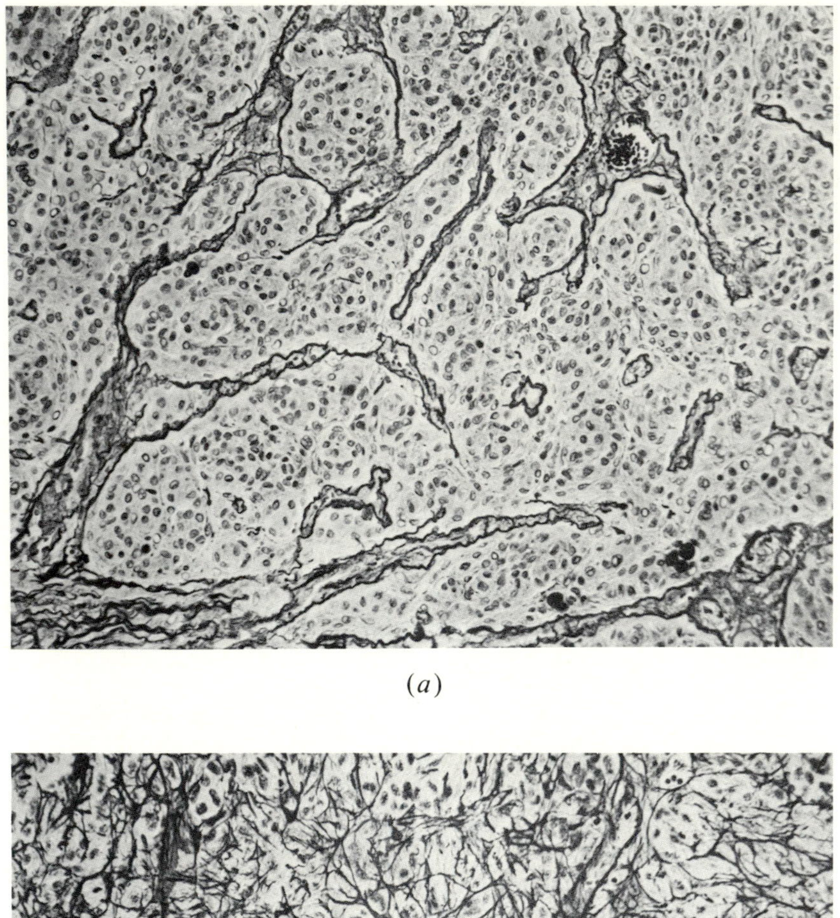

(*a*)

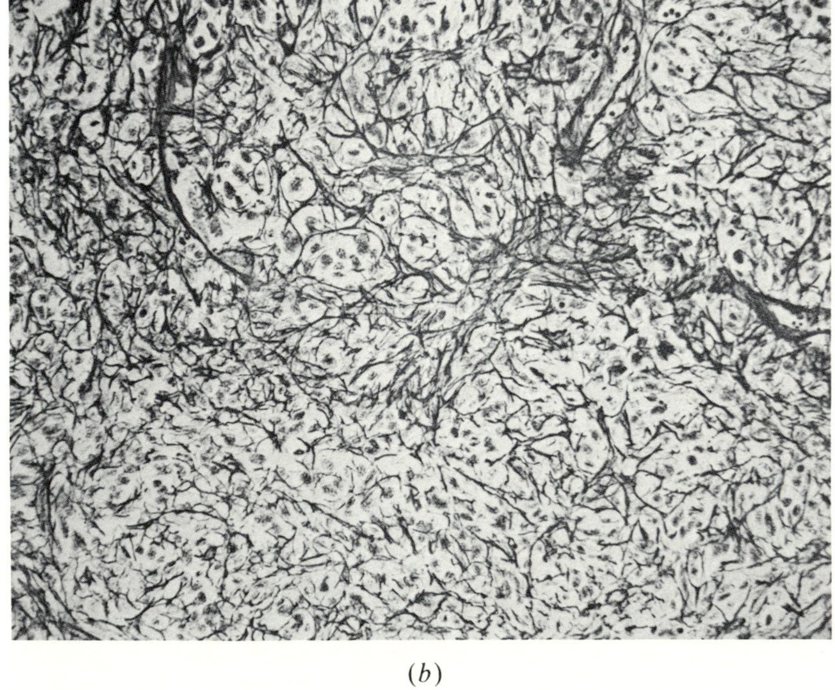

(*b*)

FIGURE 46
Reticulin fiber pattern in two different areas of meningioma. (*a*) Tumor consists of reticulin-free parenchyma and reticulin-bearing septa, containing blood vessels. (*b*) In another area of the same tumor, reticulin fibers appear between individual tumor cells as well. Wilder's reticulin stain.

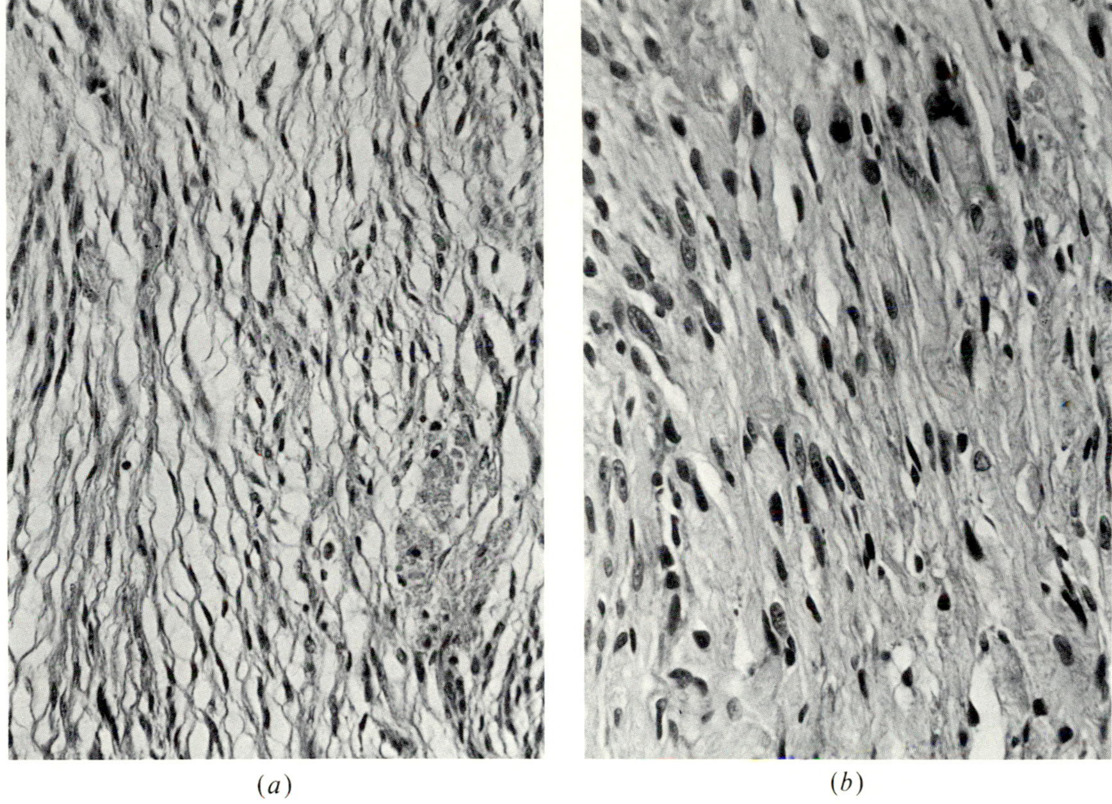

(*a*) (*b*)

FIGURE 47
Parallel bundles of elongated spindly tumor cells in two meningiomas, (*a*) without deposition of collagen; (*b*) with collagen fibers separating tumor cells.

storiform pattern actually indicates a histiocytic differentiation of the tumor is a challenging question that still awaits resolution. This problem is discussed in greater detail later.

METAPLASTIC CHANGES IN MENINGIOMAS

The preceding paragraphs discussed the classic meningothelial, psammomatous, and the partly or entirely fibroblastic types of meningiomas. The cells were arranged in variable configurations, appeared short and plump or elongated and wavy, but they still represented the same basic cell type in terms of their cytoplasmic characteristics. In cases of metaplasia, transitions to a cell type with a morphology different from that of the original cells, may be observed. One fairly common example of this is seen in the so-called lipoblastic meningiomas. Here, in an otherwise conventional meningioma, a few or many tumor cells show accumulation of fat droplets in their cytoplasm. The droplets tend to become confluent until the whole cell body becomes occupied by a large fat droplet and the remaining cytoplasm as well as the nucleus are crowded to the periphery in a signet-ring pattern (Fig. 49a,b). It is important to realize that we are not witnessing a collision, or admixture of fat tissue with a growing meningioma, but that the meningothelial cells themselves are increasingly transformed into adipocytes, at least in some areas of the tumor, with all transitions between nonlipidized and lipidized cells easily observed. These fatty cells are similar to adipose tissue elsewhere and contain mostly triglycerides.

A different type of fatty change takes place in the so-called xanthomatous meningiomas (Fig. 50a,b). Here, one encounters a few or many foamy round cells, mostly with small, dark, centrally located nuclei. The cytoplasm, rather than containing one large fat droplet as in an adipocyte, displays innumerable tiny vacuoles. The lipid material of the vacuoles can be visualized in appropriately stained frozen sections; it contains

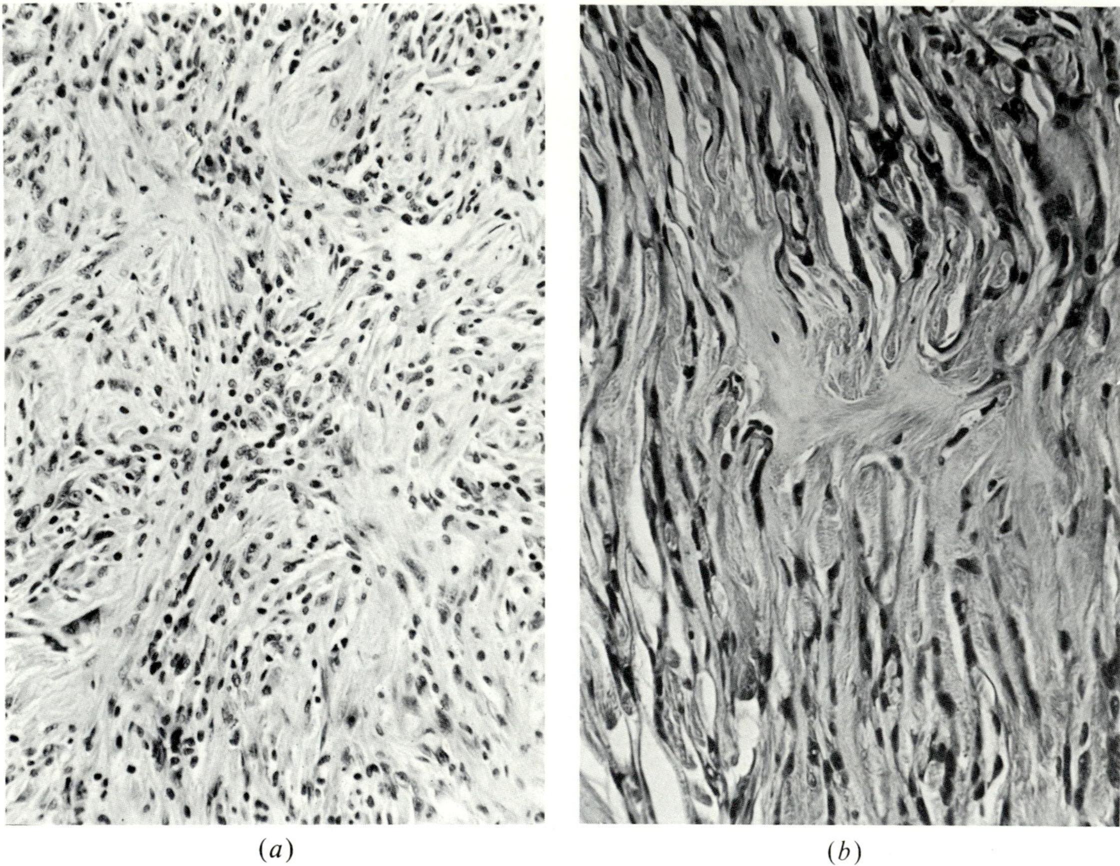

(*a*) (*b*)

FIGURE 48
Pinwheel or storiform pattern in meningioma. (*a*) Without collagen fibers in storiform area. (*b*) With collagen deposits in center of pinwheel.

much cholesterol, which appears as a birefringent substance under polarized light.

Xanthomatous cells are usually associated with histiocytes, either practicing their function as macrophages or in various histiocytic proliferative disorders. It is, of course, quite possible for meningiomas, particularly if they become necrotic or hemorrhagic, to attract migrating macrophages that will form clusters of xanthomatous appearing cells in areas where they are engaged in phagocytizing necrotic debris or breakdown products of hemorrhage. In the truly xanthomatous variant of meningiomas, however, one can observe the transformation of the meningothelial tumor cells into foamy xanthoma cells in a gradual fashion. This step-by-step change may be seen in Figure 50a, whereas in Figure 50b the xanthomatous cells dominate an area entirely. Neither lipoblastic nor xanthomatous changes of meningothelial tumor cells seem to have any implication on the prognosis of the tumor. Also, both the lipoblastic and xanthomatous transformation of the tumor cells suggest differentiation along mesenchymal lines. Myxoid and chondromatous changes in meningiomas also underline this mesenchymal differentiation potential of these tumors. Figure 51 shows an otherwise typical meningothelial meningioma with the familiar intranuclear vacuoles and some hyaline inclusions (*vide infra*). But here, the tumor cells, although still maintaining their whorling characteristics, become more distant from each other, owing to the deposition of a slightly basophilic, mucoid substance between them; the cells thus separated have a more spindly, even spidery, appearance, such as seen in Wharton's jelly and myxoid tissue in general. With reticulin stain (Fig. 52), the areas of myxoid intercellular ground substance appear to have more reticulin fibers between the cells than is seen in the neighboring unaltered tumor parenchyma. Myxoid and chon-

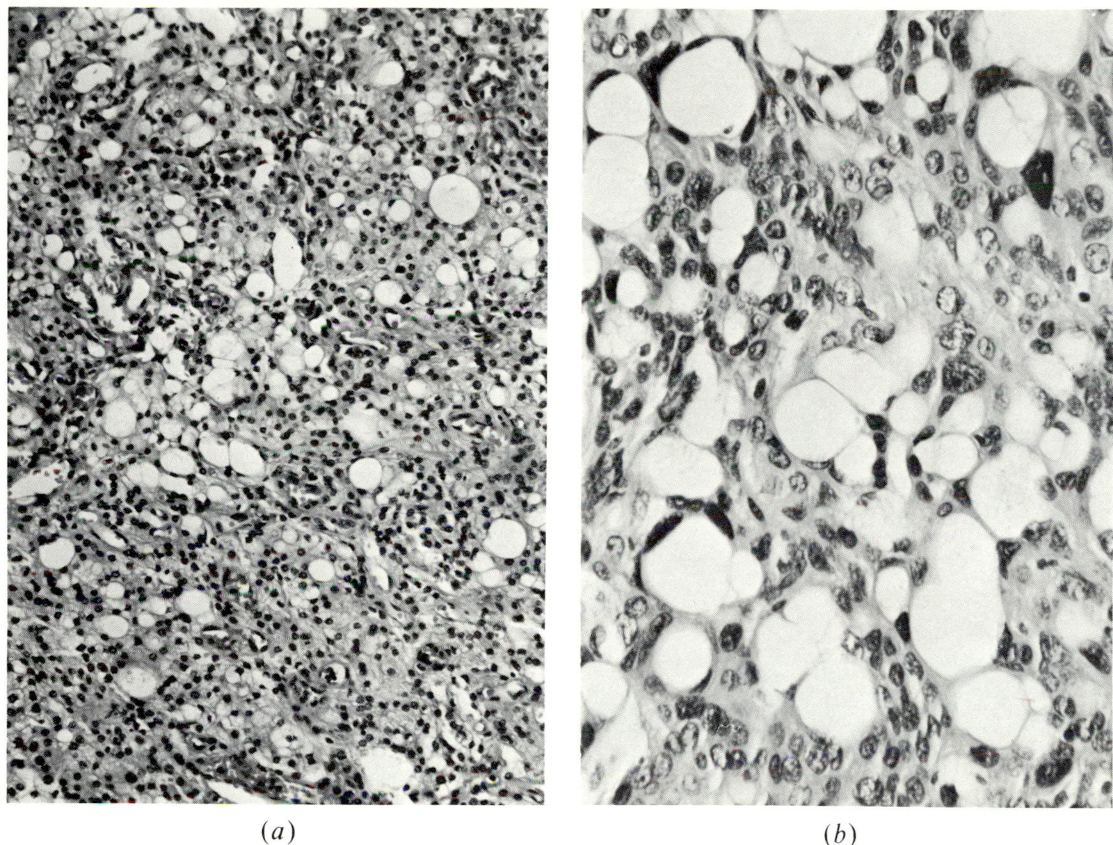

(a) (b)

FIGURE 49
Lipoblastic meningioma. (*a*) Many of the cells shown have the usual epithelioid appearance of meningothelial cells, but the tumor also contains numerous fat cells. ×100. (*b*) Higher magnification shows that the adipocytes are derived from meningothelial cells beginning with small fat droplets in some cells, progressing to the appearance of mature fat cells in others. ×400.

droid tissues are very closely related to each other in many types of proliferative processes and neoplasms in the human body (e.g., myxochondromas, chondromyxoid fibromas). Therefore, it should not be too surprising that once myxoid metaplasia has set it in a meningioma, the appearance of cartilage cannot be too far away. Indeed, in the same tumor where the cells have undergone myxoid changes, focal homogenization of the ground substance was observed and in some areas distinct hyaline cartilage made its appearance (Fig. 53a–c).

Benign meningiomas with cartilagenous areas have long been recognized as chondromatous or chondroblastic meningiomas with the basic nature of the tumor never in doubt. The same cannot be said about pure chondrosarcomas.[1,2] Of special interest is the mesenchymal chondrosarcoma, a highly malignant primitive tumor that occasionally involves the meninges. Originally thought to be essentially a tumor of the bone,[3] a number of subsequent cases have been seen in extraskeletal locations. The first case of meningeal involvement by a mesenchymal chondrosarcoma was reported by Dahlin and Henderson[4] to be followed by reports of Raskind and Grant,[5] Wu and Lapi,[6] and Guccion *et al.*[7] Scheithauer and Rubinstein[8] reviewed these cases and added eight new ones from their own material. Three of the latter were intracranial in location and five were attached to the spinal meninges. These tumors characteristically contain primitive, undifferentiated mesenchymal-like tissue, consisting mostly of closely packed, often spindle-shaped, cells. The tumor can be quite vascular, and the capillary spaces are surrounded by tumor cells in a fashion, sometimes imitating the pattern of hemangiopericytomas. Within this undifferentiated matrix, there are areas of solidified cartilage with all transitions seen from undifferentiated cells to chondroblasts. The centers of such cartilagenous areas may be calci-

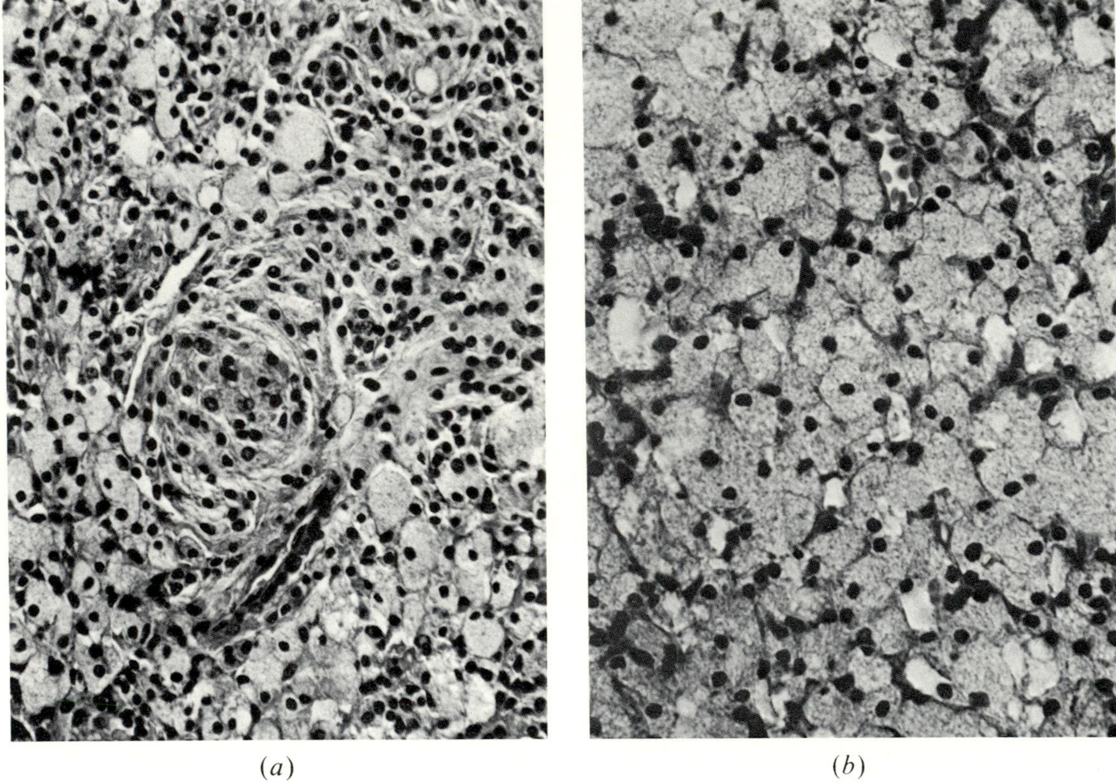

(*a*) (*b*)

FIGURE 50
Xanthomatous meningioma. (*a*) Accumulation of tiny lipid vacuoles give tumor cells a foamy appearance. Transitions between partly and fully lipidized meningothelial cells can be seen. (*b*) This portion of the same tumor is entirely composed of xanthomatous cells, and from this area alone the diagnosis of a meningioma could not be made.

fied. Throughout the tumor, including its cartilagenous portions, nuclear pleomorphism, anaplasia, and numerous mitotic figures indicate a high degree of malignancy (Fig. 54a–c). The histological structure of these tumors has a well-defined pattern, regardless whether they occur in the meninges or elsewhere in the body. It may therefore be postulated that their occurrence in the meninges is purely incidental. An alternate explanation would be that primitive meningeal cells, with a well-known potential to differentiate along other mesenchymal lines, might give rise to mesenchymal chondrosarcomas as well; but unlike in entities previously described in this chapter, no transitional forms between ordinary meningiomas and mesenchymal chondrosarcomas have been reported in the literature or observed by this author. Until such transitional forms are encountered, it is safer not to consider these tumors as variants of meningioma as such. Their gross characteristics during surgery, however, usually closely imitate an ordinary, if perhaps malignant appearing, meningioma and therefore they should be included in the discussion of morphological variants of meningeal tumors.

Whereas almost all mesenchymal chondrosarcomas of the meninges occurred as primary tumors in that location, a spinal epidural metastasis of this neoplasm originating from a primary lesion in the mandible was reported by Rengachary and Kepes.[9]

Calcification in meningiomas is not restricted to psammoma bodies or to foci of cartilage. It is not uncommon to find calcified strands of collagen (Fig. 55) and sometimes calcium is deposited in an irregular, haphazard manner within the tumor. Ossification is also a feature of some meningiomas (Fig. 56). The formation of bony spicules in a meningioma represents a form of osseous metaplasia; it should be considered separately from hyperostosis of the skull that develops as a secondary phenomenon in response to the nearby pres-

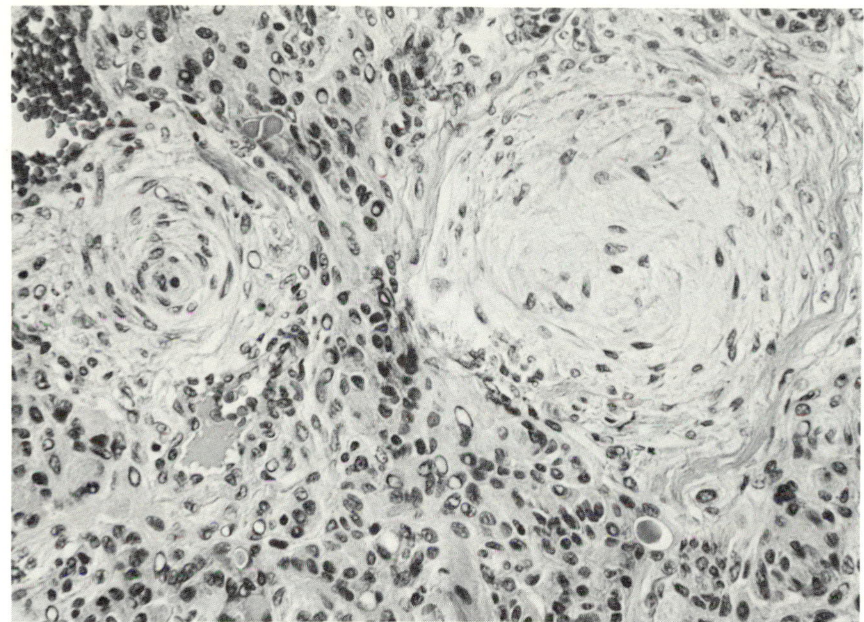

FIGURE 51
Myxochondroid changes in a meningioma. Two whorls are shown. *Left*, composed of typical meningothelial cells with vacuolated nuclei and slight loosening of intercellular connections; *right*, more advanced myxoid alterations.

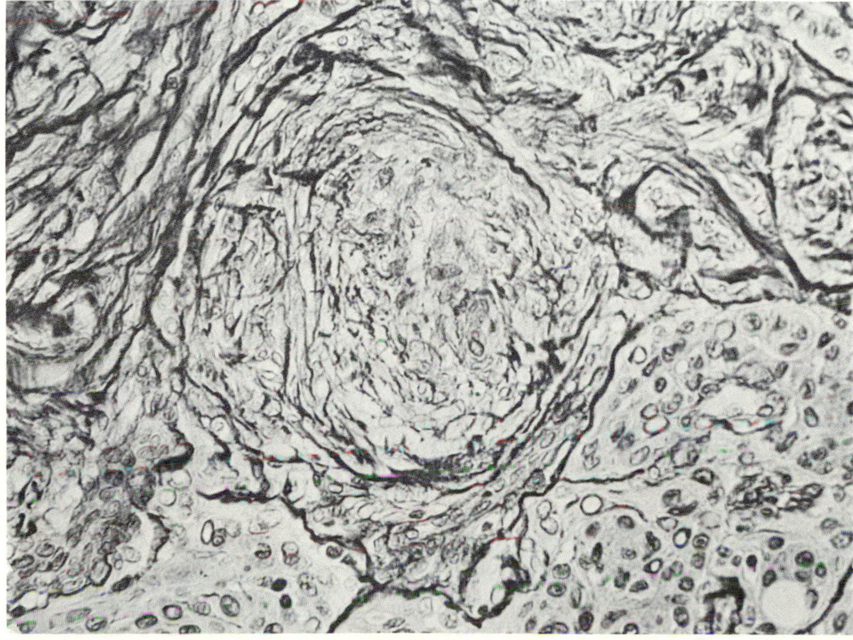

FIGURE 52
Same case depicted in Fig. 51. The whorl with myxoid changes also shows increased numbers of reticulin fibers as compared with surrounding tumor parenchyma. Wilder's reticulin stain.

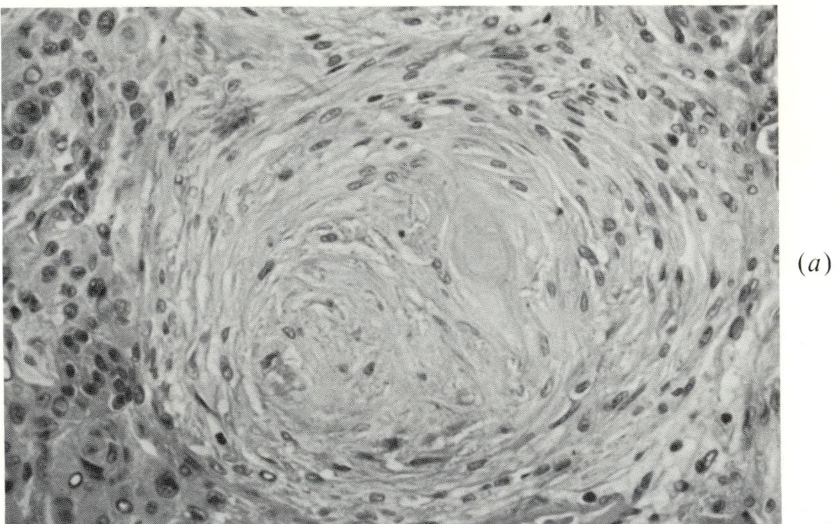

(*a*)

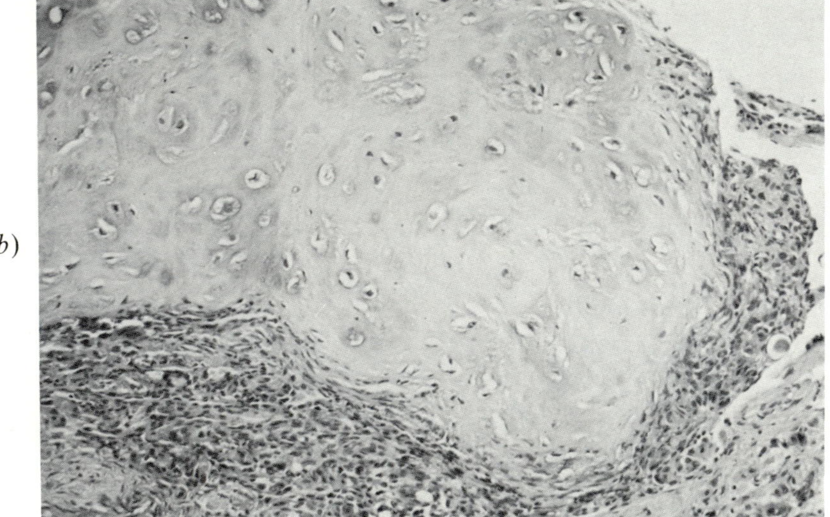

(*b*)

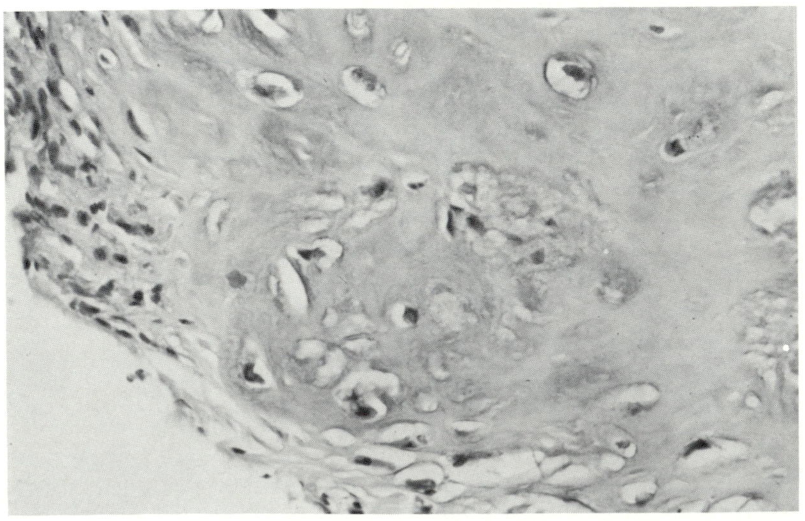

(*c*)

FIGURE 53
Same tumor shown in Figs. 51 and 52. Transition from myxoid to chondroid change. (*a*) Whorl with myxoid change and tiny focus of cartilage in center. (*b*) Large area totally transformed into cartilage. H&E. ×90. (*c*) Higher-power view of same area shows mature chondrocytes in hyaline matrix. H&E. ×260.

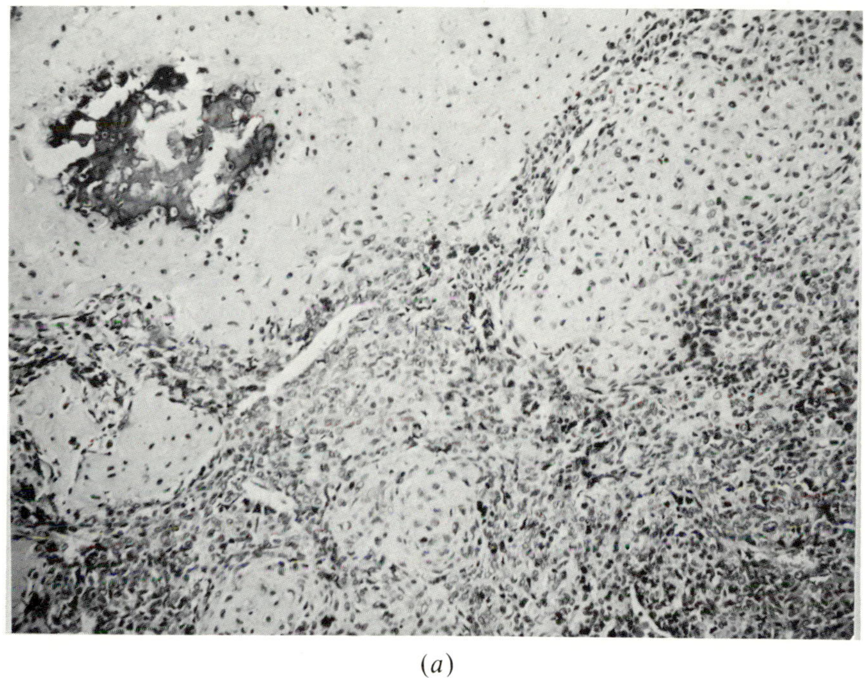

(*a*)

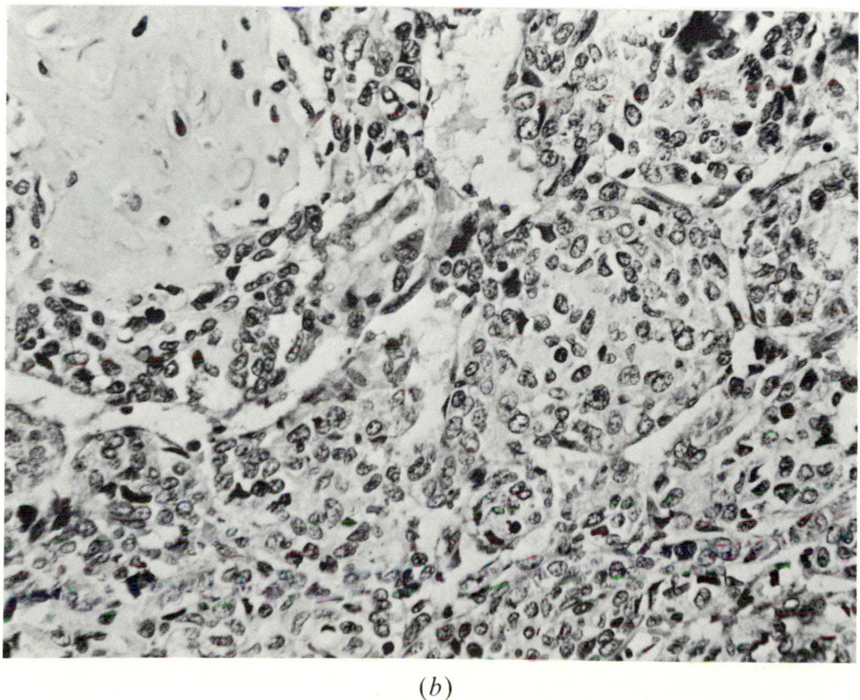

(*b*)

FIGURE 54
Mesenchymal chondrosarcoma of meninges. (*a*) Low-power view showing transition from primitive spindle-cell mesenchyme to cartilaginous foci. Largest nest (*left upper corner*) has focus of calcification. (*b*) Medium-power view showing sinusoidal spaces and pericytomalike pattern. (*c*) High-power view of cartilaginous area shows that chondrocytes are also pleomorphic and anaplastic.

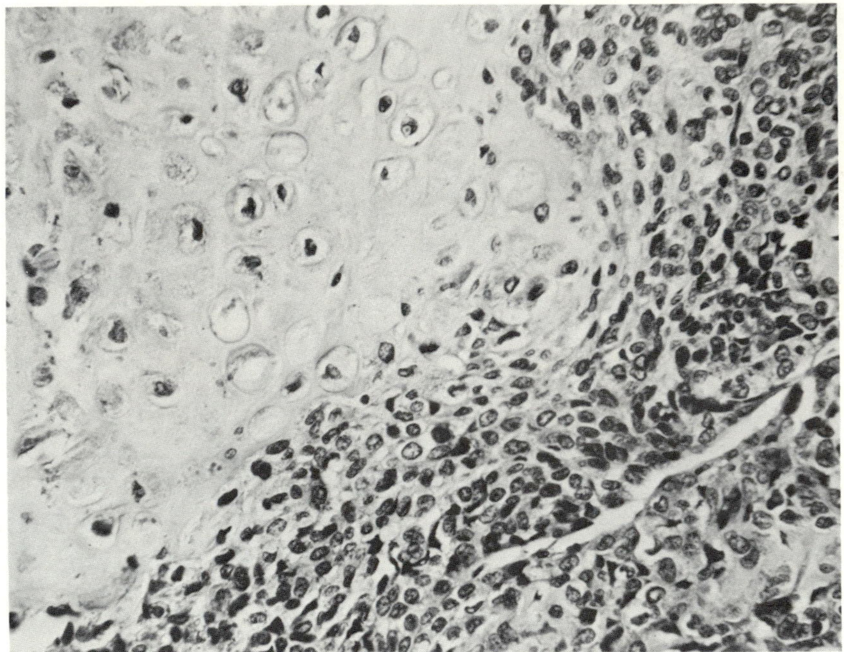

FIGURE 54c

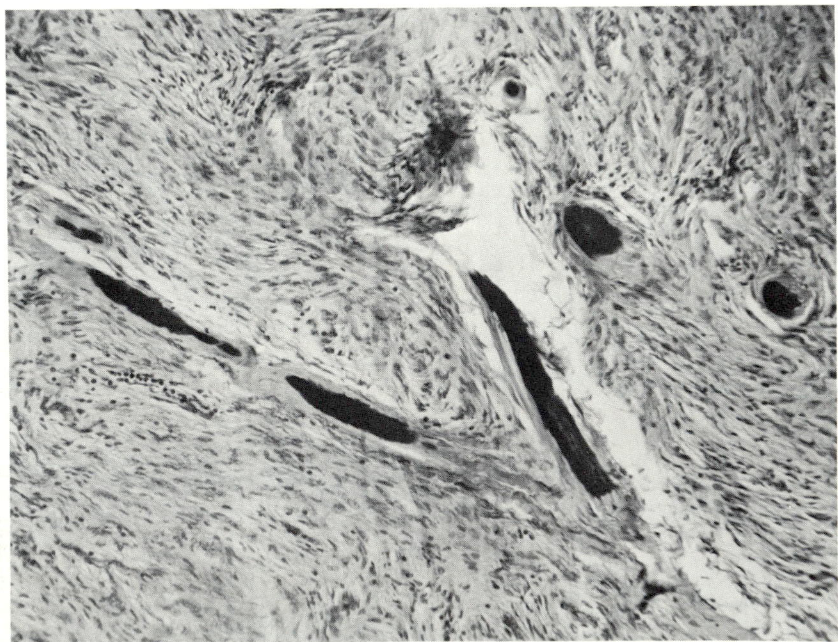

FIGURE 55
Calcification of collagen bundles in meningioma.

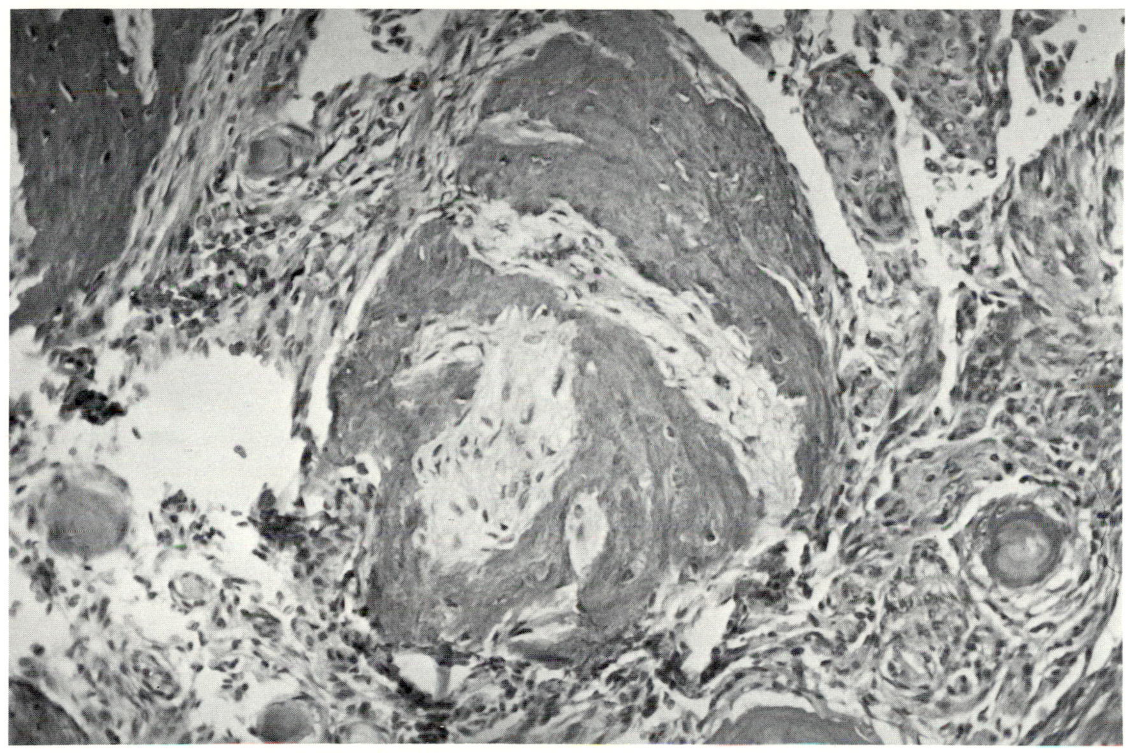

FIGURE 56
Foci of bone formation deep within meningioma, as distinct from hyperostosis of overlying cranium.

ence or invasive growth of meningiomas through the skull.

Lam *et al.*[9a] described a primary osteosarcoma of the meninges, which they regarded as a malignant counterpart of an osteoblastic meningioma. They suggested that such tumor is derived from a primitive multipotential mesenchymal cell in the meninges.

MENINGIOMAS WITH A PRONOUNCED VASCULAR COMPONENT AND ANGIOBLASTIC MENINGIOMAS

Meningeal tumors with a prominent vascular component have been the subject of much heated controversy. There appears to be agreement about at least one subgroup: tumors that have the general features of ordinary meningothelial meningiomas but are very richly vascularized. Although the blood vessels may dominate some areas, there are always regions characteristic of typical meningioma to make for an easy diagnosis (Figs. 57 and 58). This was called Variant 2 among the angioblastic meningiomas by Cushing and Eisenhardt[10] and is listed as *angiomatous meningioma* in the World Health Organization (WHO) classification.

A different type of highly vascularized meningioma is seen in Figures 59–64. Here blood vessels totally dominate the picture, but the cells between vessels are often seen to be intimately wrapped around capillaries in a concentric fashion. Some small vessels are actually totally enveloped by a single tumor cell (Fig. 61). Also, probably because of leakage of plasma lipids through thin-walled blood vessels, one often encounters lipid-laden foamy cells between the blood vessels, including those cells that are wrapped around the vessel walls (Fig. 62).

Partly because of the rich vascularity and the foamy cells seen between the blood vessels, such tumors are thought by some to be indistinguishable from hemangioblastomas of the cerebellum. In true hemangioblastomas, however, the stromal cells as a rule are forming clusters between blood vessels, but do not wrap themselves around the vascular channels as they do in this variant of angioblastic meningiomas. Also, in some meningiomas of this subtype, transitional areas to more

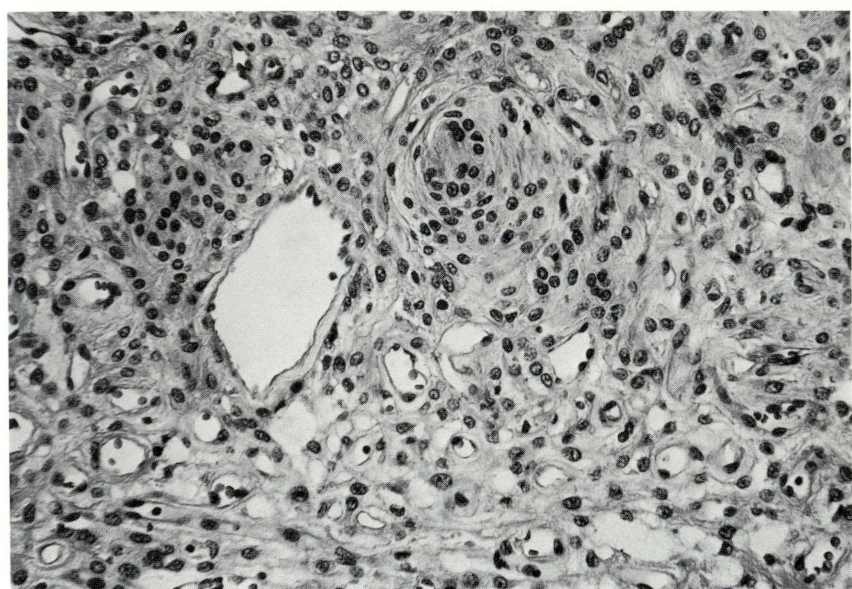

FIGURE 57
Highly vascularized (angiomatous) meningioma. The predominantly meningothelial character of this tumor can still be appreciated.

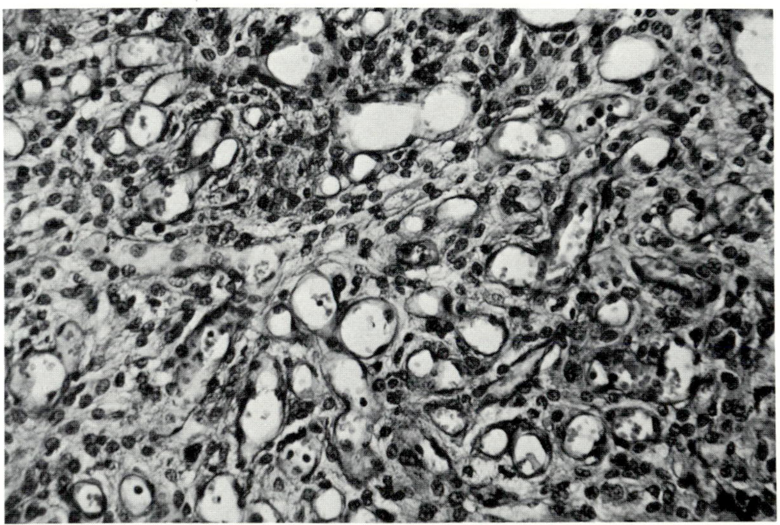

FIGURE 58
Another highly vascular meningioma. In this area the blood vessels are very prominent.

conventional angiomatous meningiomas may be found, a feature not encountered in Lindau's tumor. For these reasons, we believe that the tumor variant shown in Figures 59–64 is not a meningeal counterpart of Lindau's tumor in the cerebellum, but belongs to the meningiomas. In this particular type of tumor it is not uncommon to find bizarre hyperchromatic nuclei, suggesting atypism, but other signs of malignancy are usually not present. Tumors of this type not infrequently become partially or totally sclerosed (Figs. 63 and 64), at the same time, however, still giving the gross appearance of a meningioma. Surgeons have no problem in recognizing this tumor as a meningioma and may be quite surprised to hear the pathologist hedging over a frozen section taken from such a

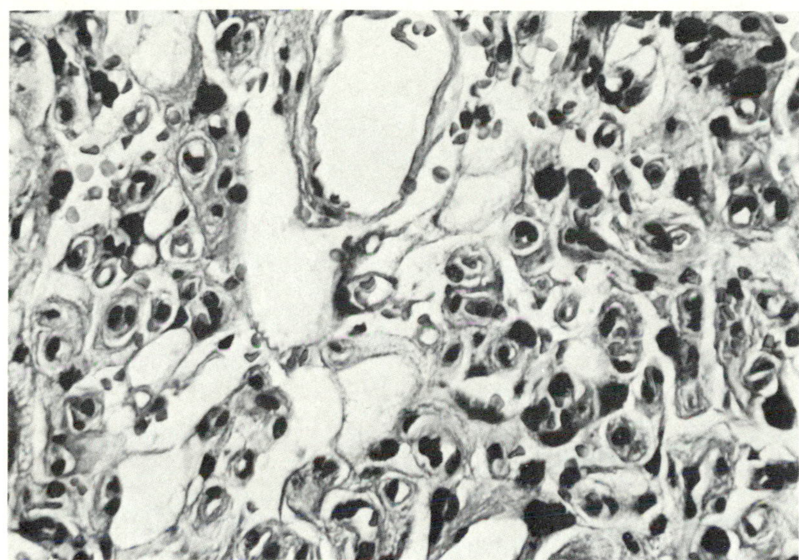

FIGURE 59
In this tumor, the blood vessels totally dominate the picture. Meningothelial cells show very little tendency to form cell clusters; instead, they are wrapped around blood vessels.

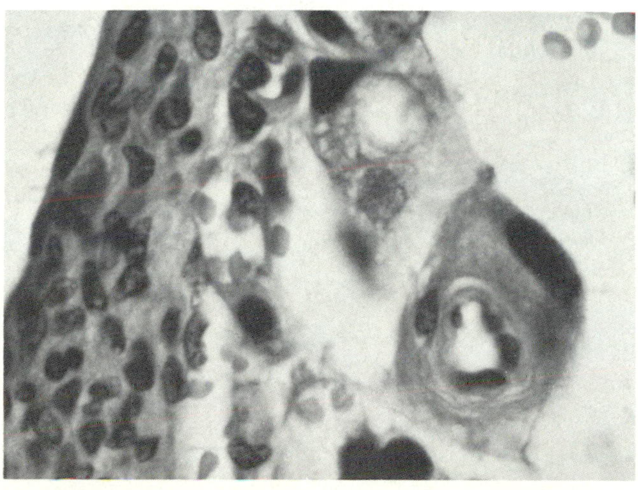

FIGURE 60
Same tumor shown in Figure 59. *Left*, a sheet of meningothelial cells; *center*, a small vessel surrounded by meningothelial cells.

tumor. Such hesitation on the pathologist's part must be understood, however, if one realizes that some areas of this tumor might consist of nothing more than thin-walled blood spaces with intervening dense fibrous tissue (Fig. 64).

Whereas we do not believe that the tumor just described is a meningeal form of a hemangioblastoma, we have seen, as others did before us,[11-14] true representatives of Lindau's tumor involving the meninges. Such a tumor is shown in Figure 65. The patient and several members of his family suffered from the von Hippel-Lindau syndrome. The patient had a cerebellar hemangioblastoma as well as a highly vascular tumor of the meninges overlying the right frontal pole.[15] Histologically, this tumor was an exact replica of his

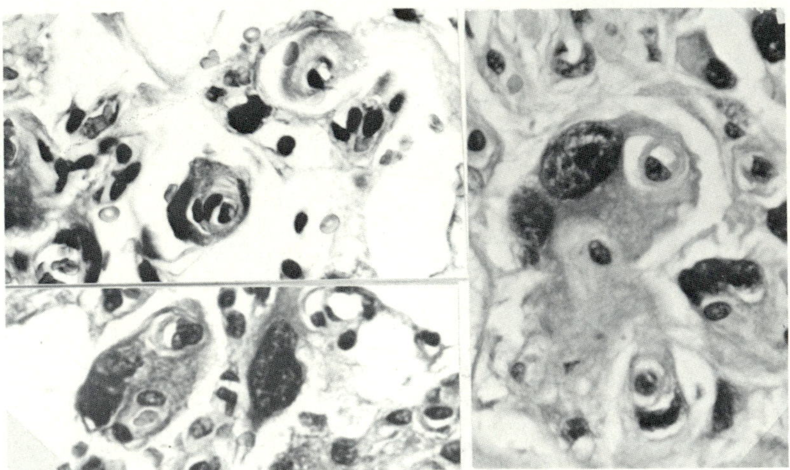

FIGURE 61
Three areas of the same tumor shown in Figures 59 and 60, exhibiting intimate relationship between meningothelial cells and blood vessels. *Right*, a single tumor cell has incorporated a capillary. Note nuclear hyperchromasia.

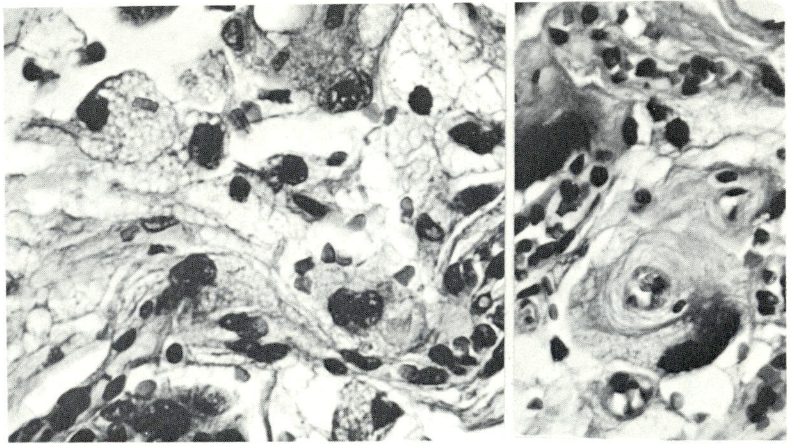

FIGURE 62
Lipid droplets are present in many meningothelial cells. *Right*, a foamy cell is wrapped around a capillary; *left*, independent clusters formed by foamy cells. The lipid material is probably derived from plasma lipids exuding from thin-walled vessels.

cerebellar hemangioblastoma, showing sprouting capillaries and large numbers of lipid-filled stromal cells in the interstices, but the stromal cells showed no tendency at all to form concentrical arrangements around vessel walls, as seen in angioblastic meningiomas.

Such a leptomeningeal form of a hemangioblastoma or Lindau tumor was listed as variant 3 of Cushing and Eisenhardt's angioblastic meningiomas and is also included in the WHO classification as a hemangioblastic form. As stated above, we do not believe that this particular tumor is interchangeable with vascular meningiomas, even if the latter happen to have many lipid-filled cells. It ought to appear strange even to the casual observer that this problem should always be raised with vascular tumors of the *meninges:* If Lindau's tumor and meningiomas were in some ways interchangeable, then the same problem of differential diagnosis ought to arise once in awhile with the classic cerebellar or the brainstem form of this tumor as well. But the fact is that cerebellar,

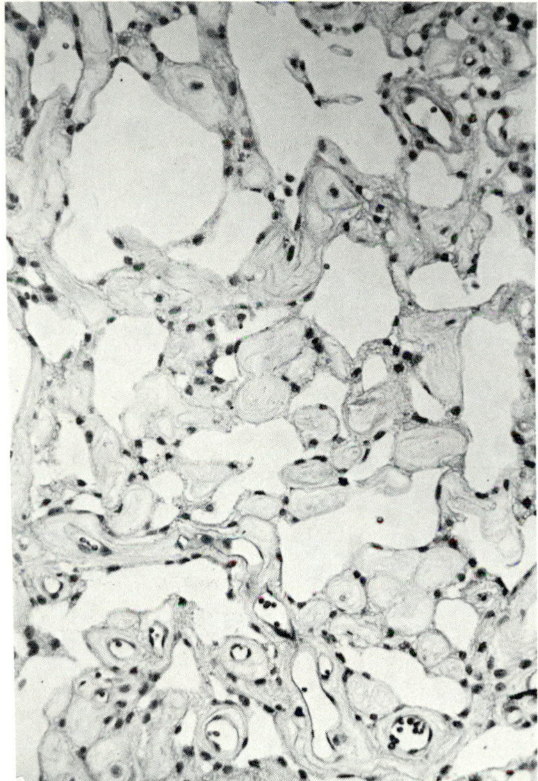

FIGURE 63
Same tumor shown in Fig. 63. Collagenization of blood vessel walls. On frozen section this tumor could easily be regarded as a sclerosing hemangioma.

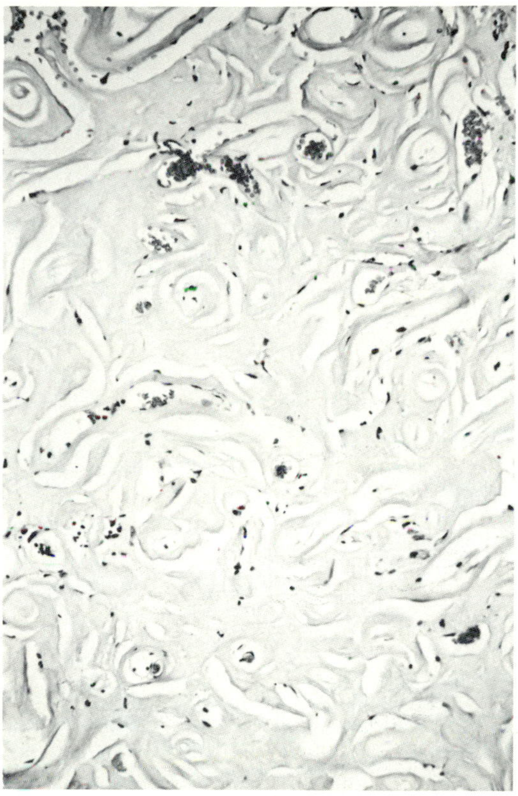

FIGURE 64
Further sclerosis as seen in this picture makes even the outlines of the blood vessels difficult to discern.

brain stem, or spinal cord hemangioblastomas are not usually mistaken for meningiomas. In fact, if there is any problem, it usually involves differential diagnosis from highly vascular *astrocytomas*. Furthermore, in the full-blown form of von Hippel-Lindau disease, patients have an assortment of associated retinal hemangiomas, pheochromocytomas of the adrenal, renal tumors, and syringomyelia, but meningiomas do not form part of this complex. This could be regarded as another argument against a close relationship between meningiomas and Lindau's hemangioblastomas.

HEMANGIOPERICYTIC MENINGIOMAS OR HEMANGIOPERICYTOMAS OF THE MENINGES

Bailey *et al.*[16] described three cases of tentorial meningiomas they called angioblastic because the histological structure reminded them of cerebellar hemangioblastomas. These workers noted nevertheless that the biological behavior of these tumors was unusually aggressive, as all three recurred after removal, eventually killing the patients. The illustrations of that 1928 article clearly show that the tumors belonged to the category later referred to as hemangiopericytomas. Indeed, in their case no. 3, these investigators' first histological diagnosis was "perithelioma." In 1938, Cushing and Eisenhardt[17] again described angioblastic meningiomas (Type IV of their classification), but now distinguished among three variants, the first of which corresponded to the three cases described in 1928. Again, they stressed that this variant had a malignant biological potential; of six operated cases so diagnosed, there was only one 5-year survivor. Begg and Garret[18] in 1954 proposed that Cushing and Eisenhardt's Type IV, variation 1 tumor was not a meningioma at all but a hemangiopericytoma that happened to develop in the meninges, no different from hemangiopericytomas

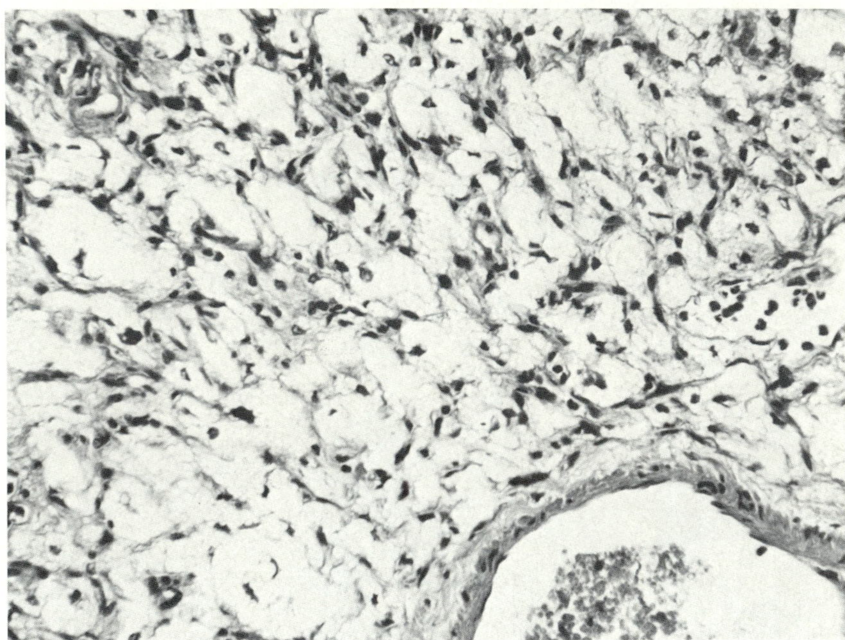

FIGURE 65
Leptomeningeal hemangioblastoma over the right frontal lobe from a patient with von Hippel-Lindau syndrome. Whereas the tumor contains many capillaries and foamy interstitial cells, the latter do not wrap themselves around the former as is seen in angioblastic meningiomas. The patient had similar tumors in the cerebellum and retina.

occurring in other locations of the body. With this, the battle lines have been drawn and today we have basically two camps locked in a lively dispute. Kruse,[19] Popoff *et al.*[20] Peña,[21] Choux *et al.*,[22] and Goellner *et al.*,[23] among others, share the view proposed by Begg and Garret that meningeal hemangiopericytomas do not truly belong to meningiomas. Jellinger and Slowik[24] also failed to find transitional forms between ordinary meningiomas and meningeal hemangiopericytomas. Peña[21] found dense bodies in the cytoplasm of tumor cells in meningeal hemangiopericytomas, which he believed indicated smooth muscle differentiation of the tumor cells, further separating them from meningiomas.

In the other camp, Rubinstein[25] and Horten *et al.*[26] believe that little is to be gained by creating a separate group of hemangiopericytomas of the meninges as totally distinct from meningiomas. There are, indeed, important data in the literature pointing to transitions between hemangiopericytomas and other forms of meningiomas. Bergstrand and Olivecrona[27] have shown the tendency for whorl formation in a hemangiopericytoma. Horten *et al.*[26] have also demonstrated such transitions between meningothelial features and hemangiopericytic pattern in one and the same tumor. Also, transitions between fibroblastic meningiomas and hemangiopericytic forms have been observed by Horten *et al.*[26] and Pitkethly *et al.*[28]

Electron microscopically, Horten *et al.*[26] observed features common to both meningothelial and hemangiopericytic tumors (e.g., fragments of basement membrane material between neighboring tumor cells in both groups). They also suggested that the above-mentioned fibrillary densities described by Peña[21] may not be specific for smooth muscle differentiation, as they have encountered them in cells of a transitional meningioma also. Muller and Mealy[29] cultured a hemangiopericytic meningioma and found whorls developing in the tissue cultures. Finally, the papillary variant of meningiomas discussed in great detail by Ludwin *et al.*[30] apparently represents a link between meningothelial and hemangiopericytic tumors, as this histologic variant has been observed to develop from both subgroups. Of these investigators' 17 cases of papillary meningiomas, five (29%) were derived from the hemangiopericytic type of angioblastic meningiomas. This would indirectly suggest a common histogenesis for these

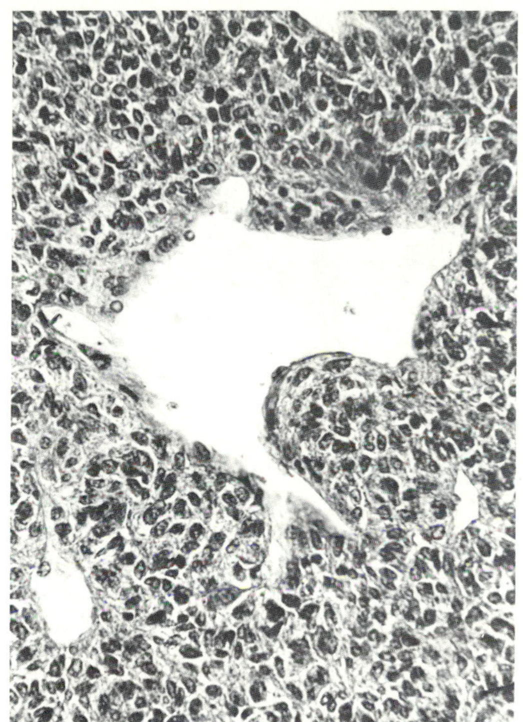

FIGURE 66
Hemangiopericytic type meningioma, or hemangiopericytoma of the meninges. In this tumor, a peritorcular mass from a middle-aged woman, thin-walled blood vessels are surrounded by closely packed primitive-appearing mesenchymal cells with cushionlike protrusions into the lumen of the vessel in center. They are, nevertheless, separated from lumen by endothelial cells.

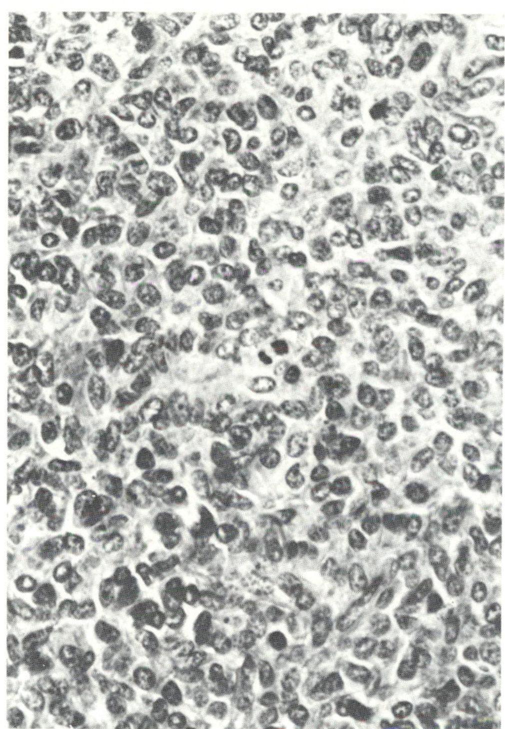

FIGURE 67
Higher-power view of same tumor shown in Fig. 66. Cells are crowded. Two mitoses are presented close to the center.

tumors. On the basis of their light, electron microscopic, tissue, and organ culture studies, Horten *et al.*[26] have concluded that hemangiopericytomas of the meninges are histogenetically related to other meningiomas.

Another interesting question relates to the possibility of hemangiopericytomas being derived from, or at least closely related to, capillary endothelium. The studies of Jellinger and Denk,[31] who were able to identify the presence of blood group isoantigens in the endothelial cells of vascular tumors of the central nervous system, but not in pericytes or meningothelial cells, would suggest that endothelial cells and pericytes are not interchangeable elements in these tumors.

In our own material, we have seen hemangiopericytic tumors that showed no transitional features to other meningiomas, but we have also seen examples where transitions to both meningothelial and fibroblastic meningiomas existed.

Some of our cases of hemangiopericytic meningiomas are shown in Figures 66–75. The pure hemangiopericytic form is shown in Figures 66–67. A tendency for fibroblastic differentiation is noted in Figure 68 and 69, whereas Figures 70 and 71 show areas indistinguishable from a cellular fibroblastic meningioma.

We found a few cellular whorls in otherwise typical hemangiopericytic meningiomas (Figs. 72 and 73). We also found that some hemangiopericytomatous meningiomas have a tendency to have their cells arranged in a trabecular pattern (Fig. 74a,b). Between such trabeculae, a basophilic myxoid material is sometimes deposited, creating a similarity to chordomas (Fig. 75a,b).

Of great theoretical interest are cases of otherwise typical meningothelial meningiomas which contain apparently non-neoplastic proliferation of pericytes around blood vessels described by Mirra[32] (Fig. 76a). Although these cells were apparently distinct from surrounding meningothelial tumor cells, their very presence in a meningothelial meningioma gives rise to interesting speculations as to the relationship between the two elements. In

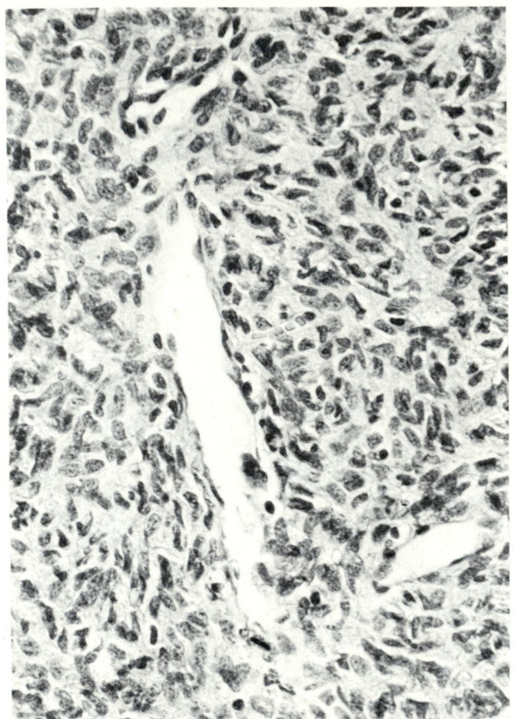

FIGURE 68
Another hemangiopericytic tumor of the meninges. The same relationship between tumor cells and blood vessels exists as in the previous case, but the cells are more elongated, resembling primitive fibroblasts.

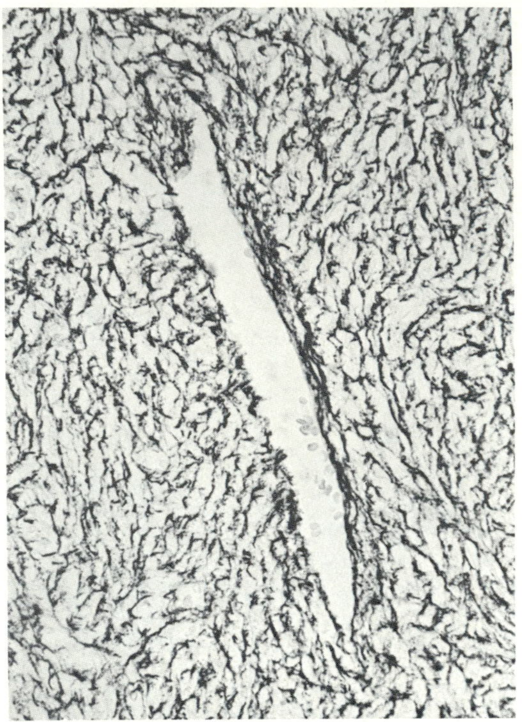

FIGURE 69
Same tumor shown in Fig. 68. A very rich reticulin network, continuous with the adventitia of blood vessel in center, is seen. Wilder's reticulin stain.

3 cases of Challa,[33] and Challa *et al.*[33a] somewhat similar cell proliferation was observed in the media of arterioles. These cells appeared somewhat less distinct from the meningothelial tumor cells in the surrounding areas (Fig. 76b,c). In the three cases of this nature described by these investigators, the meningiomas, although small, provoked massive cerebral edema around them. This was attributed to the increased vascular component in these tumors.

It cannot be emphasized too strongly that the above considerations are primarily of academic interest. Whether meningeal hemangiopericytomas represent a variant of meningiomas or are tumors histogenetically independent from other meningiomas, the most important fact about them is their unfavorable biological and clinical behavior. As stated above, this was already recognized in the very first paper that dealt with these tumors, and the intervening years have done nothing to improve the reputation of this tumor. Relatively low in incidence compared with other forms of meningiomas, these hemangiopericytic tumors are leaders in statistical data dealing with local recurrences and distant metastases. All eight patients of Kruse[19] who had this tumor either died from the tumor or at least needed reoperation for local recurrences, with one of them developing distant metastases in the skeletal system. Distant metastases from this tumor were also reported by Kepes *et al.*[34] Petito and Porro,[35] Lowden and Taylor,[36] and others. Clinicopathological correlations by Pitkethly *et al.*[28] Skullerud and Löken,[37] and Jellinger and Slowik[24] also attest to the aggressive course, with recurrence in 80% of patients and metastases in 23% in the series of the last-mentioned investigators.

Whereas the above discussion mostly centered on intradural cranial forms of hemangiopericytomatous tumors, the same neoplasm may occur epidurally in the cranium,[38] as well as in the spinal canal (intradural[39] and extradural[40,41]).

UNUSUAL CELLULAR PATTERNS IN MENINGIOMAS

The variations of histological patterns in meningiomas are almost endless. Some of them are mor-

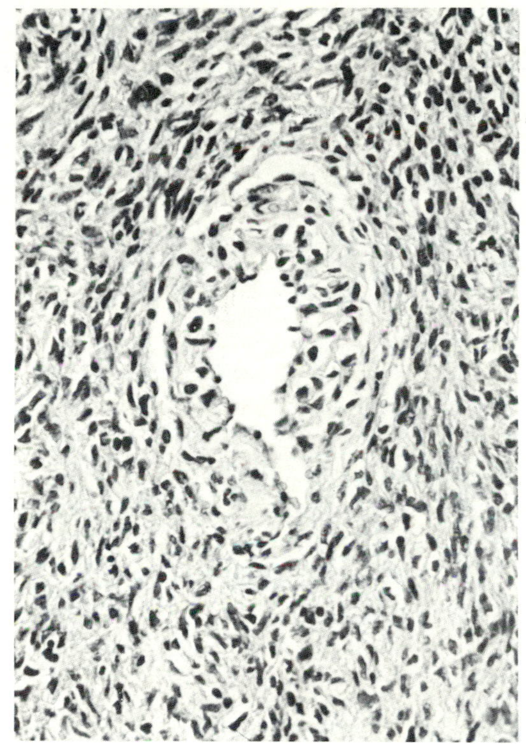

FIGURE 70
This area found in a hemangiopericytic meningioma could not be differentiated from a highly cellular fibroblastic meningioma.

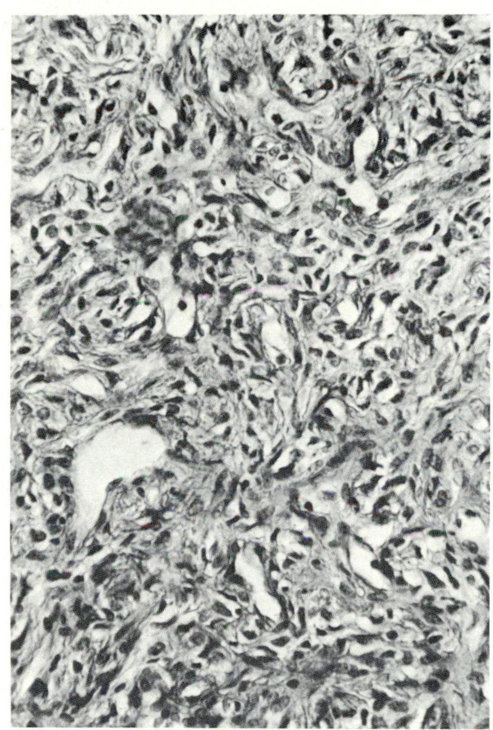

FIGURE 71
Still another variant of this entity. The vascularity is very high and the arrangement of cells suggestive of a hemangiopericytoma, but the cells appear more like fairly mature fibroblasts.

phologic curiosities, others have recognized biologic significance. As examples of the former, one occasionally finds rosettelike structures in meningiomas (Fig. 77) (see also Bertrand *et al.*[42]), but there is little danger of these tumors being mistaken for neuroblastomas. A rare pattern of structures resembling primitive renal glomeruli is shown in Figure 78.

Papillary formations in meningiomas seem to have important prognostic significance. First observed in Cushing and Eisenhardt's[43] famous patient, Dorothy M. Russell, these structures were absent from the patient's original peritorcular meningioma, but became increasingly evident in subsequent recurrences and finally came to dominate the tumor and its pulmonary metastases. First there were a few doubters; Hamblet,[44] Christensen *et al.*[45] and Ringsted[46] suspected that the pulmonary foci of Cushing and Eisenhardt's case represented an unrelated papillary carcinoma of the lung. Subsequently, however, Russell,[47] Russell and Rubinstein,[48] Kepes *et al.*[34] Miller and Ramsden,[49] Ludwin and Conley,[50] and Ludwin *et al.*[30] demonstrated beyond any doubt the existence of transitions between nonpapillary and papillary forms of meningiomas. The changes usually begin with some tumor cells surrounding blood vessels or connective tissue cores in a perpendicular fashion. Loosening of surrounding tumor tissue will make the papillary pattern more conspicuous. Most interestingly, Russell,[47] and later Ludwin *et al.*,[30] found some of the cells in papillary formations to have argyrophilic cell processes; in addition, Ludwin *et al.*[30] found cells with fibrils staining positively with phosphotungstic acid hematoxylin. Figures 79–86 illustrate the evolution and presence of a papillary pattern of several meningiomas and of the pulmonary metastases of one.

Undoubtedly, the primary significance of recognizing a papillary configuration in any given meningioma lies in the biologically aggressive behavior this pattern is often associated with. The rate of local recurrences and distant metastases is

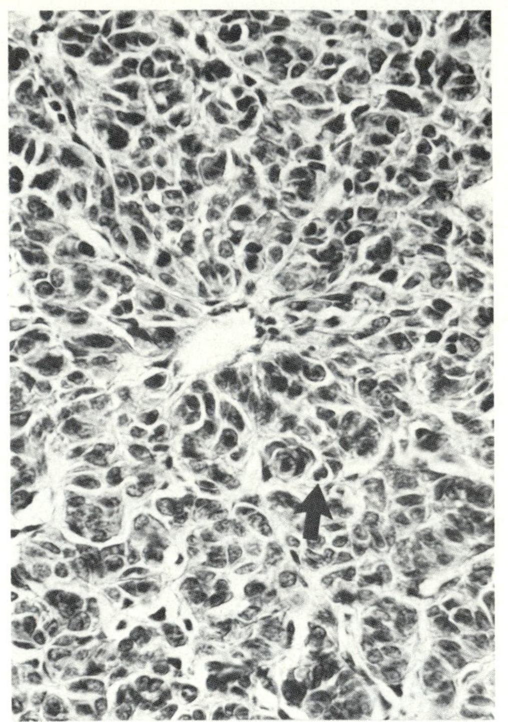

FIGURE 72
Hemangiopericytic meningioma with sinusoidal vascular pattern. Note formation of small cellular whorl (*arrow*).

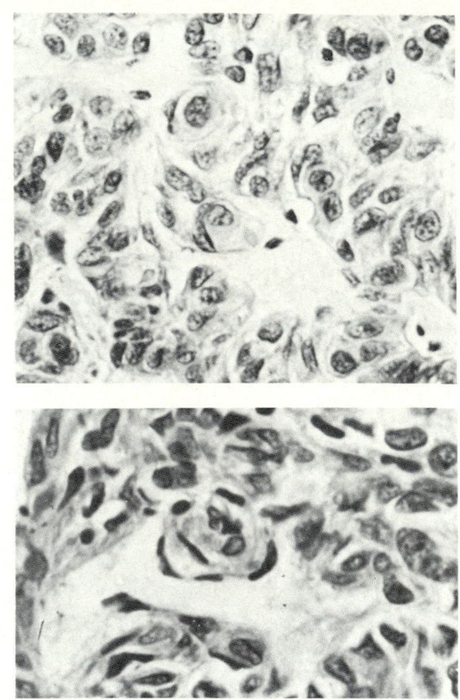

FIGURE 73
Other areas from same tumor shown in Fig. 72. Multiple whorls (*top*). A whorl (*bottom*) is protruding into vessel, separated only by endothelial cells from lumen.

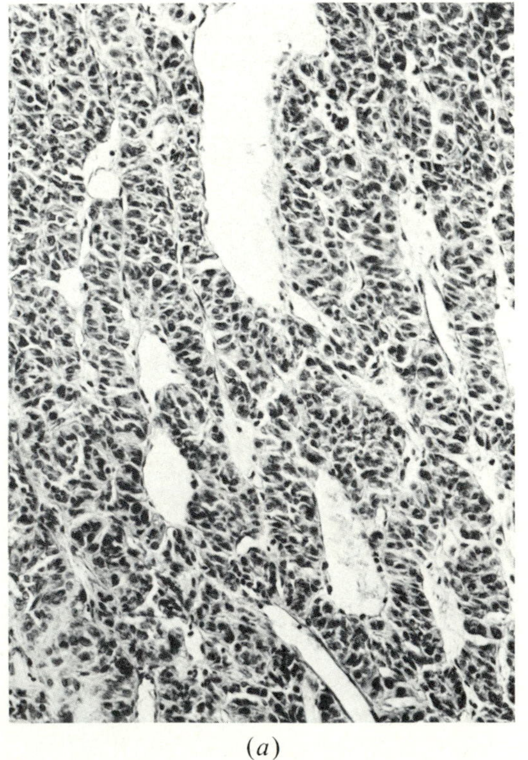

(*a*)

(*b*)

FIGURE 74
Hemangiopericytic meningioma with trabecular pattern. (*a*) Trabeculae surrounding sinusoids are reminiscent of a hepatoma. (*b*) In another area of tumor, in addition to trabeculae, cellular whorls can be observed (*arrows*).

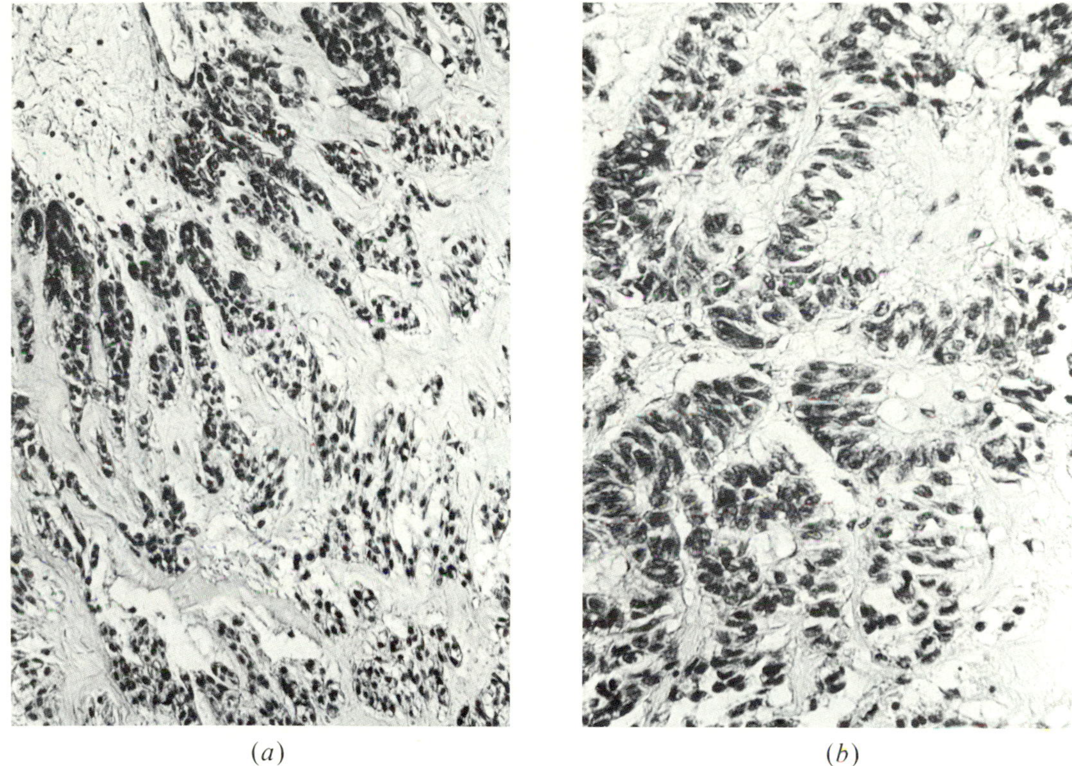

(*a*) (*b*)

FIGURE 75
Trabecular pattern in another meningioma with myxoid metaplasia of stroma between tumor cells causing resemblance to chordoma. (*a*) H&E. ×160. (*b*) H&E. ×280.

unduly high in this subgroup of meningiomas, which was therefore designated by Ludwin *et al.*[30] as a malignant variant of meningioma.

MENINGIOMAS WITH PATTERN OF FIBROUS HISTIOCYTOMAS

The focal presence of a storiform pattern and of foamy xanthomatous cells in meningiomas was alluded to earlier. In some meningeal tumors, however, this pattern predominates all over the tumor, and the problem arises whether one is dealing with still another variant of meningiomas or with a fibrous histiocytoma incidentally located in the meninges. Some investigators, to be sure, preferred the latter interpretation. Gonzalez-Vitale *et al.*[51] described a malignant fibrous histiocytoma involving the base of the brain, that developed following irradiation of a pituitary tumor. Lam and Colah[52] observed a fibrous histiocytoma with a myxoid stroma, apparently originating from the basal cranial dura.

In our material we have seen meningeal tumors with the appearance of fibrous histiocytomas. In addition to a storiform pattern and xanthomatous cells, these tumors also had some cellular atypia, large ganglioid cells, and multinucleated giant cells (Figs. 87–91). One case seen in consultation from the Mayo Clinic, a meningeal tumor from the parietal area of a young woman, had marked infiltration of acute inflammatory cells in the tumor otherwise showing the features of a fibrous histiocytoma (Figs. 92–93). According to Kyriakos and Kempson,[53] such inflammatory fibrous histiocytomas carry a very grave prognosis, but so far—3 years after surgery—our patient is still doing well. Another case of a meningeal tumor with the histologic hallmarks of a malignant fibrous histiocytoma, superficially invading the brain is shown in Figures 94–100. Although by light microscopy this tumor had all the characteristics of a fibrous histiocytoma, electron microscopically it had features of a meningioma (interdigitating cell membranes, tight junctions, and others) (see Chapter 26).

(*a*)

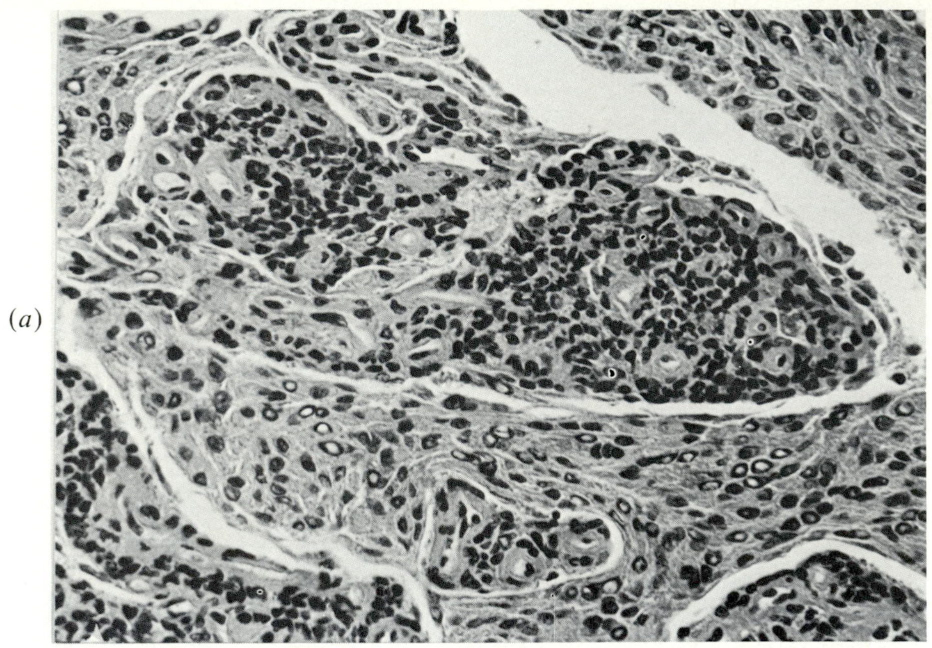

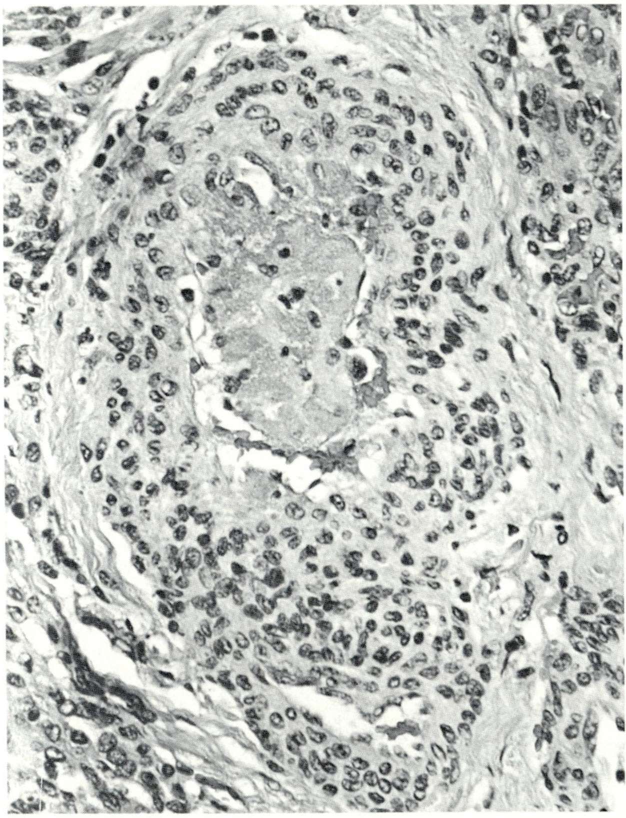

(*b*) 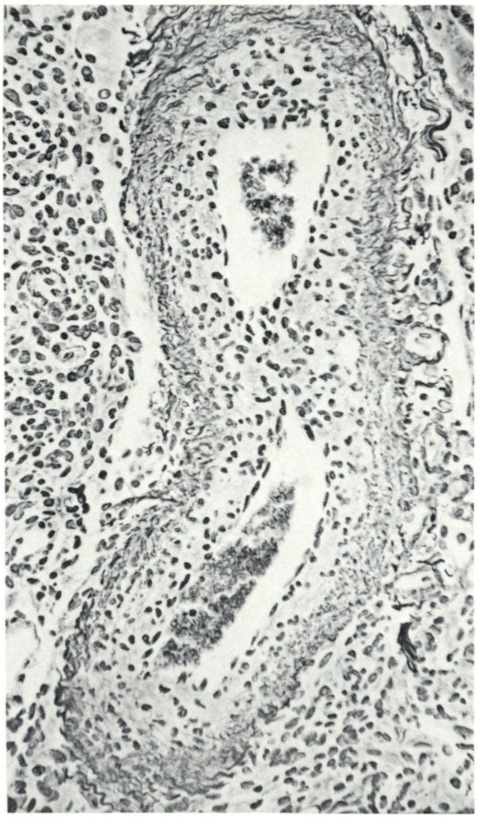 (*c*)

FIGURE 76
Pericytes and pericytelike cells in meningothelial meningioma. (*a*) Meningothelial meningioma composed of typical tumor cells with intranuclear vacuoles. Blood vessel in center is surrounded by clusters of smaller and darker pericytes. (Courtesy Dr. S. Mirra.) (*b*) Proliferation of glomuslike cells within wall of small artery in meningioma. H&E. (*c*) Same area with reticulin stain indicating adventitia separating proliferating cells from the tumor outside the blood vessel. Wilder's reticulin stain. (*b* and *c* courtesy of Dr. V. R. Challa.)

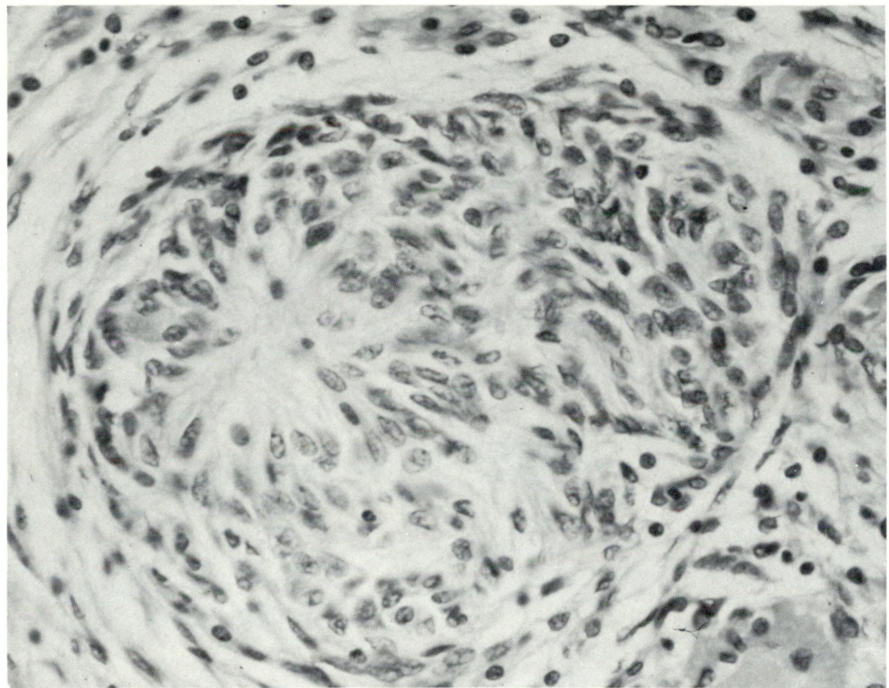

FIGURE 77
Rosettelike arrangement of tumor cells in predominantly fibroblastic meningioma.

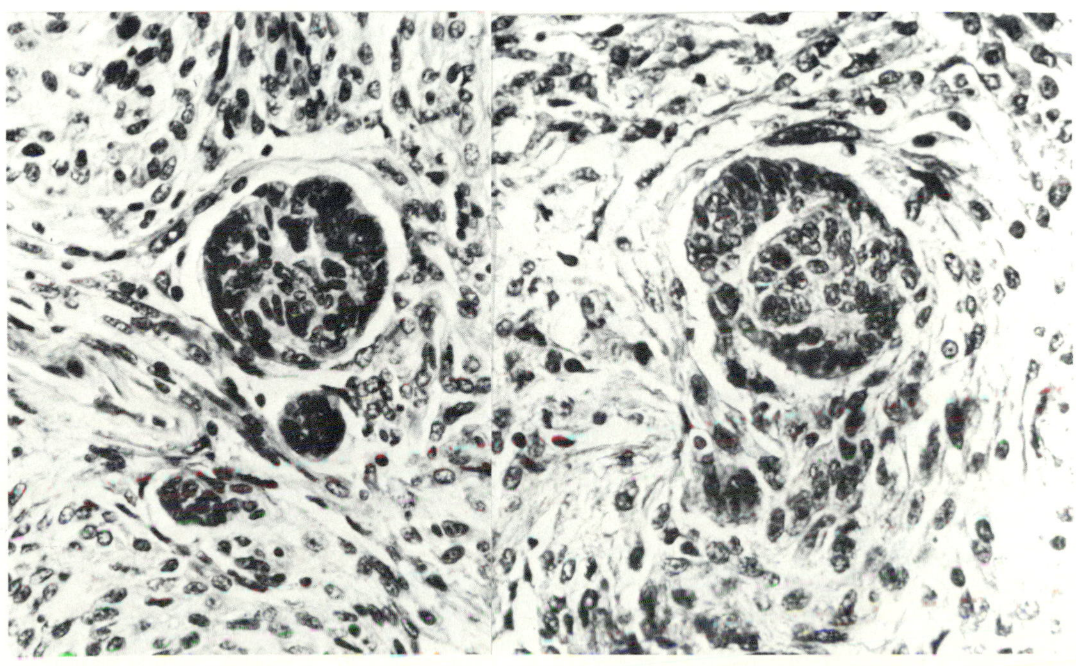

FIGURE 78
Cell clussters closely resembling primitive glomeruli of developing kidneys (cellular fibroblastic meningioma).

FIGURES 79–86
Papillary pattern in meningiomas.

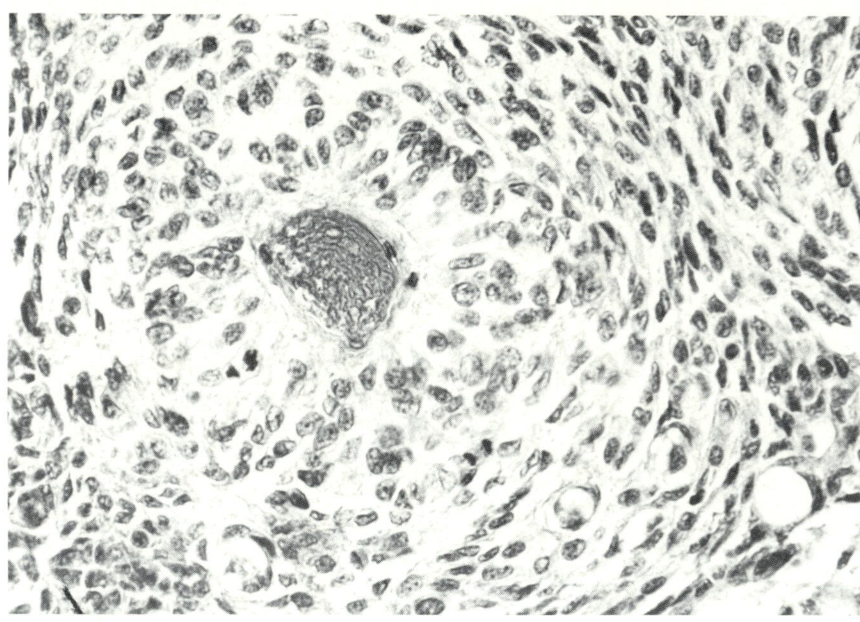

FIGURE 79
Perivascular radial arrangement of tumor cells in meningioma is often the first step to formation of papillary structures.

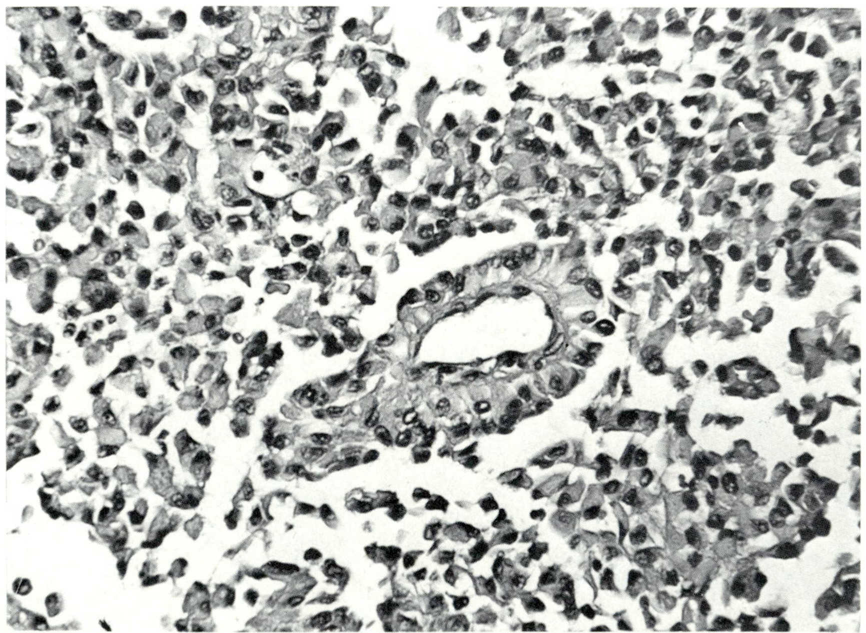

FIGURE 80
Loosening of a tumor such as seen in Figure 79 will result in perivascular rosettelike structures, resembling those seen in some ependymomas.

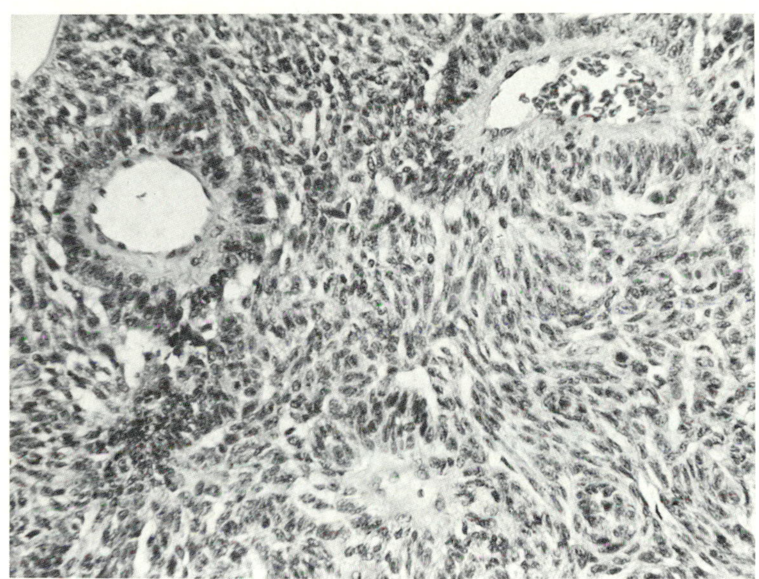

FIGURE 81
Cellular meningothelial meningioma with perivascular pallisading cells.

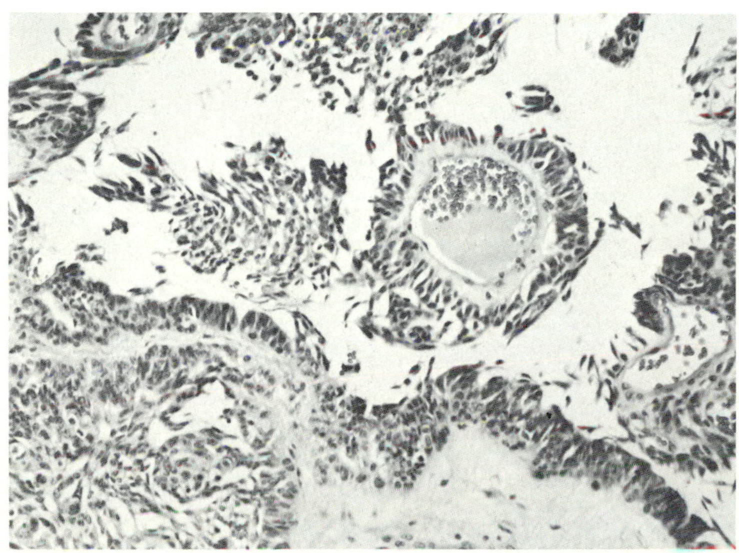

FIGURE 82
Same case shown in Fig. 81. Edematous loosening of tumor results in papillary arrangement of perivascular cells.

Ferrer and Aceves[54] reached the same conclusion with regard to a highly xanthomatous meningeal tumor of the left frontal area. Although the tumor resembled a fibrous xanthoma by light microscopy, ultrastructurally the presence of extensive interdigitation of cell membranes, desmosomes, and hemidesmosomes, as well as 100 Å-diameter cytoplasmic filaments convinced these investigators that they were dealing with a variant of a meningioma.

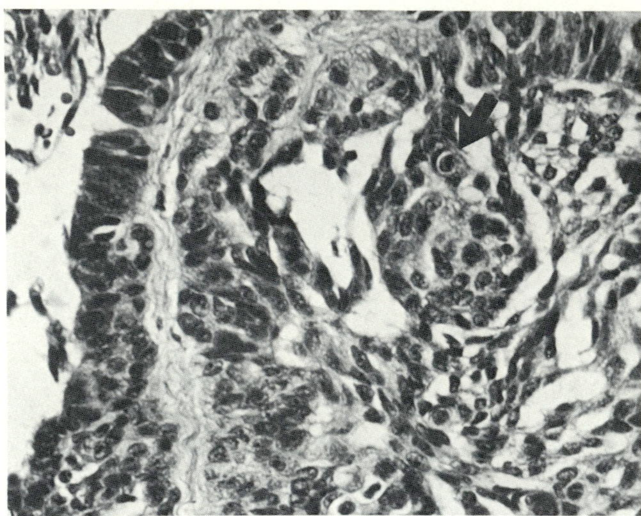

FIGURE 83
Same case shown in Figs. 81 and 82. Papillary arrangement (*left*); meningothelial whorl (*center*, *arrow*).

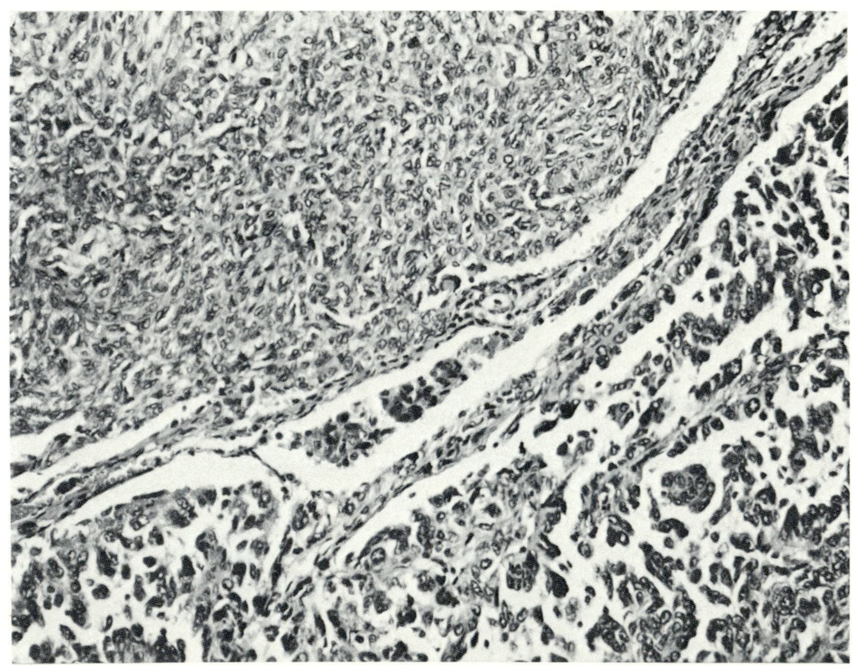

FIGURE 84
Pulmonary metastasis of a peritorcular fibroblastic–hemangiopericytic meningioma: dense, closely packed cells (*upper left*); looser area (*lower right*).

NONLIPID SUBSTANCES STORED IN OR SECRETED BY MENINGIOMA CELLS

Some meningiomas appear grossly dark brown because they contain large amounts of *hemosiderin.* This pigment likely is derived from previous hemorrhage within the tumor, although such cannot always be documented clinically or pathologically. The iron granules may be located primarily in the fibrous septa of the tumor (Fig.

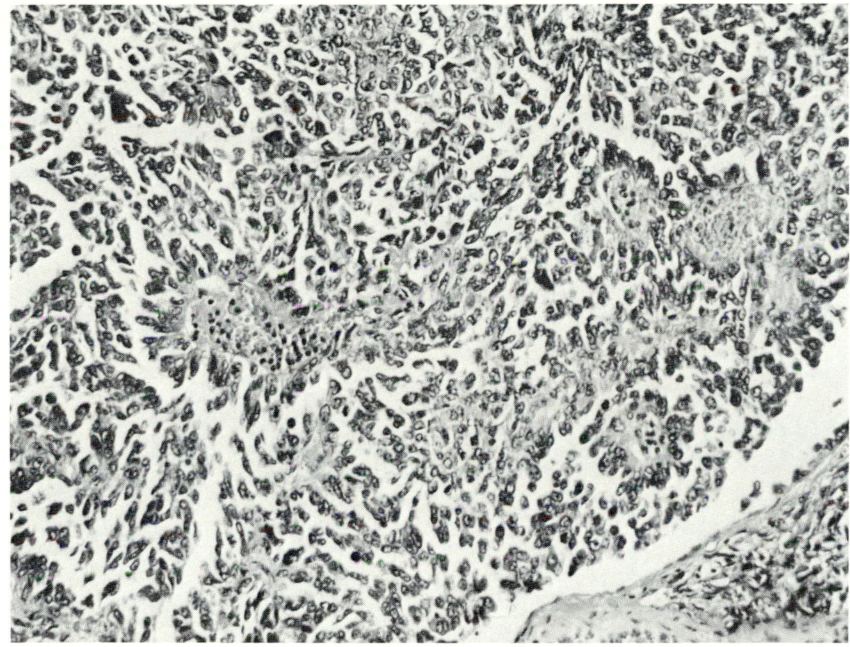

FIGURE 85
Further loosening in the part of the metastatic mass shows beginning outlines of papillary formations.

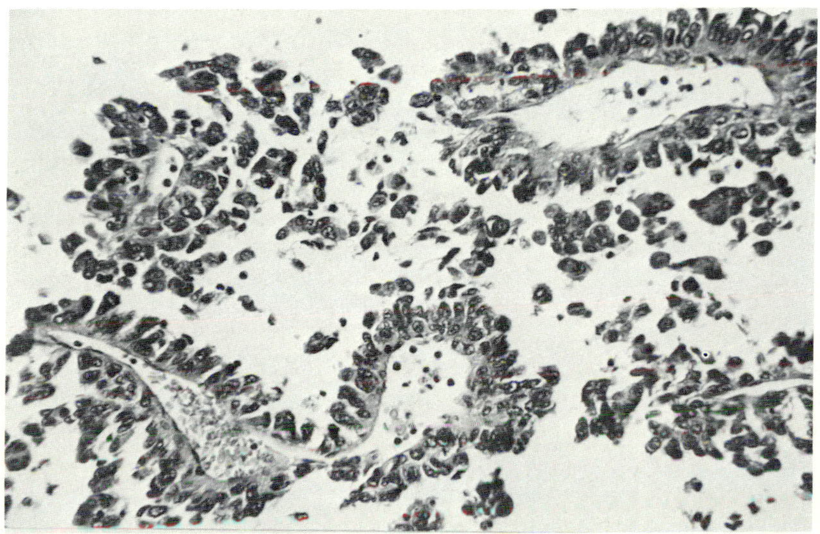

FIGURE 86
Same lesion, pure papillary areas.

101), but in other instances they may be found in the tumor cells themselves (Fig. 102).

A number of meningeal tumors with *melanin* contained in tumor cells have been reported in the literature. Most of these occurred in the posterior fossa or in the spinal canal. Grossly, such tumors may be light or dark brown, or even pitch black. Limas and Tio[55] suggested that such tumors are not true meningiomas, but rather represent melanocytomas, that is, benign nevoid tumors of the

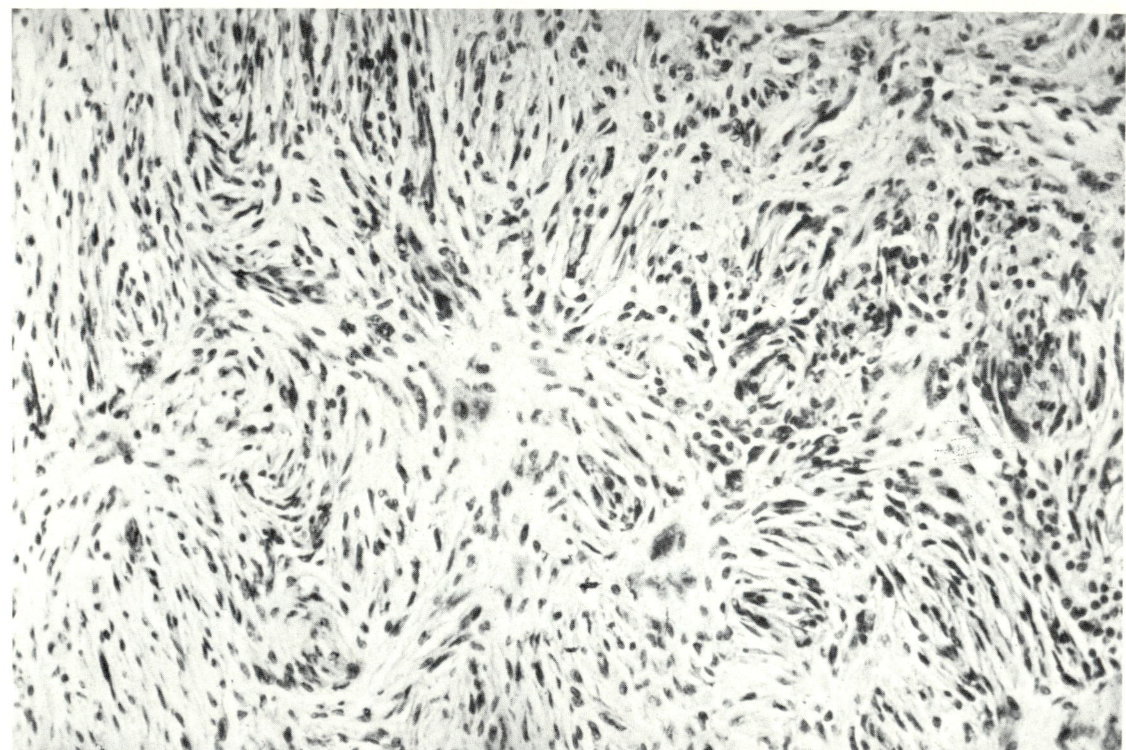

FIGURE 87
Meningeal tumor with fibroblastlike cells arranged in storiform pattern.

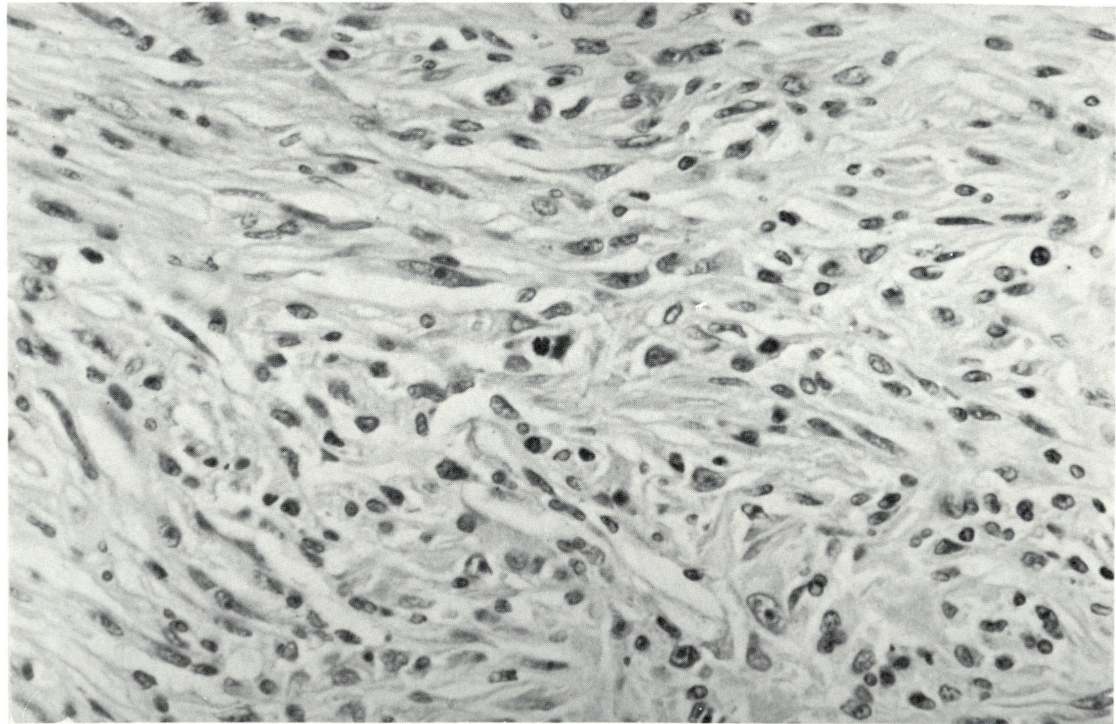

FIGURE 88
Same tumor shown in Fig. 87 with fibroblasts, collagen formation, and a few plasma cells. Note mitosis (*center*).

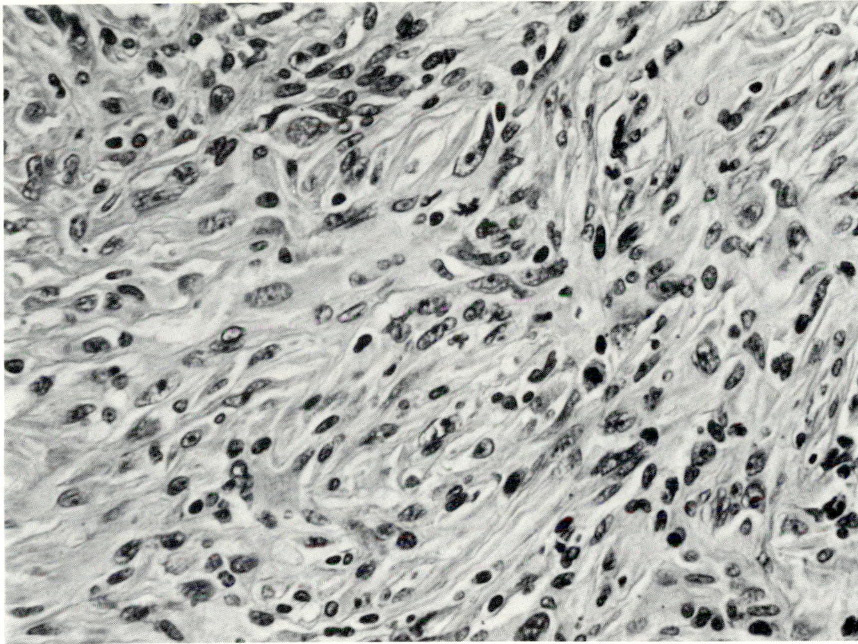

FIGURE 89
Same tumor with pleomorphic, anaplastic-appearing fibroblasts.

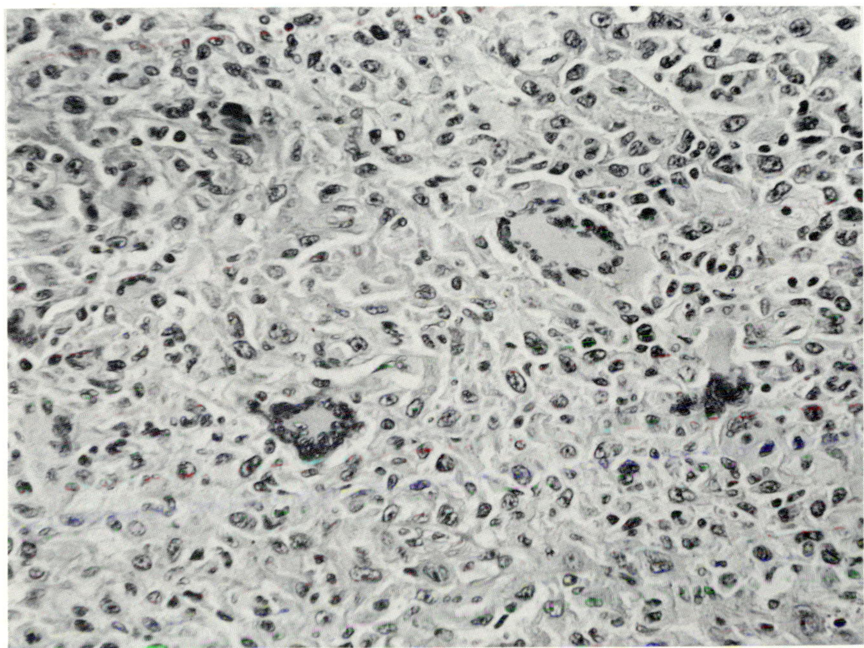

FIGURE 90
In this area of the same tumor, the cells appear more like histiocytes, with a few multinucleated giant cells.

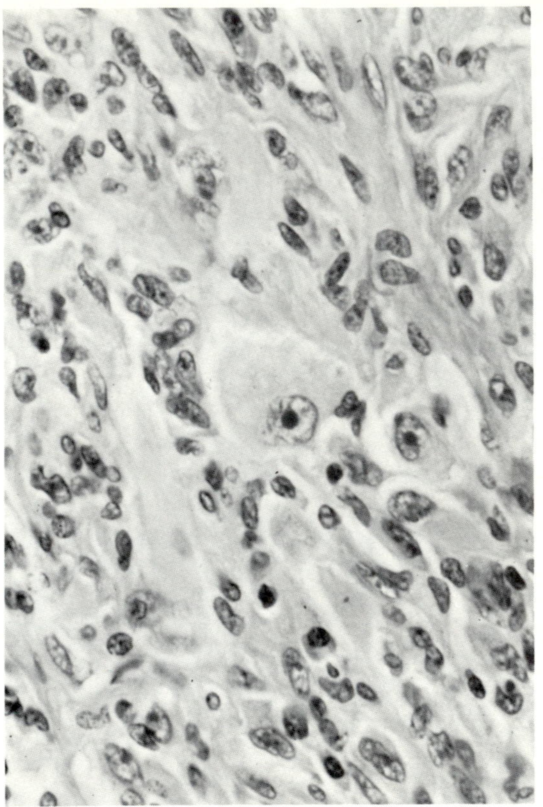

FIGURE 91
Some histiocytes have large pale nuclei with prominent nucleoli (ganglioid cells).

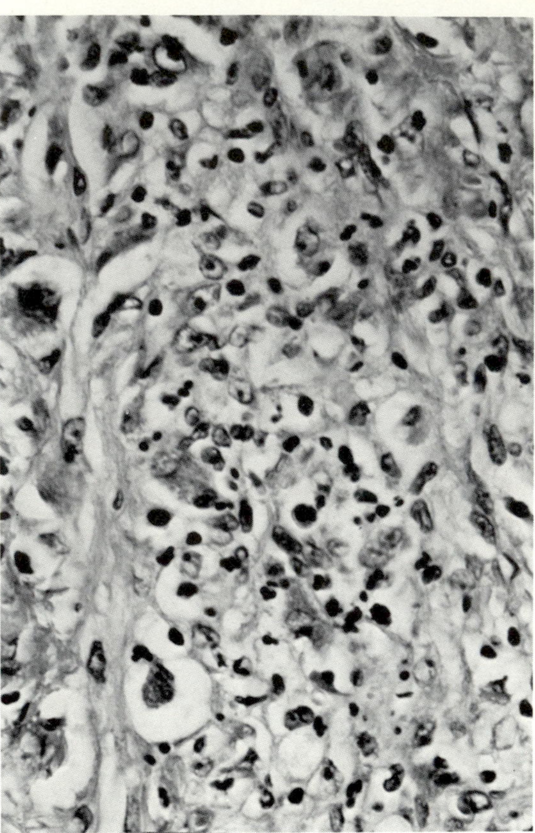

FIGURE 92
Inflammatory fibrous histiocytoma of the meninges (parietal lobe in 24-year-old woman).

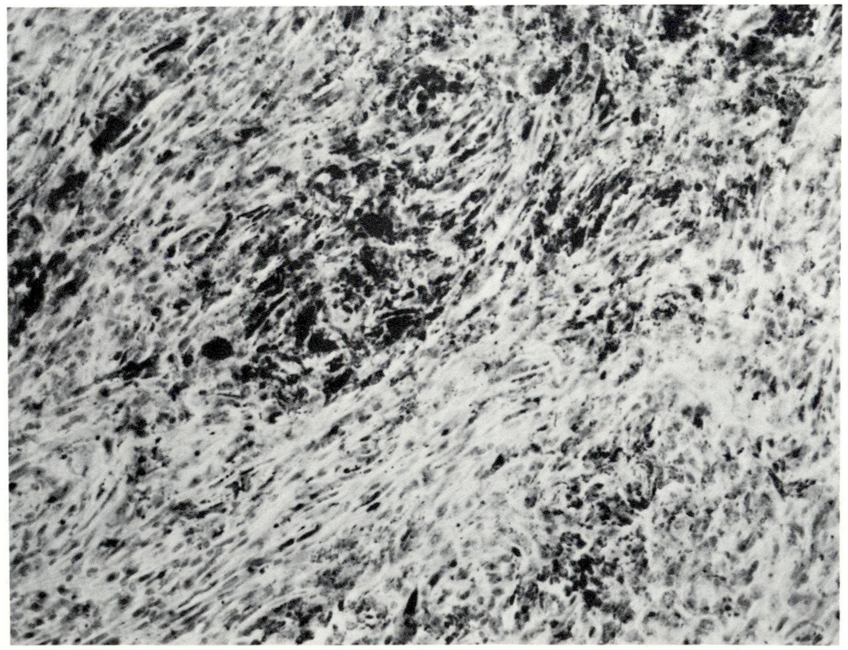

FIGURE 93
Same case shown in Figure 92, showing abundant lipid droplets in histiocytes. Oil-red-O stain.

FIGURES 94–100
Meningeal tumor. Clinically meningioma, by light microscopy malignant fibrous histiocytoma (electron microscopy showed features of meningioma).

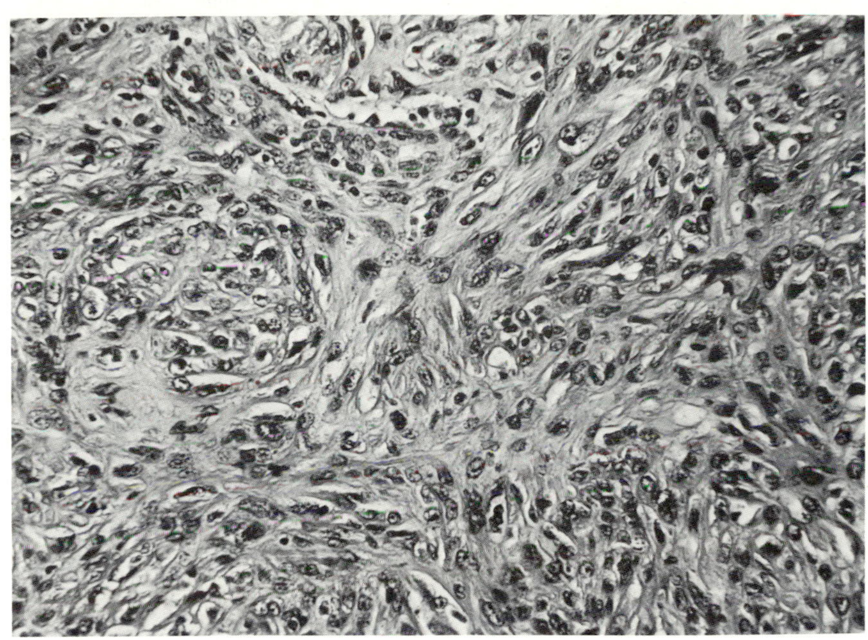

FIGURE 94
Storiform pattern.

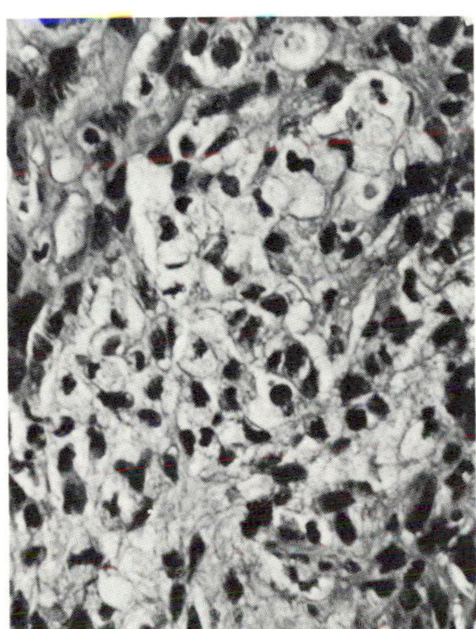

FIGURE 95
Foamy cells in tumor.

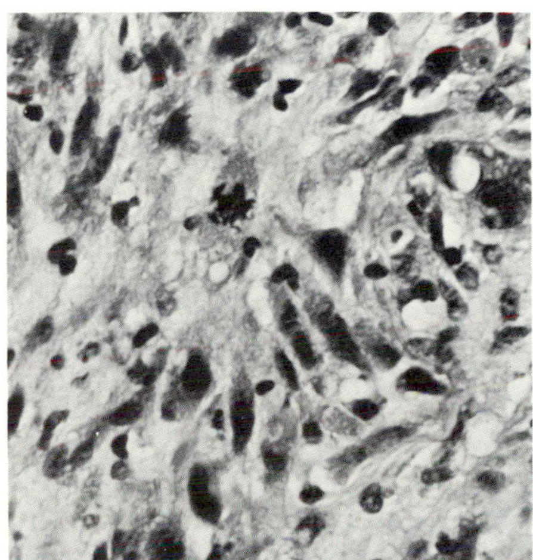

FIGURE 96
Nuclear pleomorphism and atypical mitoses.

leptomeninges. They pointed out that nevocellular lesions may have a fasciculated and whorling pattern; nevertheless, ultrastructurally they are different from meningiomas. Their own case, a pigmented tumor of the foramen magnum area, had the light- and electron-microscopic features of a melanocytic rather than those of a meningothelial neoplasm. Limas and Tio[55] thought this would apply to all previously reported cases of melanotic meningiomas.

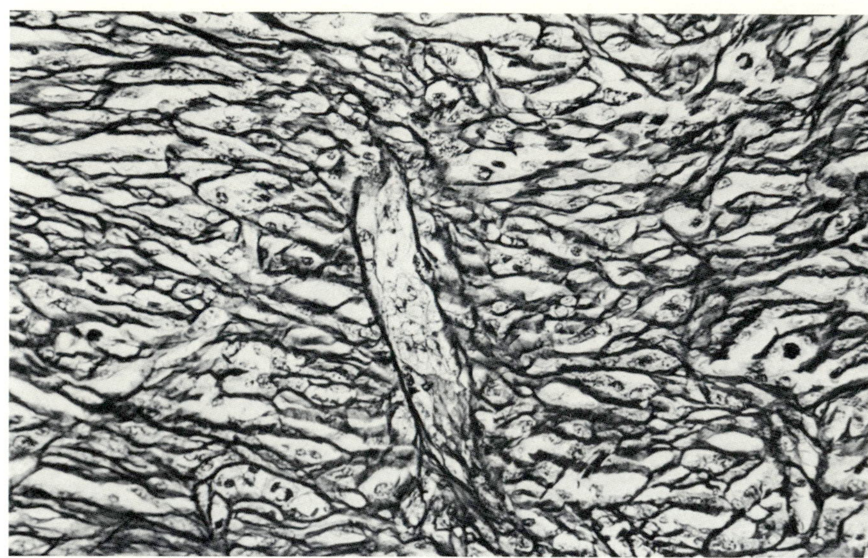

FIGURE 97
A dense reticulin network connected to central vessel surrounds individual tumor cells.

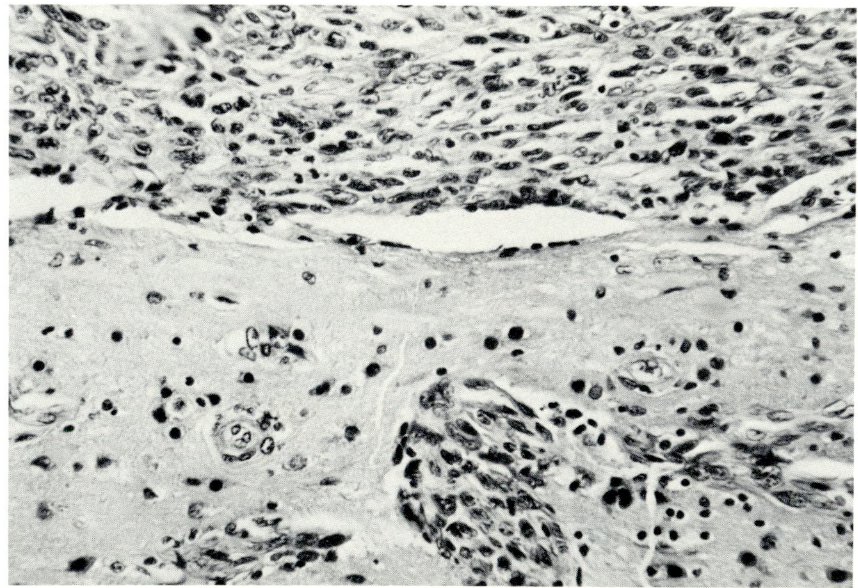

FIGURE 98
The malignancy of the tumor is manifested by invasion of underlying cortex, mostly via perivascular spaces.

A careful analysis of these cases, however, seems to indicate that melanotic tumors of the meninges may have more than one type of basic character. Quite apart from the localized and diffuse primary malignant melanomas of the leptomeninges, and the pigmented neurofibromas, which are not discussed here, the circumscribed solid benign melanotic tumors themselves seem to belong to two

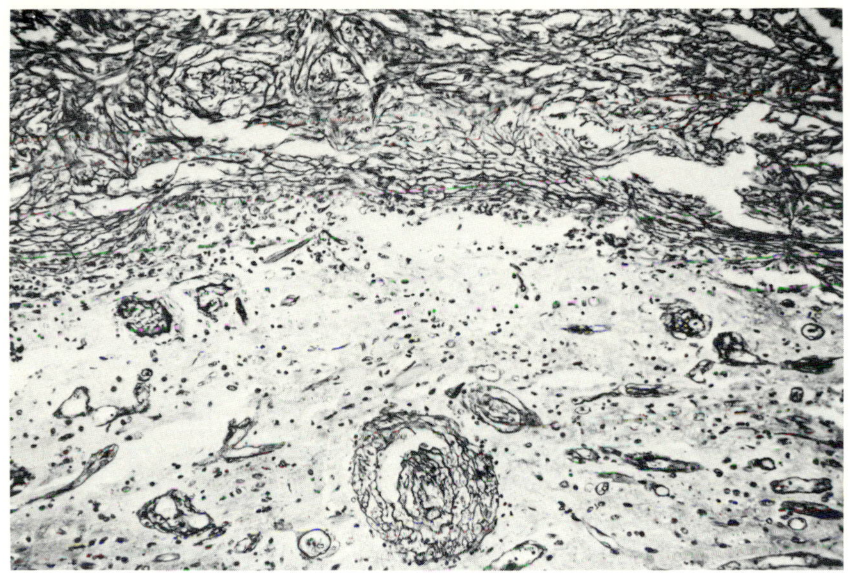

FIGURE 99
Same area shown in Fig. 98. Rich reticulin network in tumor (*top*) and in cortical perivascular spaces invaded by tumor. Wilder's reticulin stain.

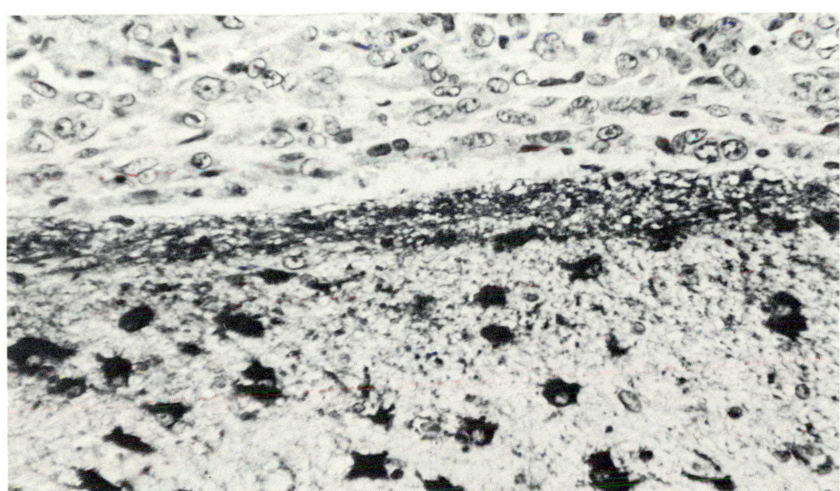

FIGURE 100
Interface between tumor and brain. Tumor (*top*); hypertrophic reactive astrocytes (*bottom*). Immunoperoxidase stain for glial fibrillary acidic protein in astrocytes.

different groups. The case of Limas and Tio seems to have been a melanocytoma, as was the spinal mass of Steinberg *et al.*,[56] and quite possibly the multiple cervical cord tumors of Scott *et al.*[57] and case 2 of Ray and Foot.[58] From studying the illustrations one cannot be absolutely sure about the cases of Abbot *et al.*[59] and the pigmented meningioma reported by Keegan and Mullan,[60] which seem to have been meningiomas rather than melanocytomas. There can be no doubt, however, about two reported cases of melanin-containing tumors. Both the case of Bakody *et al.*[61] and the one described by Turnbull and Tom[62] are classic meningiomas. In the latter case, bleaching of the

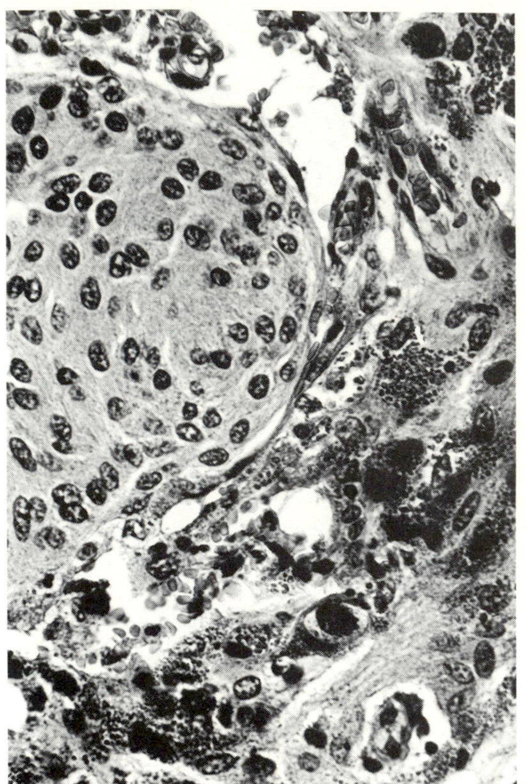
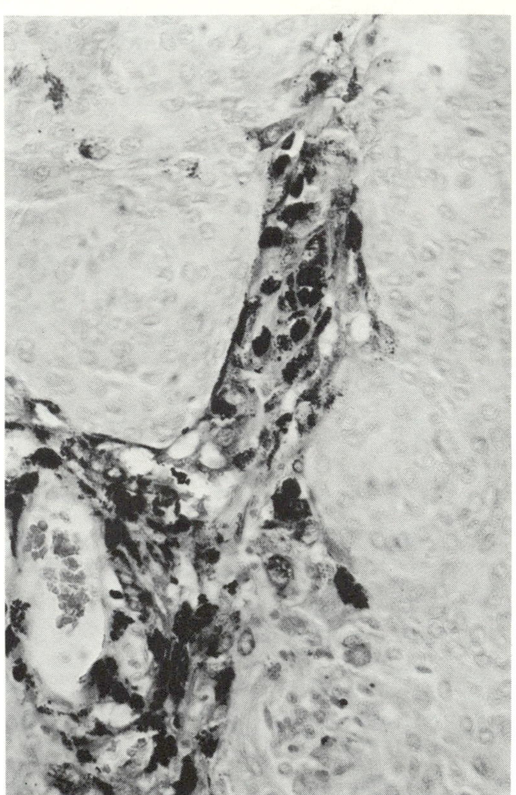

FIGURE 101
Iron (hemosiderin) granules in fibrous septa of meningioma. The tumor parenchyma is free of iron. (*Left*) H&E stain. (*Right*) Perls' iron stain.

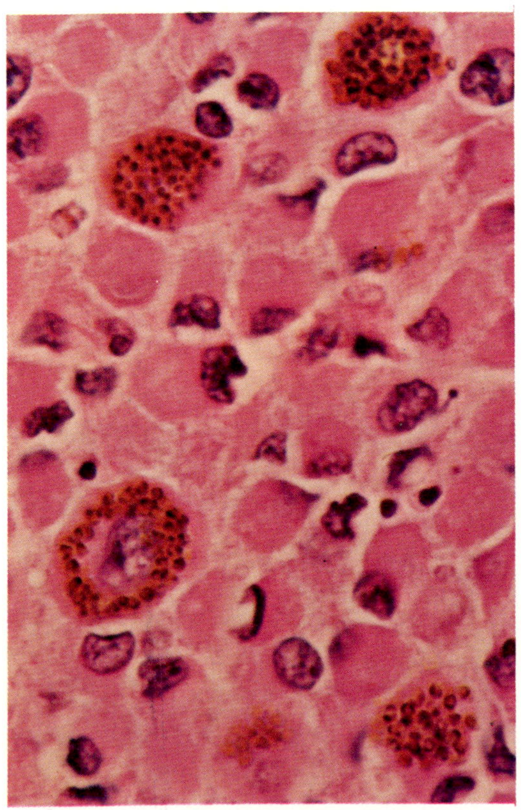
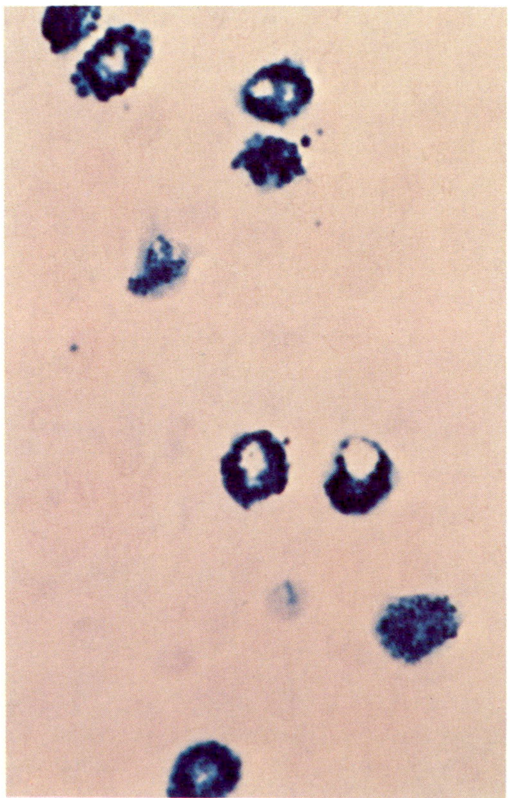

FIGURE 102
Iron granules in tumor cells of meningioma. (*Left*) H&E stain. (*Right*) Perls' iron stain.

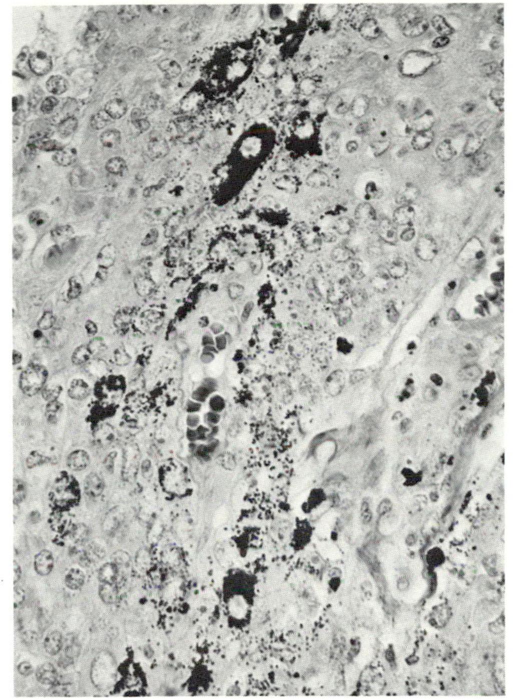

FIGURE 103
Melanin granules in cells of meningioma. Fontana's silver stain. (Courtesy Dr. Horoupian).

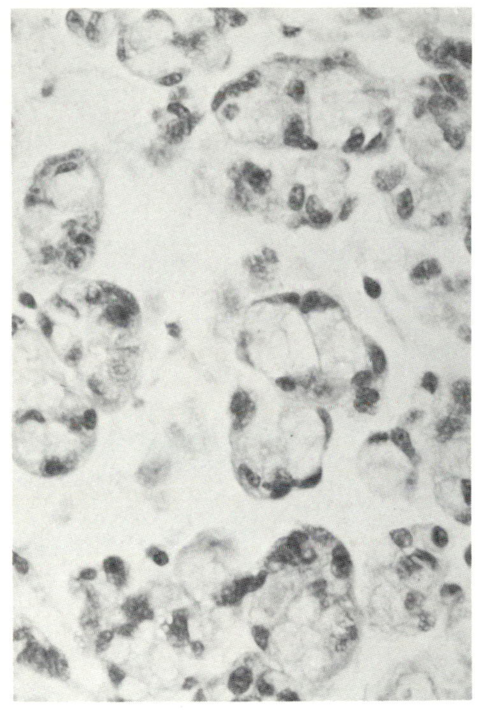

FIGURE 104
Mucus droplets in meningioma cells. Note resemblance to mucus-producing or colloid carcinoma.

melanin pigment with hydrogen peroxide reveals a pathognomonic underlying picture of a mengiothelial meningioma, as was also confirmed in their case by J. Olczewski.

Russell and Rubinstein[63] have also seen a spinal and a cerebellar example of a pigmented meningioma and we have also encountered it in material reviewed by us (Fig. 103). Such presence of melanin granules in an otherwise typical meningioma may be of considerable theoretical importance with regard to the ultimate embryological derivation of arachnoidal cells. The possibility exists, of course, that neighboring melanin granules have been ingested by tumor cells, as suggested by Turnbull and Tom. If, however, the pigment can be shown in some future case to have been produced by neoplastic meningothelial cells, such finding would go a long way to support neuroectodermal origin of meningiomas, as melanin is a substance closely associated with cells derived from the early ectoderm, but not from other germinal layers.

Some meningiomas have cells with a mucoid substance in their cytoplasm. Whether this represents a form of mucoid degeneration or secretion is not known, but meningiomas with this type of change may closely resemble a metastatic mucus-producing (colloid) carcinoma (Fig. 104). A very unusual granulofilamentous type cytoplasmic inclusion was observed in a meningioma by Goldman *et al.*[64] (Fig. 105a,b). Under the electron microscope, these proved to be closely packed desmosomal filaments.

HYALINE INCLUSIONS (PSEUDOPSAMMOMA BODIES) IN MENINGIOMAS

Cushing and Eisenhardt[65] examined a meningioma of the clivus and found it to contain "numerous peculiar cellular inclusions of highly refractive glassy hyalinoid material." Kepes[66] described similar inclusions in five additional meningiomas. The bodies ranged in size from 3 to 100 μm. They were eosinophilic; strongly positive on PAS stain, even after diastase treatment; and histochemically appeared to contain basic proteins, such as histons. They did not contain amyloid or fibrin, and they never showed a tendency for calcification. Because of their globular shape and a superficial similarity to hyalinized psammoma bodies, the term *pseudopsammoma body* was

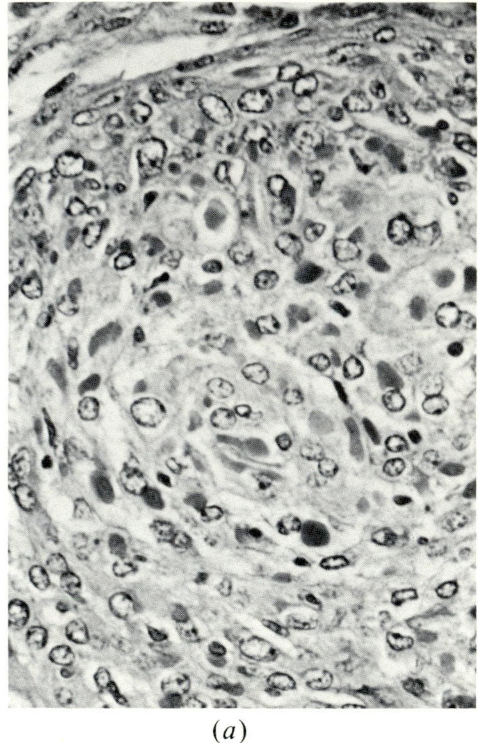

(*a*)

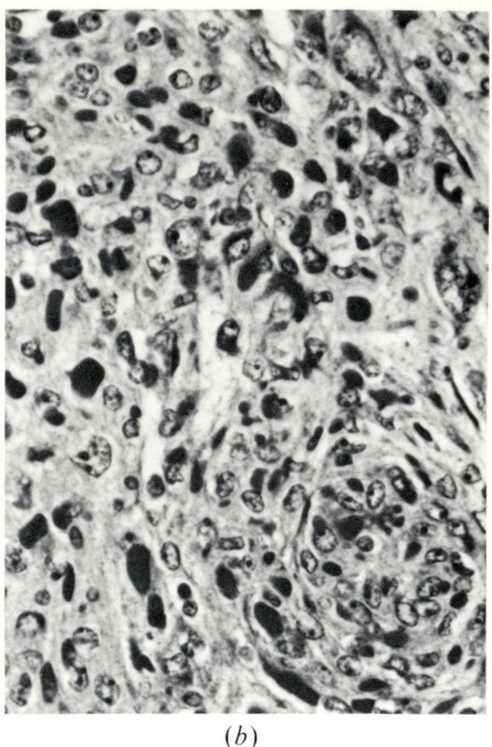

(*b*)

FIGURE 105
Granulofilamentous inclusions in meningioma cells, composed of filaments of desmosomal origin. (*a*) H&E stain. (*b*) Gomori's trichrome stain. (Courtesy Dr. Horoupian.)

suggested for them. Subsequently, an electron microscopic study[67] demonstrated that these structures were located within the tumor cells in what appeared like intracytoplasmic lumina, lined by microvilli. Similar intracellular ductules or intracellular neolumen formations have been described in breast cancer[68] and in mesotheliomas.[69] In the meningiomas, these changes may well represent a form of glandular metaplasia. In some instances, the hyaline inclusions actually stained positively with mucicarmine. By electron microscopy the intraluminal material was described as fine granular or droplet like by Kepes,[67] and Berard *et al.*[70] found additional components, such as lamellar structures with a triple linear density, vesicles, and dense bodies in them. The latter structures may be derived from the microvilli. Eventually, according to Berard *et al.*, the microvilli disappear and the inclusions will lie in a smooth-walled cavity. Hyaline inclusions do not seem to have a bearing on the prognosis of a given meningioma, except that, so far at least, they have always been seen in histologically benign meningiomas of the meningothelial type (Figs. 106–112).

CYSTIC MENINGIOMAS

Protein-rich fluid sometimes accumulates between cells of a meningioma, causing their separation and the formation of microcysts (Fig. 113). At times, such fluid-filled spaces become confluent and grossly visible cystic spaces develop (Fig. 14). Moraci and Cioffi[71] referred to this development as cyst formation from Masson's[72] *forme humide* of meningiomas. Cushing and Eisenhardt[73] illustrated two cases of this type. A more peripherally located, but still intratumoral, cyst was exemplified by the case of Lake *et al.*[74] As cystic changes are most often associated in the minds of neurosurgeons and pathologists with gliomas, it is not surprising that cystic meningiomas may be mistaken

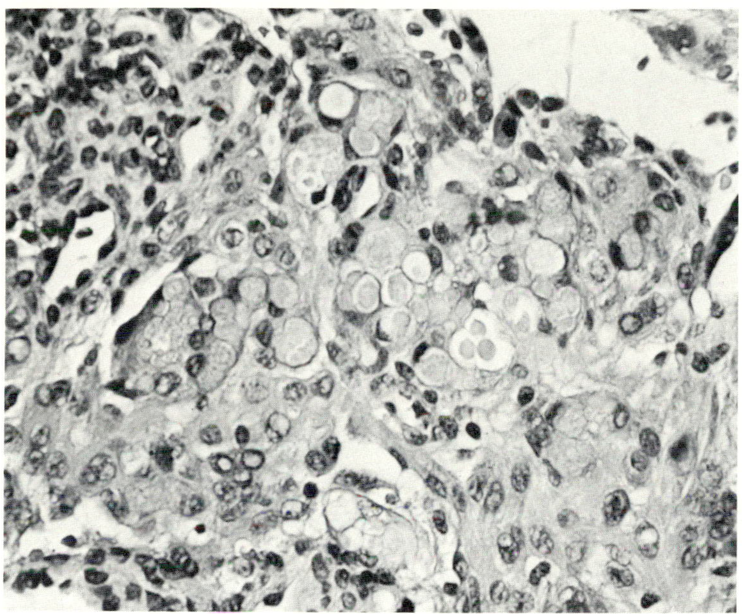

FIGURE 106
Hyaline inclusions (pseudopsammoma bodies) in meningothelial meningioma.

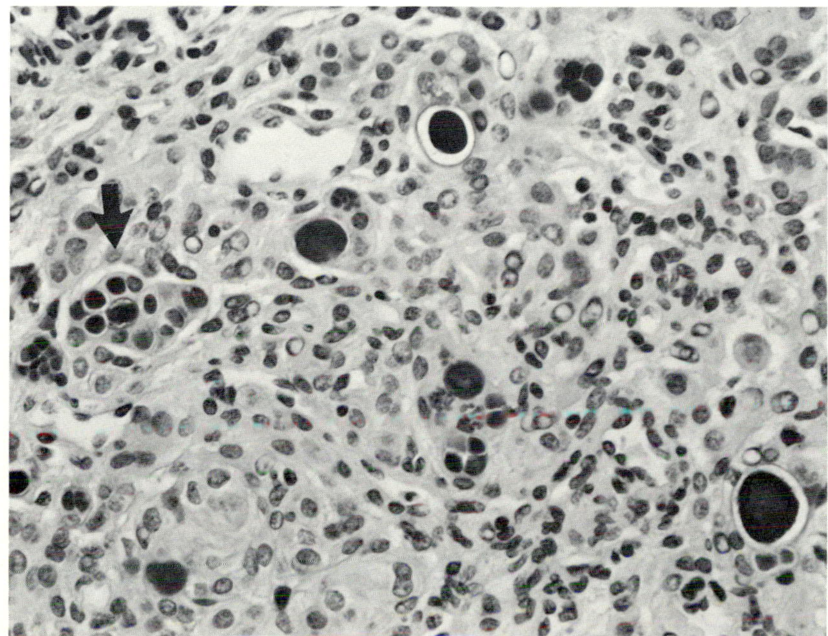

FIGURE 107
Same tumor shown in Fig. 106. The inclusions stain positively (here dark) on PAS stain. Note small droplets (left, *arrow*), which are clearly intracellular in location.

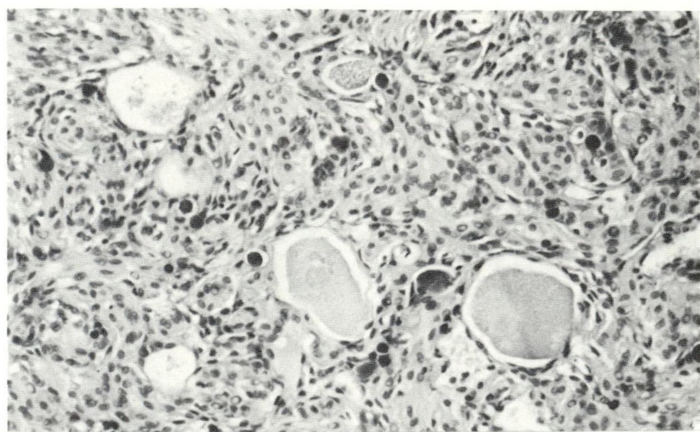

FIGURE 108
Low-power view of another meningioma showing very large hyaline inclusions. After attaining such large size, the inclusions usually become less homogeneous and consist of loosely packed tiny droplets or granules.

for astrocytomas during surgery as reported by Henry *et al.*[75]

Brain tissue next to, and compressed by, a meningioma not infrequently becomes edematous and, as a result, may eventually undergo cystic degeneration. Large cysts next to a meningioma have been encountered by David *et al.*,[76] Cushing and Eisenhardt,[73] Olivecrona,[77] Russell and Rubinstein,[78] Nauta *et al.*,[79] and others. Rengachary *et al.*[80] reported three cases of large peritumoral cysts next to intracranial meningiomas. As astrocytic proliferation was observed in the cyst wall—in one case even with some degree of cellular atypism—the possibility of such alterations potentially being precursors of a glioma developing next to the meningioma was considered.

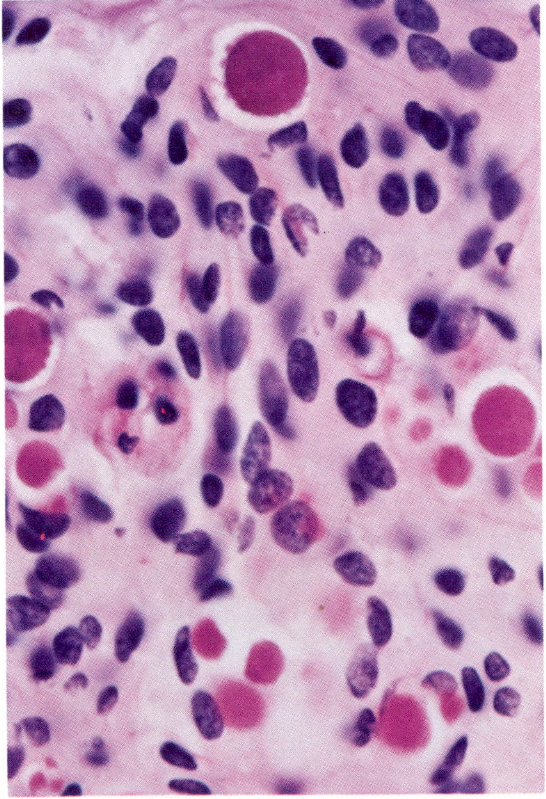

FIGURE 109
Hyaline inclusions (pseudopsammoma bodies) staining homogeneously positive with PAS stain.

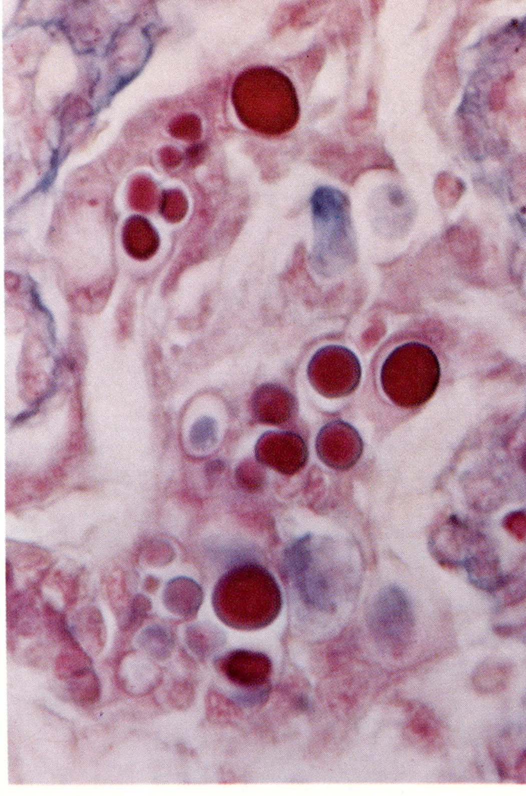

FIGURE 110
With Heidenhain's azan stain, the inclusions appear less homogeneous, with red and blue staining areas alternating.

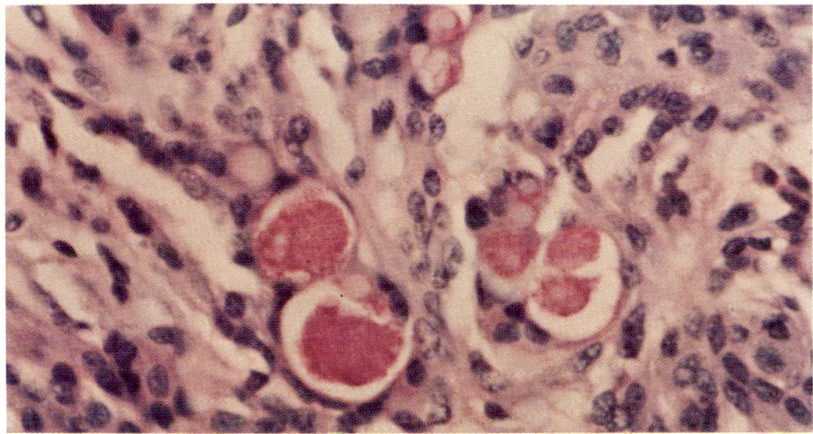

FIGURE 111
Many hyaline inclusions also contain mucus and stain positively for this substance. Mucicarmine stain.

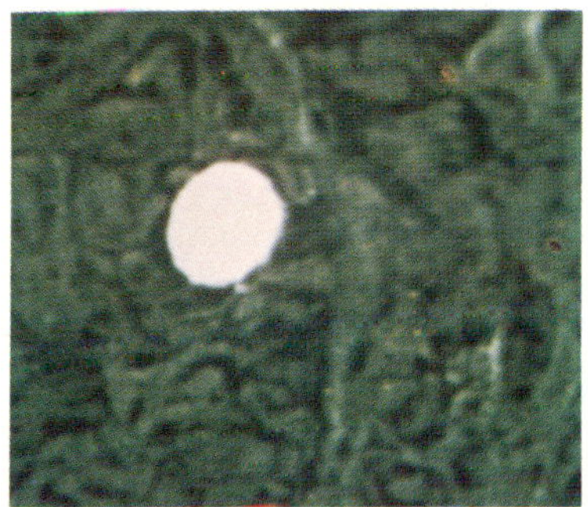

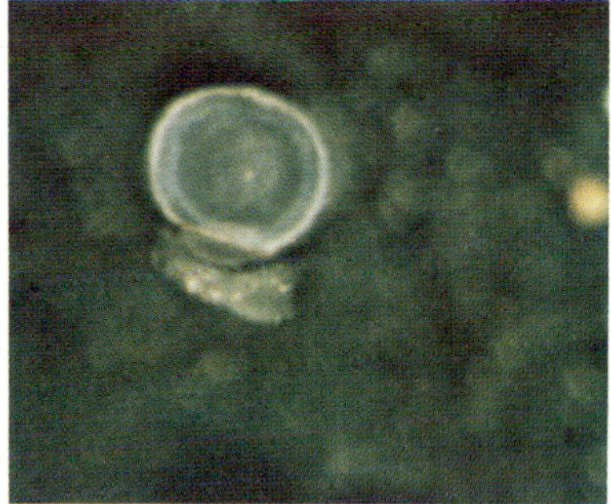

FIGURE 112
(*a*) Hyaline inclusions as a rule show very bright autofluorescence. (*b*) A lesser degree of autofluorescence is also seen in hyalinized cellular whorl.

LYMPHOPLASMACELLULAR INFILTRATES IN MENINGIOMAS

It is not uncommon to find foci of lymphocytes or plasma cells, or both, in meningiomas in a perivascular arrangement (Fig. 114) or diffusely scattered (Figs. 115a,b). An interesting group of meningiomas is distinguished, however, by the presence of very large numbers of lymphocytes and plasma cells within the tumor. These cells may be present in such large numbers that they totally overshadow the underlying meningioma, and it is only after examining several microscopic fields that the true nature of the neoplasm will become evident. The first such tumor in the meninges was described by Banerjee and Blackwood,[81] who considered the possibility of this representing a collision tumor between a meningioma and a plasmacytoma. Russell and Rubinstein,[82] who studied three examples of this tumor, favored the interpretation that the infiltration of plasma cells was of a secondary character. Horten *et al.*[13] described five additional cases with similar histologic features, and we also had the opportunity to examine two examples of this entity (Fig. 116a,b). To us, too, it seemed that the lymphocytes and plasma cells were reactive rather than neoplastic in nature, partly because of their bland appearance and partly because they represented a varied type of infiltrate including, in addition to lymphocytes and plasma cells, phagocytic elements (histiocytes) as well. Stam *et al.*[84] examined a tumor of this kind and, applying immunohistochemical analysis, were able to demonstrate the polyclonal nature of the plasma cell population, indicating that they represented a non-neoplastic component. It is proba-

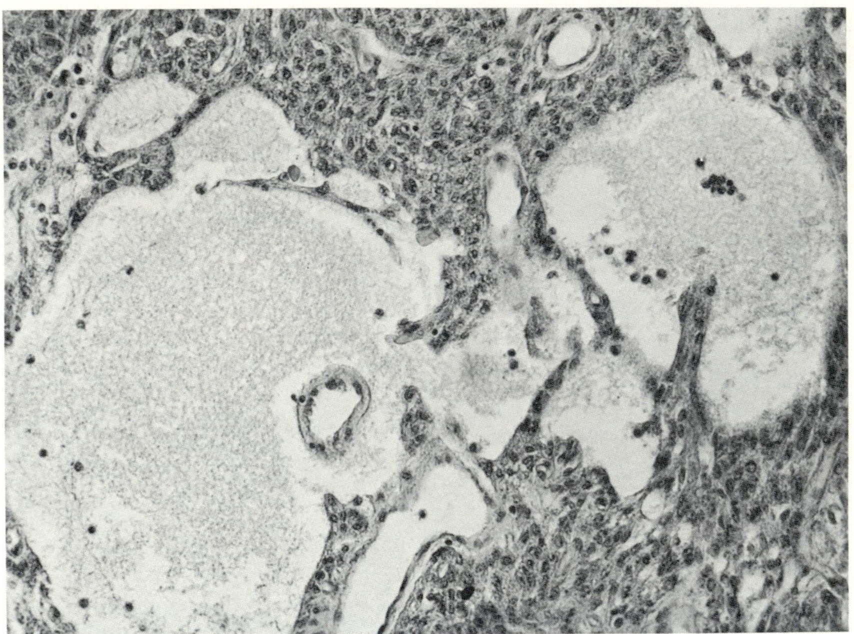

FIGURE 113
Protein-rich edema fluid in microcystic changes. Confluence of such fluid-filled spaces may give rise to grossly cystic meningiomas.

ble that the lymphocytes and plasma cells invade these meningiomas in response to some kind of antigen stimulus from the meningioma tissue itself. None of these patients thus far has shown indications of having a systemic immune disorder affecting the body defenses, but the first case of Horten *et al.* did have associated polyclonal hypergammaglobulinemia. West *et al.*,[85] who described a case of an intracranial plasma cell granuloma without a meningioma component, considered the possibility that the previously reported meningiomas with conspicuous plasma cell–lymphocytic components might also actually represent plasma cell granulomas with only incidental inclusion of meningeal elements. This view will probably be challenged in the future. Our material showed meningothelial islands exceeding both in size and cellularity what one might consider inclusions of non-neoplastic arachnoidal cell nests.

INVASION PATTERN OF MENINGIOMAS

By far most meningiomas are well-circumscribed tumors, but it is not at all unusual, even for benign meningiomas, to grow into and through the dura mater, to partially or completely fill a venous sinus of the dura, to penetrate the overlying bone, and even to enter the temporalis muscle or the soft tissues of the scalp. At the base of the brain, meningiomas sometimes surround and incorporate vascular structures. All this is likely to make total surgical removal that much more difficult, if not impossible, but by itself is not an expression of biological malignancy. On the other hand, benign meningiomas as a rule will compress, but not infiltrate, the underlying brain. Figures 117–119 show various relationships between meningioma and overlying dura, from simple contiguity (Fig. 117) to massive invasion of the pachymeninx (Figs. 118 and 119). The walls and mucosa of paranasal sinuses may be invaded by meningiomas from neighboring structures (Fig. 120), although occasionally they may even originate within the sinus from ectopic arachnoidal cell nests. Fat tissue is sometimes involved by meningioma (Fig. 121) and the bones of the skull may become deeply invaded with or without secondary hyperostosis (Fig. 122a,b). Invasion of the temporalis muscle was alluded to earlier. When it comes to peripheral nerves—most often cranial nerves at the base of the skull—meningiomas are likely to push them aside, but occasionally they infiltrate a nerve and

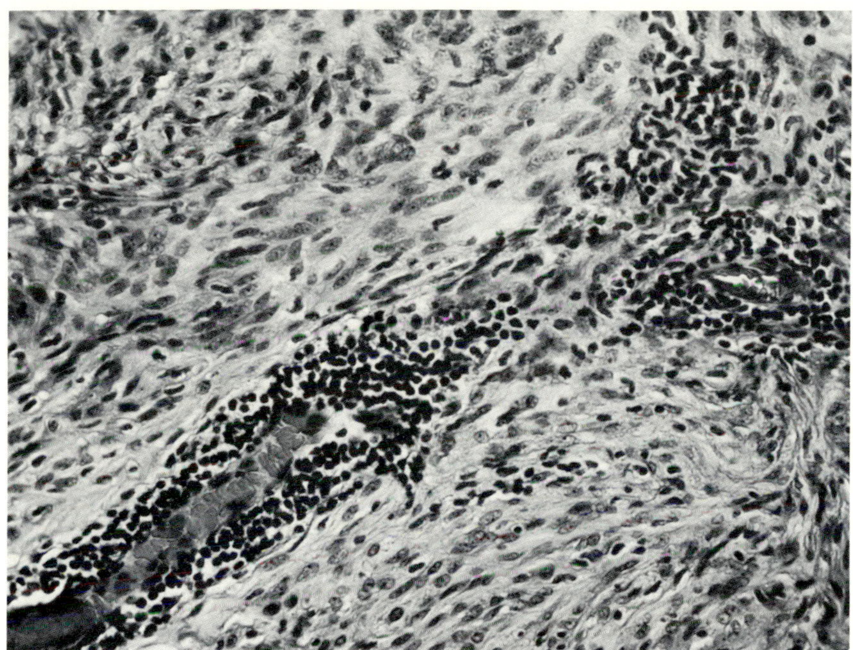

FIGURE 114
Perivascular lymphocytic/plasmacellular infiltration in meningioma.

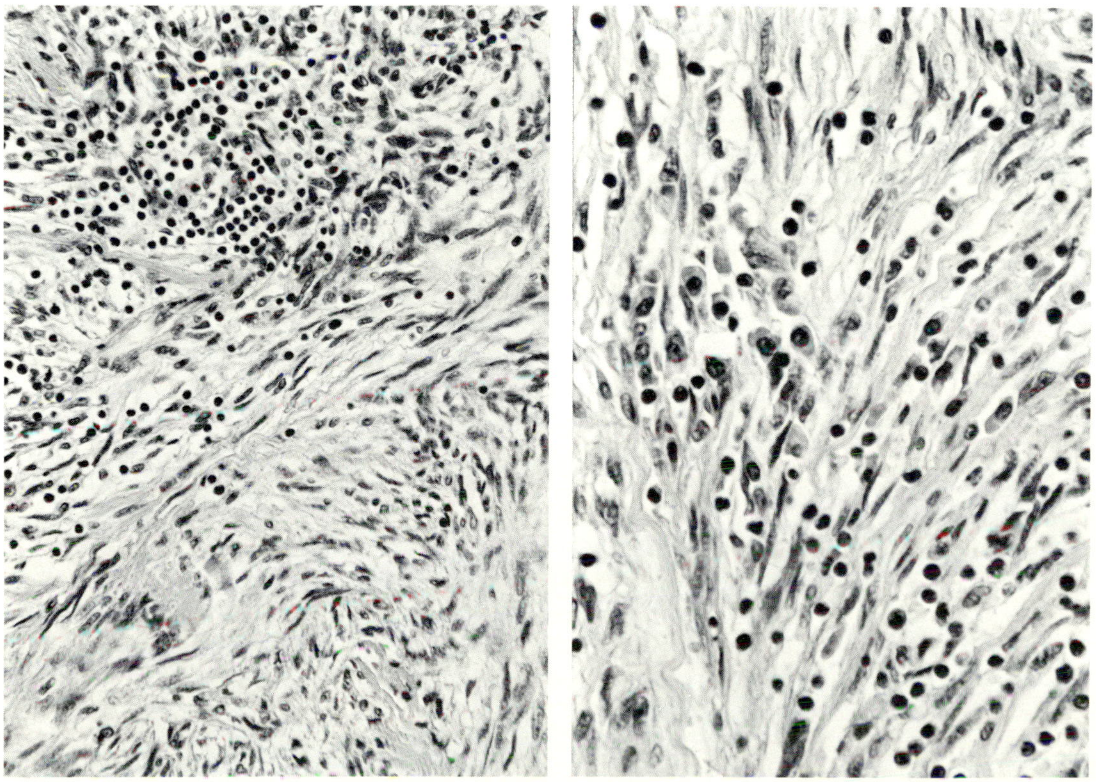

FIGURE 115
Infiltration of tumor parenchyma of a fibroblastic meningioma by lymphocytes and plasma cells. (*a*) ×90. (*b*) ×220.

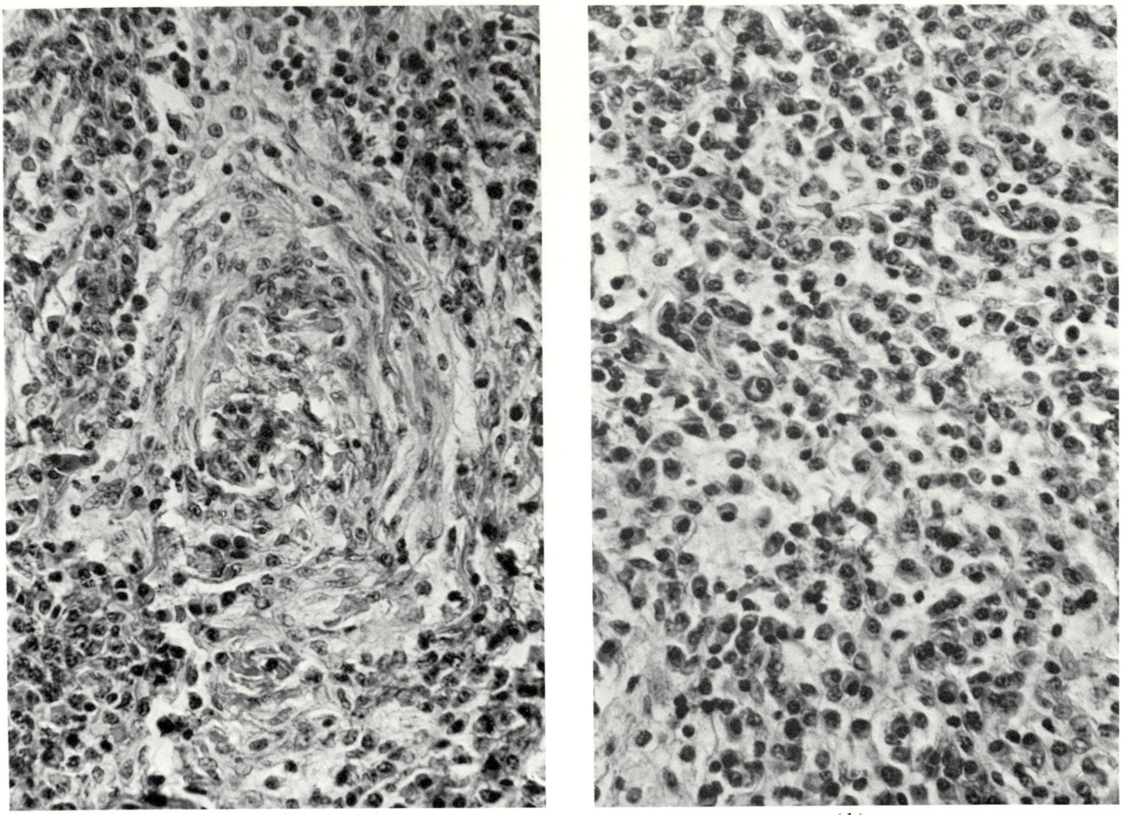

(*a*) (*b*)

FIGURE 116
Meningioma with massive lymphoplasmacytic infiltrates. (*a*) Concentric arrangement of elongated meningothelial cells can be recognized in center, amidst infiltrates of plasma cells. (*b*) This area of the mass consists entirely of plasma cells, making diagnosis of meningioma impossible if other areas were not examined.

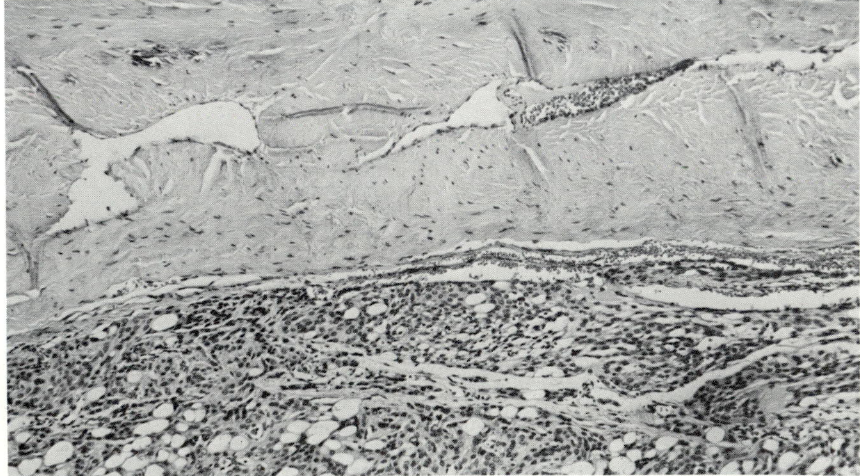

FIGURE 117
Meningioma attached to inside of cranial dura. The demarcation between dura and tumor is sharp—no invasion of the dura has taken place.

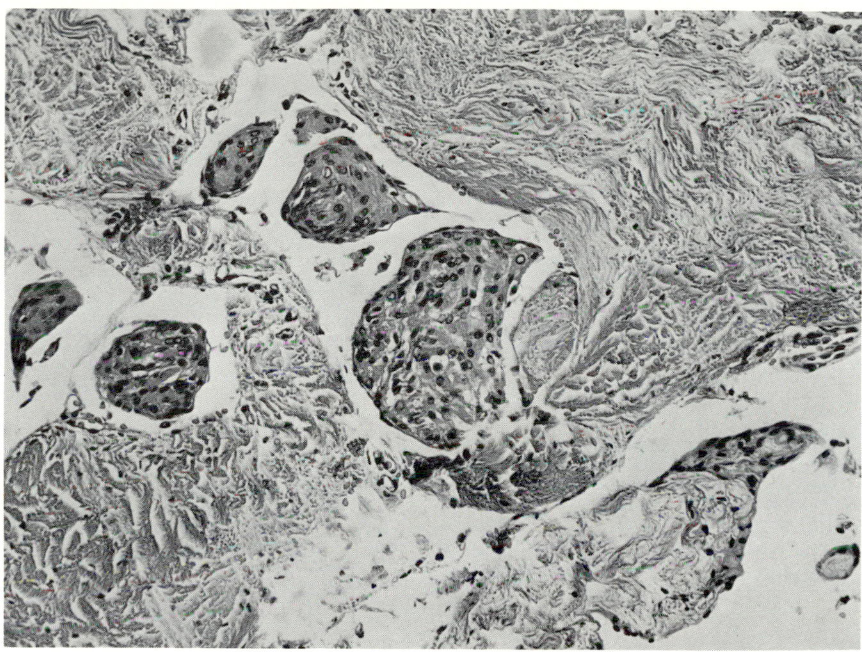

FIGURE 118
Another meningioma, showing tumor cell clusters within tissue spaces of the dura.

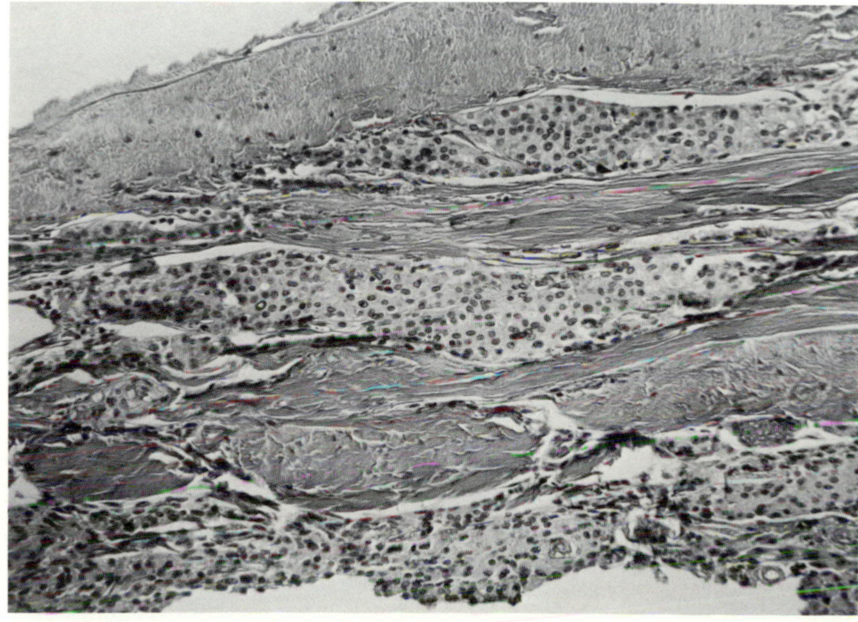

FIGURE 119
Alternating layers of collagen bundles and meningioma cells in this diffusely invaded dura mater.

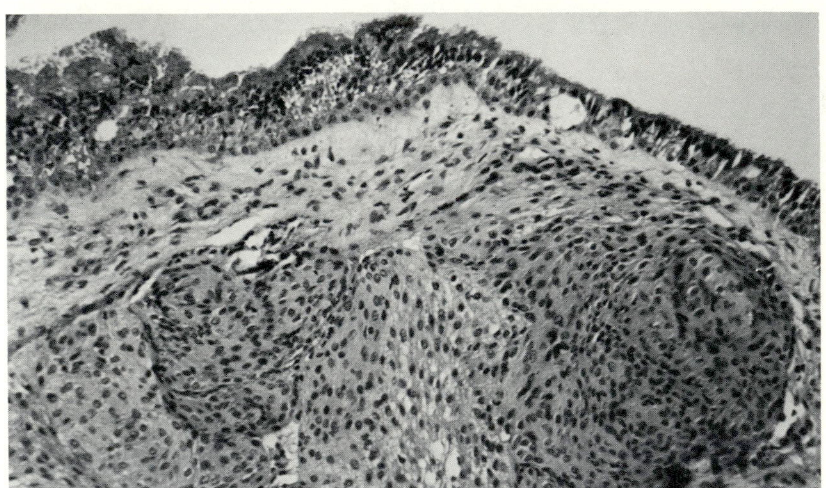

FIGURE 120
Meningioma invading wall of sphenoid sinus. Note tumor cell clusters immediately beneath ciliated columnar epithelium of the sinus mucosa.

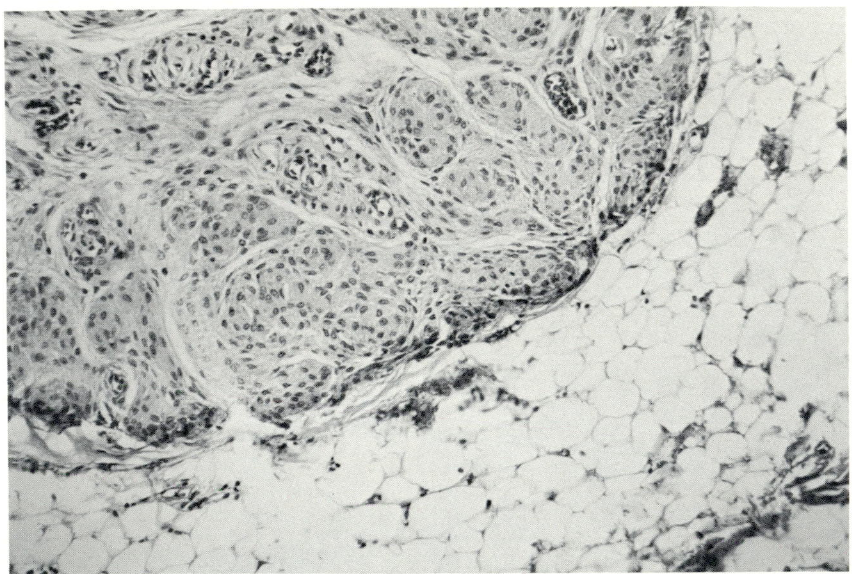

FIGURE 121
Meningioma invading fat tissue in area of foramen lacerum.

even penetrate the perineurial space (Fig. 123a,b). Meningiomas of the orbit rarely extend into the eyeball.[86] Such a case from a 14-year-old girl is also shown in our Fig. 124a–d. Meningiomas involving the optic nerve sheath often proliferate both intra- and extradurally and cause severe pressure atrophy of the optic nerve (Fig. 125).

HISTOLOGICAL AND CYTOLOGICAL FEATURES IN THE CONSIDERATION OF MALIGNANCY

It has already been pointed out that meningeal tumors of a hemangiopericytic pattern and papillary meningiomas are likely to behave in an ag-

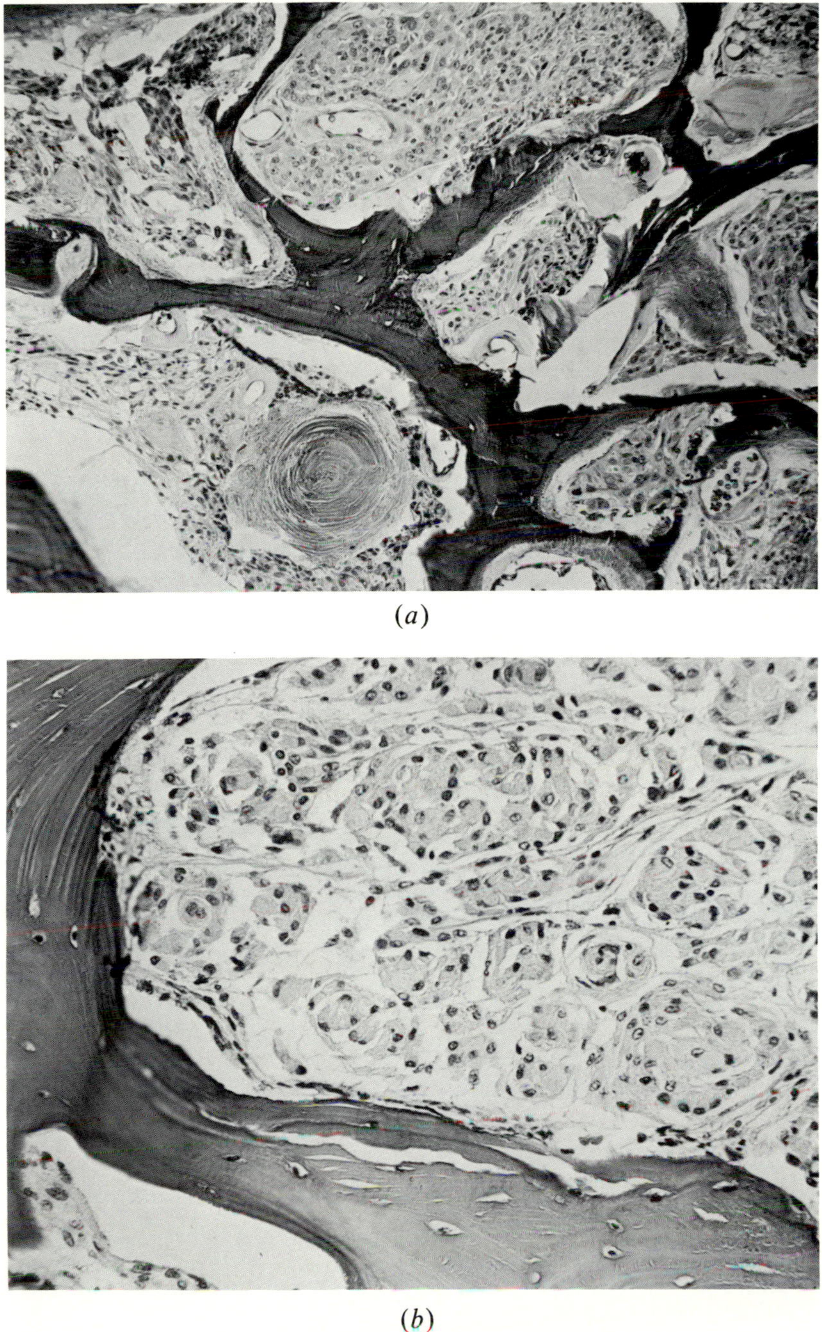

(*a*)

(*b*)

FIGURE 122
Meningioma growing through diploë of calvaria filling marrow spaces. (*a*) ×100. (*b*) ×200.

gressive fashion, calling for a guarded prognosis in terms of local recurrences and distant metastases. There is much less agreement on the significance of other histological features, suggesting anaplasia. It would seem, and this is our experience too, that the presence of large, hyperchromatic bizarre nuclei in meningiomas is by itself not a sign of malignancy (Fig. 126). By contrast, Skullerud

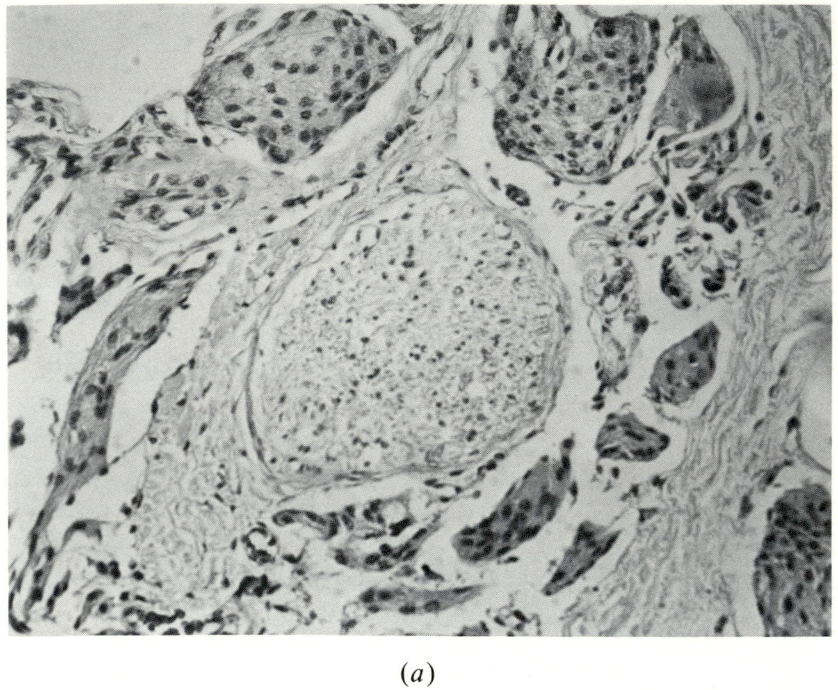

(*a*)

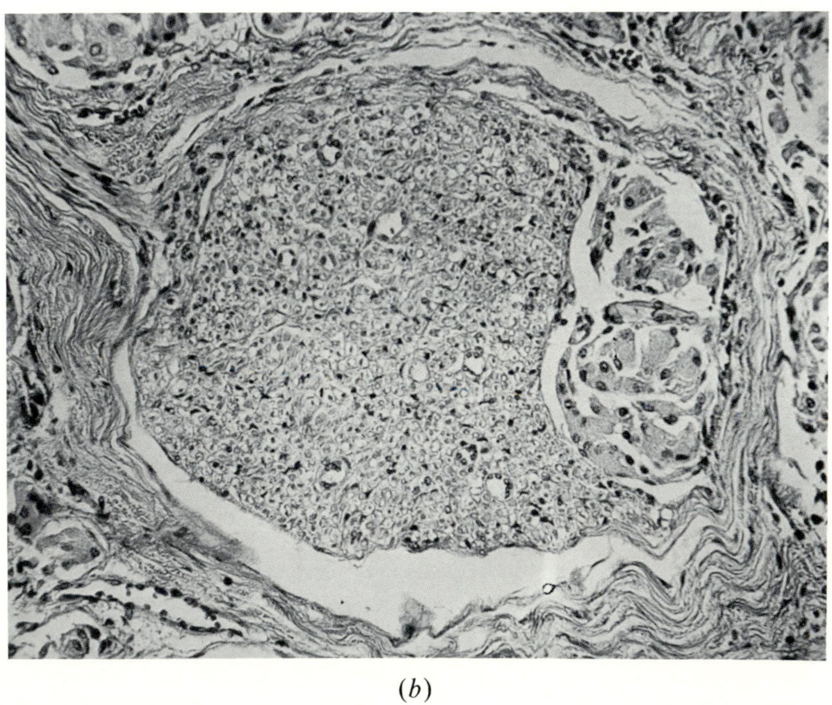

(*b*)

FIGURE 123
Branch of glossopharyngeal nerve invaded by meningioma at base of skull. (*a*) Perineural invasion. (*b*) Invasion within perineurial space.

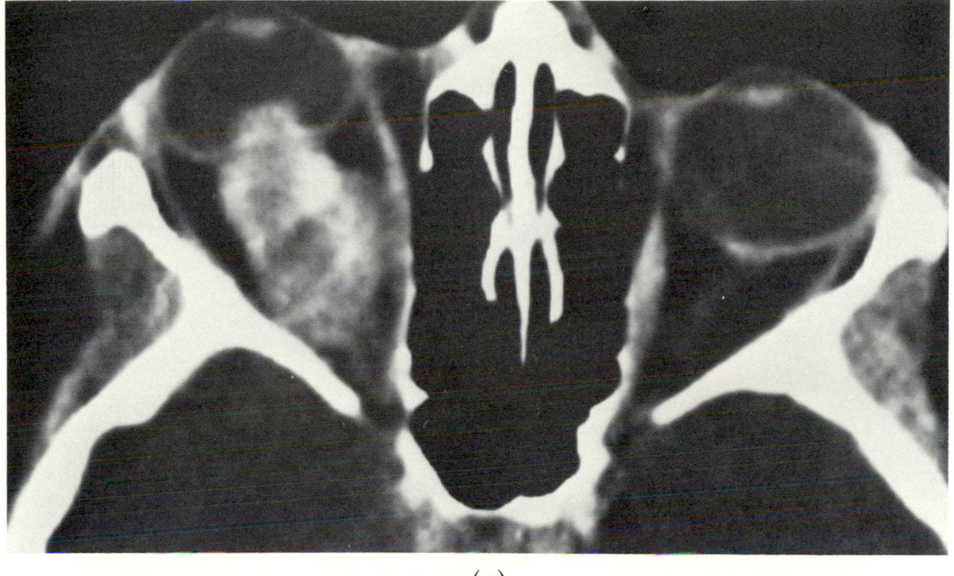

(*a*)

(*b*)

FIGURE 124
Orbital meningioma invading the globe. (*a*) CAT scan view of tumor behind and within left eyeball. (*b*) Sagittal section of gross specimen shows invasion of optic disc with lifting of retina. (*c*) Same as (*b*), microscopic slide. H&E. ×2. (*d*) Finger-like projections of meningioma invade retina and provoke reactive gliosis.

and Löken,[37] as well as Jellinger and Slowik,[24] believed that areas of markedly increased cellularity (Fig. 127), combined with increased mitotic activity, indicated malignant behavior. On occasion, such features become pronounced in recurrent tumors. Jellinger and Slowik suggested that invasion of the cerebral cortex probably was also more common among recurrences, although they were not convinced of the significance of mitotic figures or focal necroses by themselves. Fabiani *et*

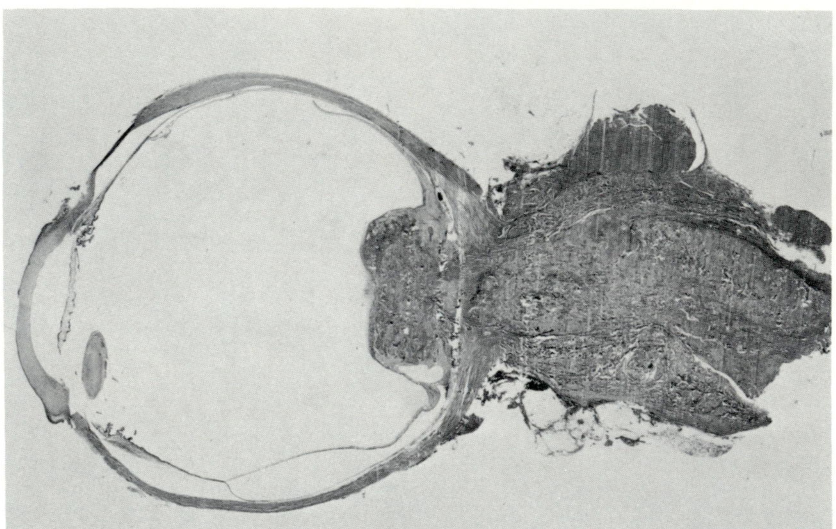

FIGURE 124c

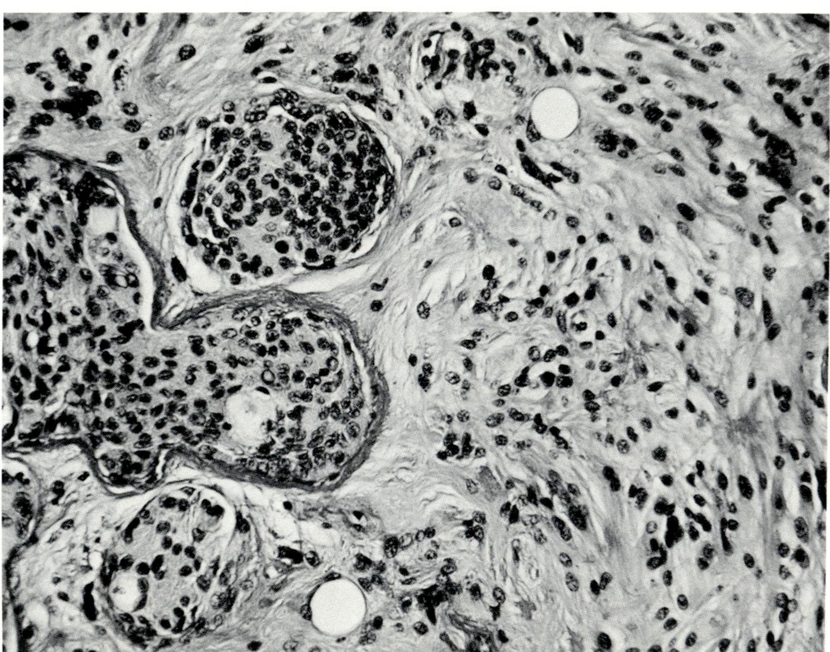

FIGURE 124d

al.[87] singled out five meningiomas as histologically malignant from their material of 568 meningiomas (hemangiopericytic type was excluded). All five tumors had areas of necrosis, high cellularity, and typical and atypical mitoses, and they infiltrated neighboring tissues, including the brain. Despite what seemed to be total surgical removal, all five patients died from the tumor within a period of 4 months to 7.5 years. The patients' ages ranged from 21 to 61 years and, interestingly, all were males.

Whereas some of these features may not be statistically significant, it is probably worth noting in terms of a closer follow-up if a meningioma displays mitotic figures (Fig. 131), invades the cortex (Fig. 128), or has foci of necrosis in it (Fig.

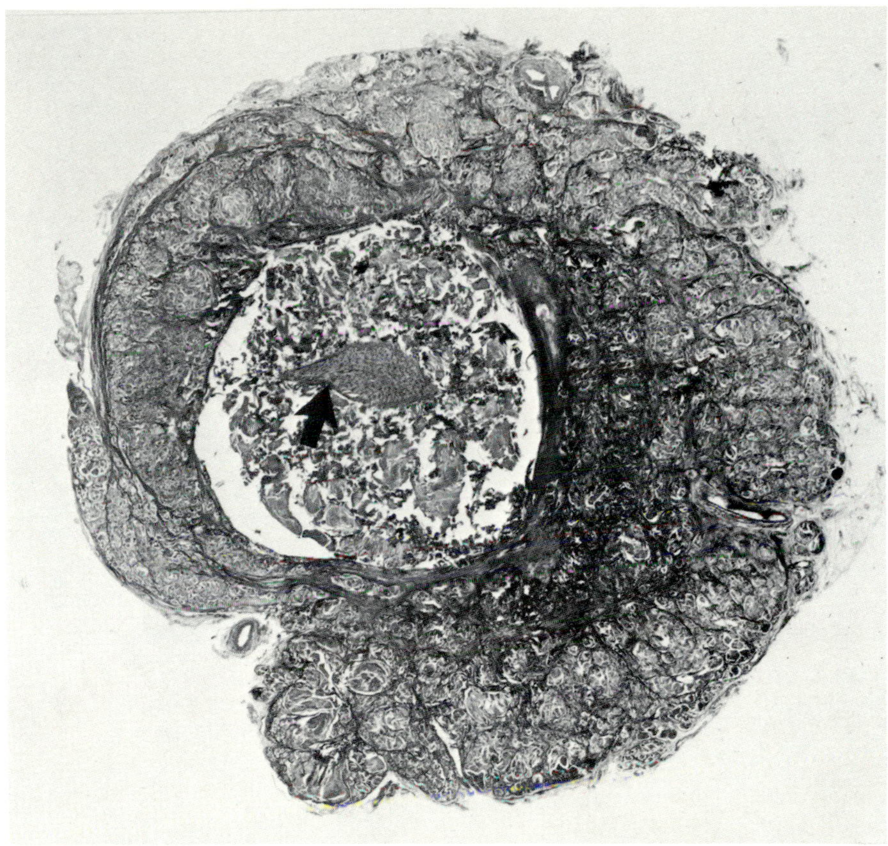

FIGURE 125
Meningioma of the optic nerve sheath. Tumor has invaded the dural sheath, as well as the subdural space. The optic nerve (*arrow*) suffered severe pressure atrophy. H&E. ×20.

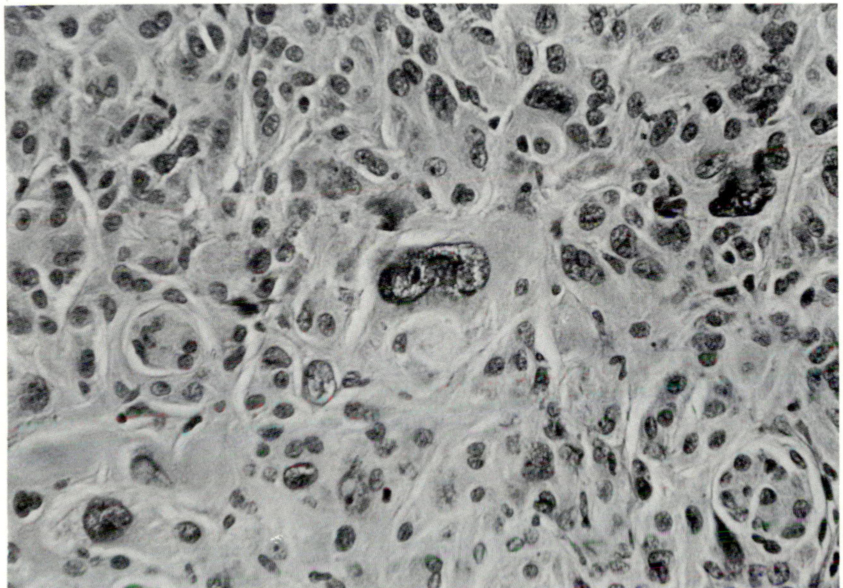

FIGURE 126
Large, bizarre nuclei in meningothelial meningioma. These nuclear alterations by themselves do not necessarily signify malignancy.

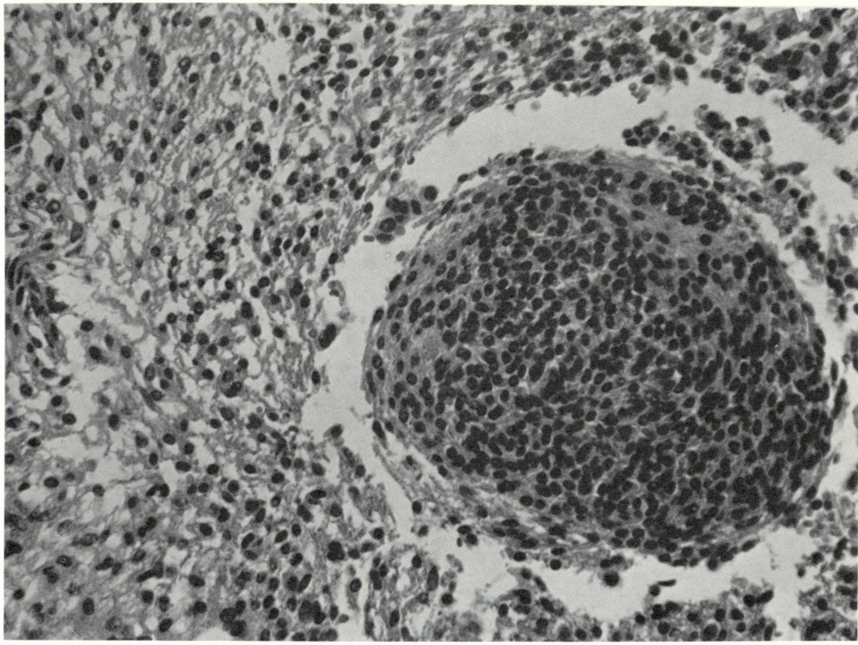

FIGURE 127
Focal increase in cellularity in meningioma. This phenomenon often indicates increased biological activity of tumor.

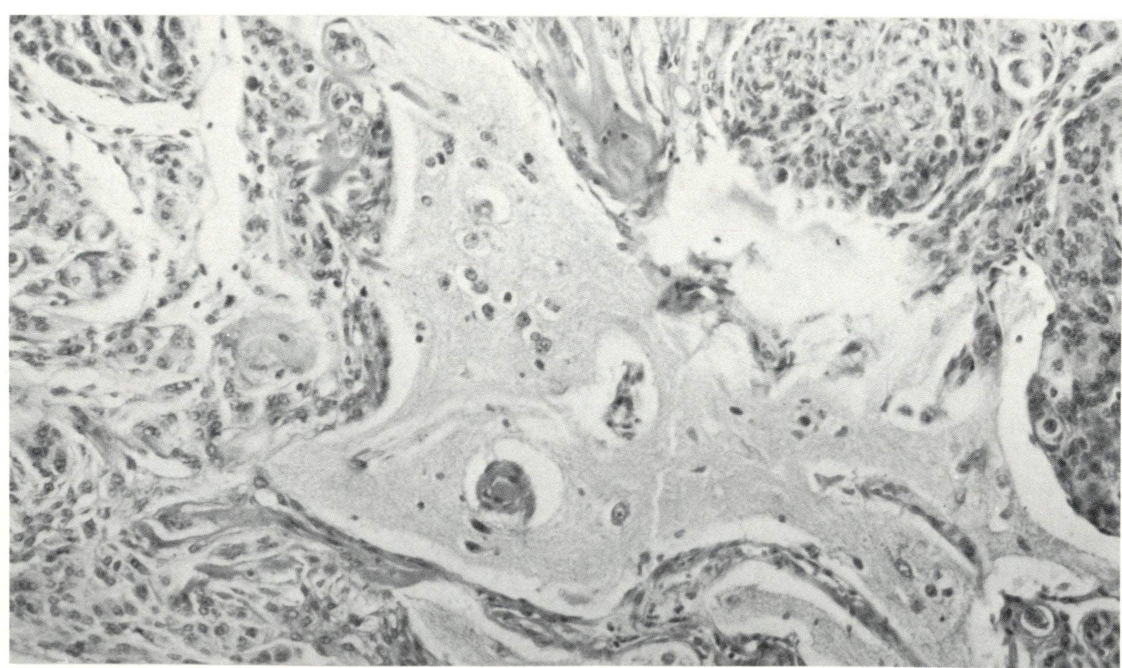

FIGURE 128
Invasion of brain by malignant meningioma with pinched-off islands of cortex.

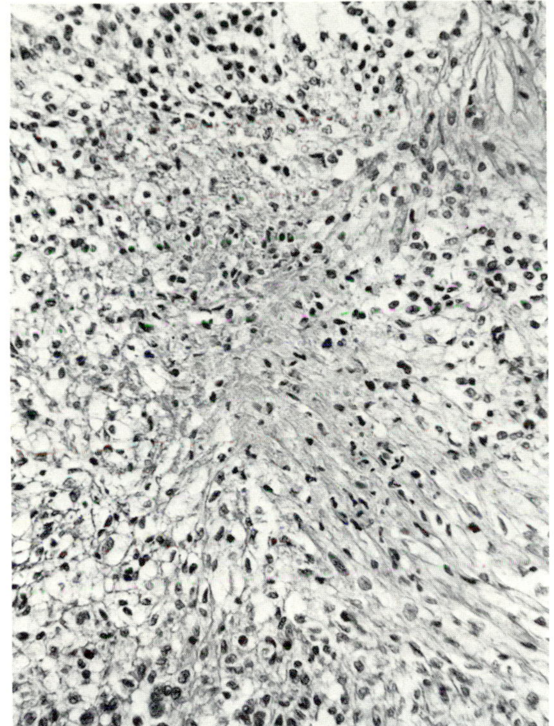

FIGURE 129
Focus of coagulation necrosis in meningioma.

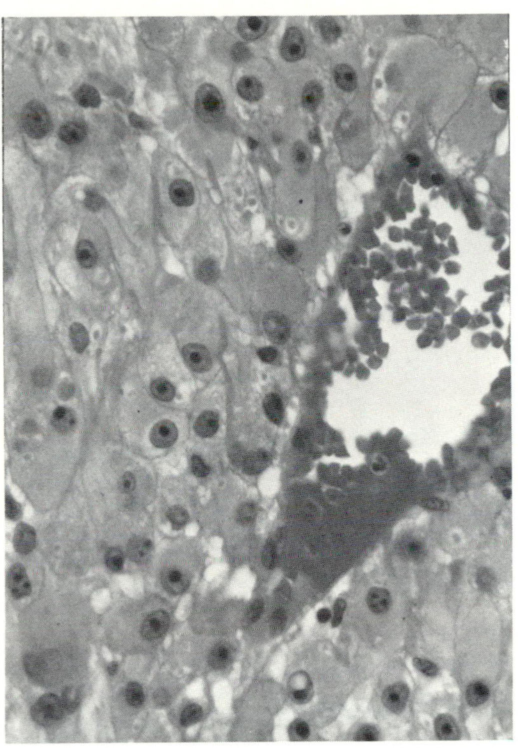

FIGURE 130
Prominent nucleoli in a recurrent malignant meningioma. (Courtesy Dr. W. Schoene.)

129). In one case, a recurrent and apparently clinically aggressive meningioma referred to us by Dr. William Schoene, impressed us by the presence of very prominent nucleoli in the tumor cells (Fig. 130). Naturally, metastatic implants via the cerebrospinal fluid attest to the aggressivity of a meningioma (Figs. 132a,b) as does invasion of *small blood vessels* within the tumor (Fig. 133), as contrasted to penetration of dural venous sinuses. Distant blood-borne metastases are, of course, the strongest proof of malignant behavior of a meningioma (Fig. 134).

PROBLEMS OF HISTOLOGICAL DIFFERENTIAL DIAGNOSIS

Most meningiomas are easily recognized under the microscope for what they are, and in general, pathologists usually have fewer problems with them than with gliomas. There exist, however, a not insignificant number of meningiomas that have areas which are hard to distinguish from other unrelated neoplasms.[88,89,89a]

Some meningiomas of the epithelioid variety undergo a fine granular–floccular change of their cytoplasm, resulting in a close resemblance to granular cell tumors (Fig. 135). Lapresle *et al.*[90] described such cells in a meningioma, but thought that they actually represented an admixture of a myoblastoma (i.e., a mixed tumor). Edematous and myxoid loosening of the tumor parenchyma will make a meningioma resemble a myxoma (Fig. 136). When the tumor is permeated by edema fluid as well as intra- and extracellular lipid material (the *forme humide* of Masson), even the components of cellular whorls will lose their cohesiveness, making the diagnosis of meningioma that much more difficult (Figs. 137 and 138). Particularly in fibroblastic meningiomas, nuclear palisading reminiscent of Verocay bodies (Fig. 139) is sometimes seen. This would not be a problem in a meningioma of the convexity where neurilemmomas are unlikely to occur, but may lead to some

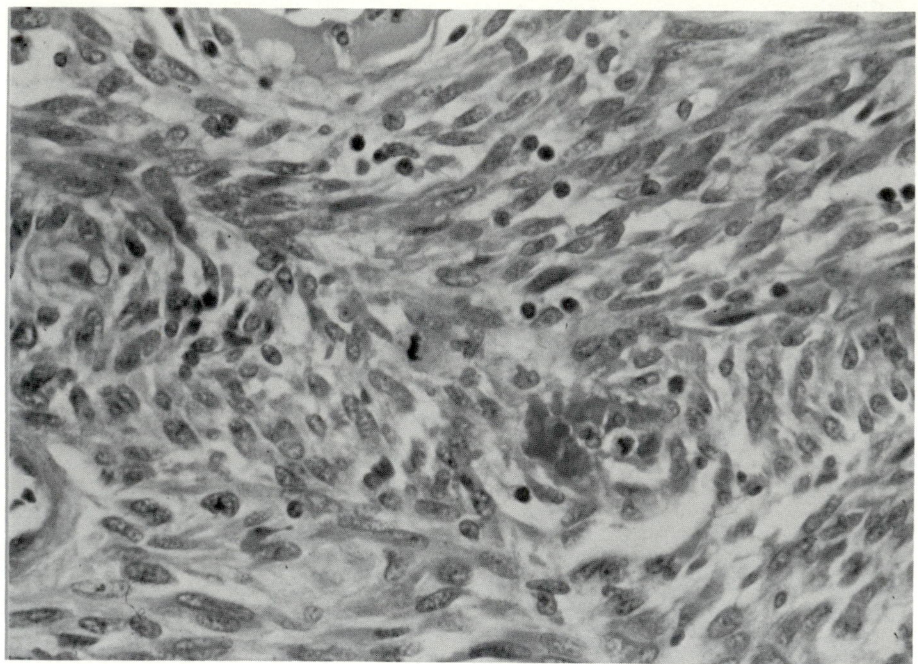

FIGURE 131. Mitotic activity in meningioma that has metastasized to spinal subarachnoid space and lungs.

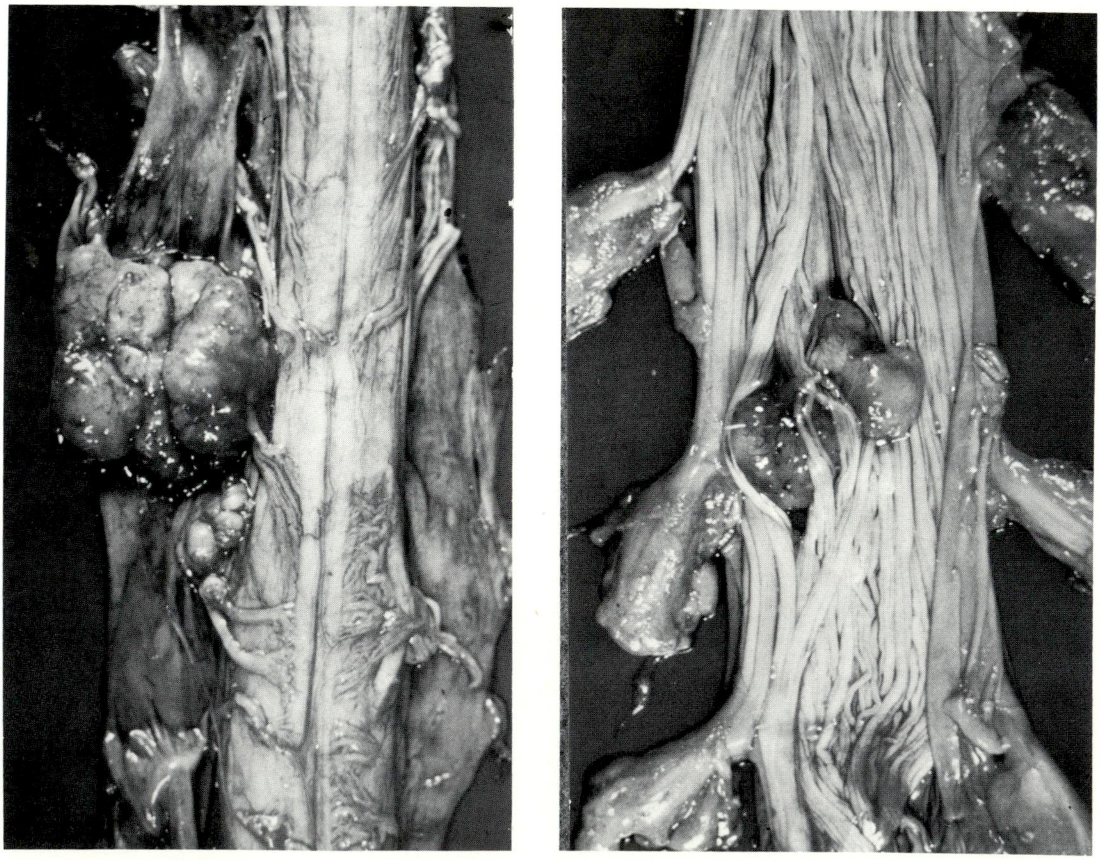

(*a*) (*b*)

FIGURE 132. Same tumor shown in Fig. 131. (*a*) Subarachnoid tumor deposits compressing thoracic spinal cord. (*b*) Tumor implants involving cauda equina.

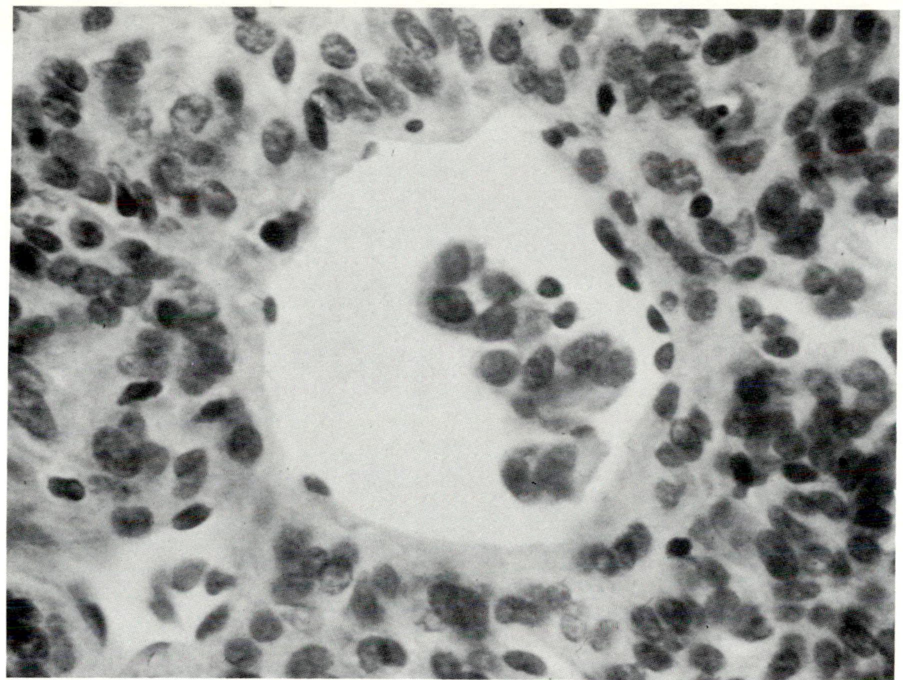

FIGURE 133
Malignant meningioma arising from tentorium cerebelli with tumor cells invading the neoplasm's own small blood vessels.

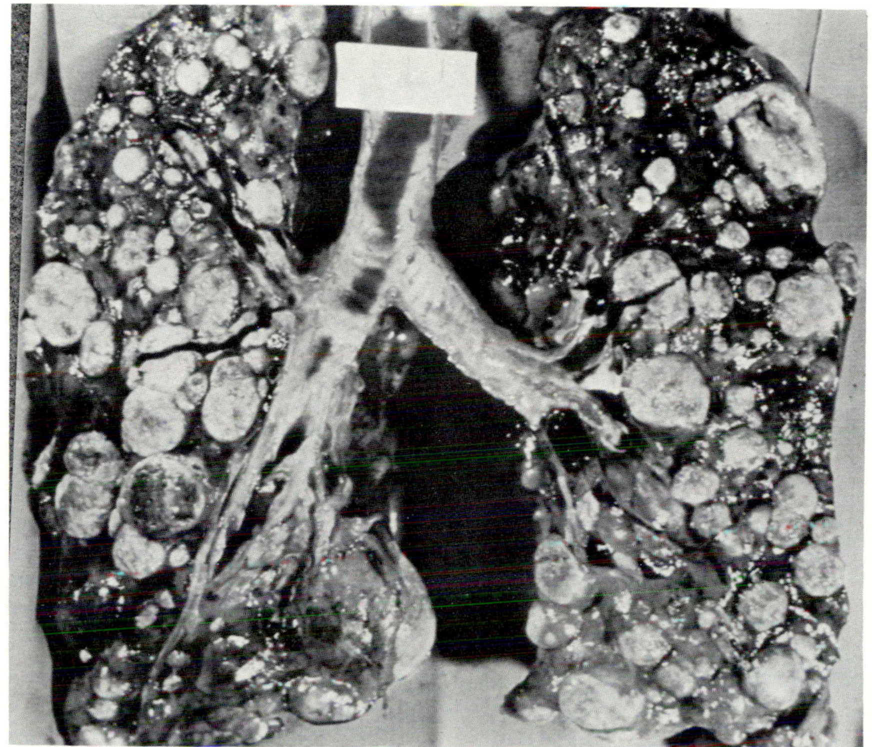

FIGURE 134
Same case shown in Figs. 133 and in 84–86. Multiple metastases in lungs. (From Kepes, J J., *et al.:* Malignant meningioma with extensive pulmonary metastases. *J. Kans. Med. Soc. 72: 315, 1971.* Reproduced with permission.)

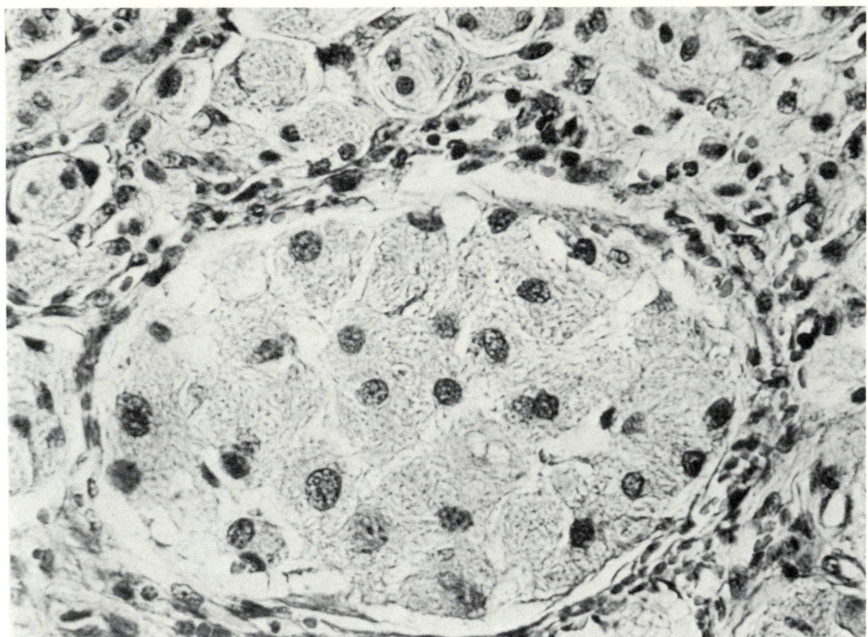

FIGURE 135
Granulofloccular transformation of cytoplasm of meningothelial cells creating similarity to granular cell tumor.

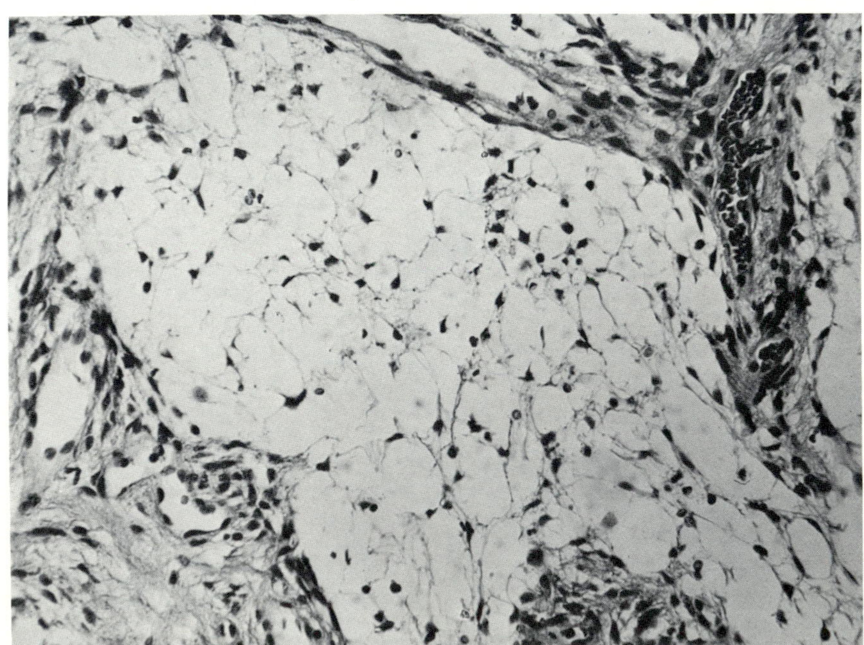

FIGURE 136
Myxoid changes in this meningioma resemble pattern of myxoma or myxosarcoma.

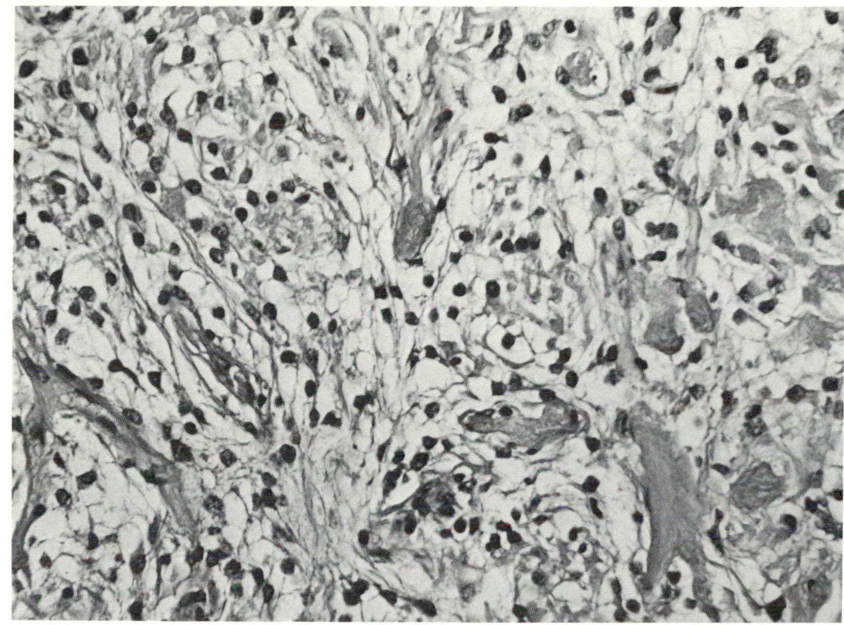

FIGURE 137
Edematous meningioma with mucoid degeneration (*forme humide* of Masson) from lower spinal canal. Diagnosis from this area is difficult.

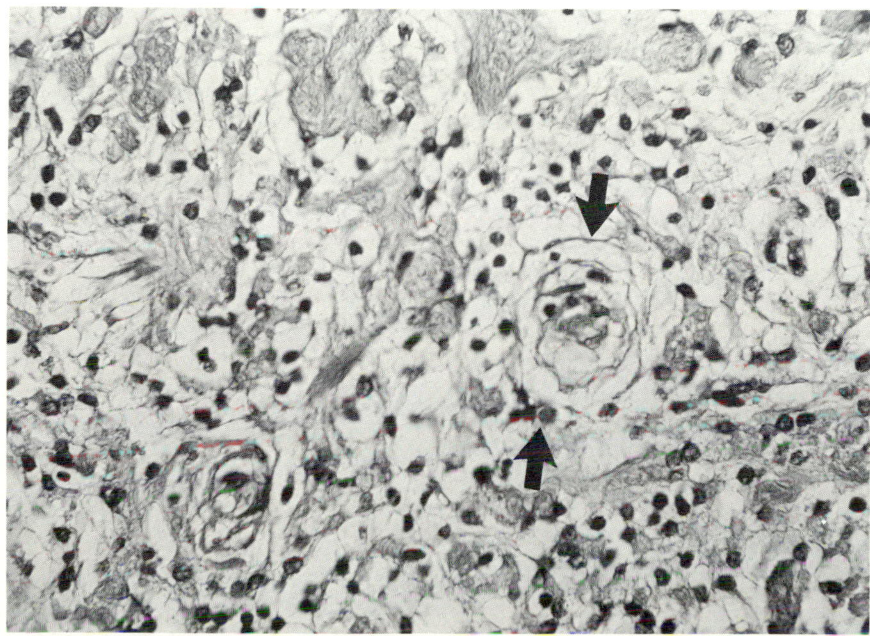

FIGURE 138
Same case shown in Fig. 137. *Arrows*, point to very loosely structured whorl. (See also E.M. Figs. 204–205.) (Courtesy Dr. B. W. Scheithauer.)

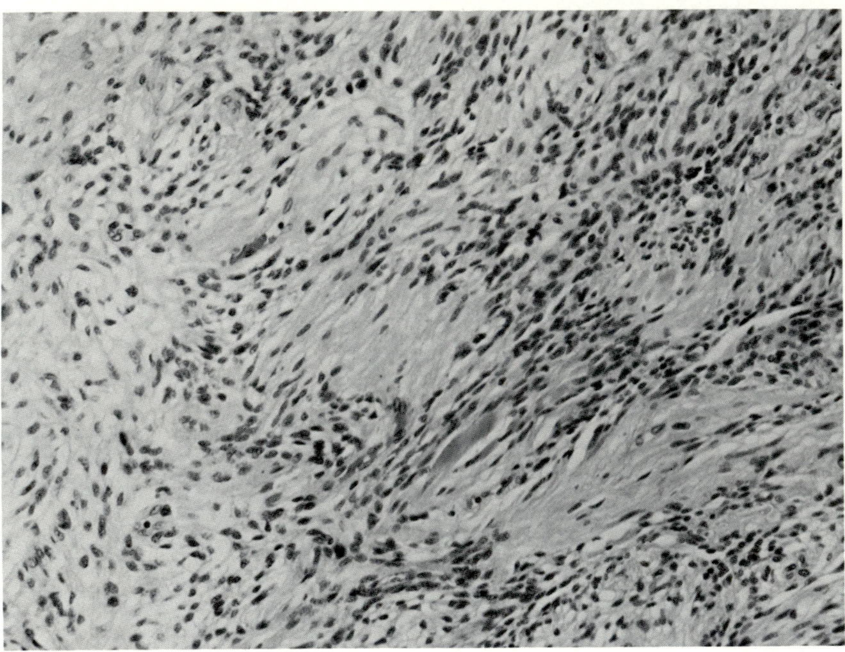

FIGURE 139
Nuclear pallisading in otherwise typical transitional meningioma resembles pattern of neurilemmoma.

confusion if it is found in a meningioma of the pontocerebellar angle or the spinal canal. On reticulin stain neurilemmomas more often have fibrils in a parallel arrangement, whereas in fibroblastic meningiomas they are likely to form interlacing bundles instead.

Gliomas, including astrocytomas, may involve the cerebral cortex and on occasion may grow into the leptomeninges.[90a] They may elicit a desmoplastic reaction in doing so and grossly may begin to resemble meningiomas. It may therefore become a problem during surgery to differentiate a superficially located astrocytoma from a meningioma. Unfortunately, some meningiomas have features that closely resemble those of astrocytomas. On the one hand intercellular edema and myxoid degeneration may cause meningioma cells to become multipolar (stellate), thus closely imitating astrocytes (Figs. 140 and 141), whereas the plump epithelioid forms of meningioma cells may bear a very close resemblance to gemistocytic astrocytes (Figs. 142 and 144). Immunoperoxidase staining for glial fibrillary acidic protein (GFAP) may be most helpful, because gemistocytic astrocytes will stain positively with this method (Fig. 143a,b), but the plump cells of the meningioma remain unstained (Fig. 144).

Rosettes with central lumina, reminiscent of ependymal canaliculi, are very rarely seen in meningiomas (Figs. 145–146). (Papillary meningiomas, of course, may closely resemble papillary ependymomas or carcinomas and occasionally may even have a pseudoglandular pattern.)

Burger and Vogel[91] noted the occasional close resemblance between meningiomas with hydropic changes of the tumor cells and oligodendrogliomas. We have also encountered this phenomenon in our series (Figs. 147a,b).

As meningioma cells infiltrate the dura mater they may become compressed into narrow spaces between collagen fibers and may come to imitate the single-file pattern of a metastatic scirrhous carcinoma (Fig. 148a). Unless a deeper biopsy is taken to verify the true nature of the tumor (Fig. 148b) the surgeon may decide against continuing the operation, particularly if the tumor is in a poorly accessible area that makes removal technically difficult.

INTRACRANIAL AND INTRASPINAL NEOPLASMS WITH HISTOLOGIC FEATURES IMITATING MENINGIOMAS

The tendency of whorl formation is a well-known histological hallmark of many meningiomas, but

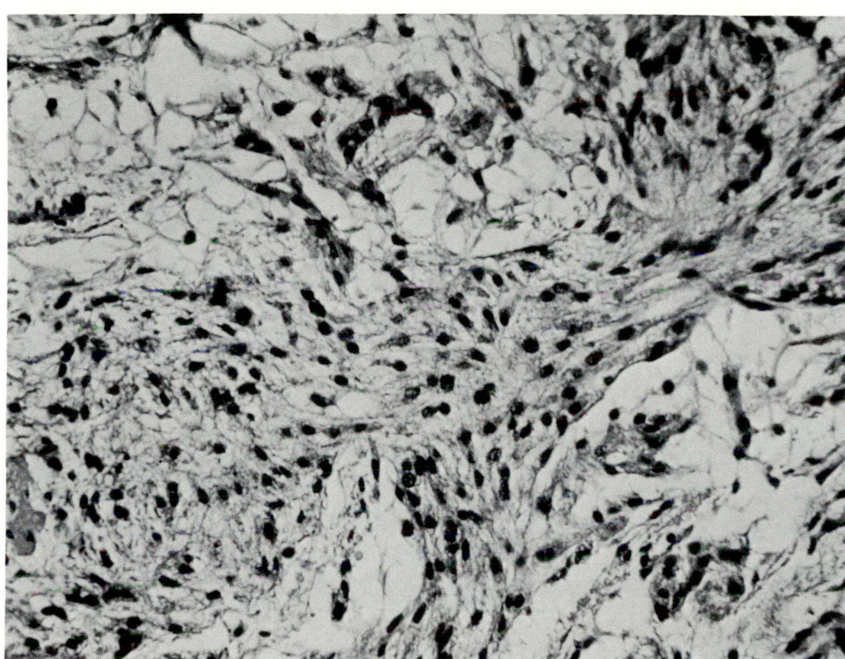

FIGURE 140
Edema and myxoid changes make for close resemblance to microcystic astrocytoma in this detail of a meningioma.

it must be recognized that tumors other than meningiomas occasionally form cellular whorls.[92] A whorling pattern many sometimes be seen in metastatic squamous carcinomas, in malignant melanomas, medulloblastomas, and even in glioblastomas (Figs. 149–153). Obviously, it is necessary to examine the general architecture and cytology of such tumors beyond the fact that they contain whorled arrangement of cells.

It has been mentioned earlier that nuclear palisading in some meningiomas results in occasional resemblance to Schwannomas. It should be mentioned here that, conversely, the tendency for the formation of cellular whorls in some Schwannomas causes a similarity to meningiomas. Figure 154 shows a detail from an intraspinal, otherwise histologically typical, Schwannoma with areas of whorl formation. Bodian stain demonstrated axons between the tumor cells, further attesting to the peripheral nerve origin of this neoplasm (Fig. 155). Characteristic wavy bundles of reticulin fibers were also present both within and outside the whorls (Fig. 156). This tumor was in many respects similar to the ones reported by Feigin[92a] and regarded by that author as mixed mesenchymal tumors of the spinal canal.

Electrocautery is widely used in neurological surgery; a neoplasm with a tendency to bleed profusely during operation might invite a particularly vigorous use of this method of hemostasis. Unfortunately, the heat generated by cautery is likely to cause structural alterations in the tumor being biopsied. Most commonly, the affected cells become elongated and wavy, sometimes imitating the whorling pattern of a meningioma (Fig. 157a), which can result in the mistaken frozen section diagnosis of meningioma, when subsequent examination of areas unaffected by the heat of the cautery may reveal a totally different tumor pattern, in this case a metastatic carcinoma (Fig. 157b).

METASTATIC TUMORS IN MENINGIOMAS

Fried[93] was the first to report deposits of metastatic carcinoma within a meningioma, in 1930. The primary tumor was a bronchogenic carcinoma with signet-ring cells. Subsequently other instances of carcinomas metastasizing to meningiomas were recorded. Some, as Fried's case, originated from the lung,[94–100] to two meningiomas in the case

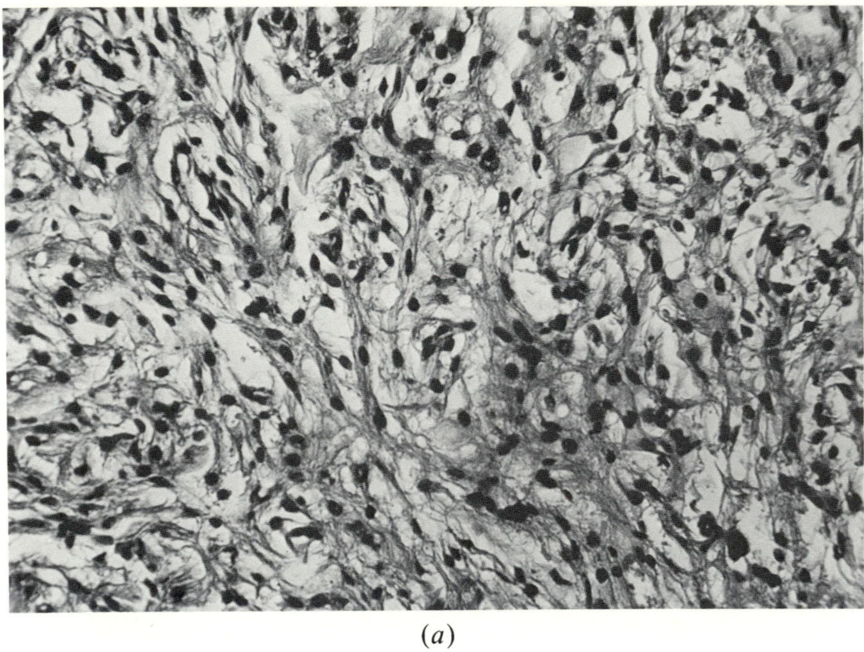

(*a*)

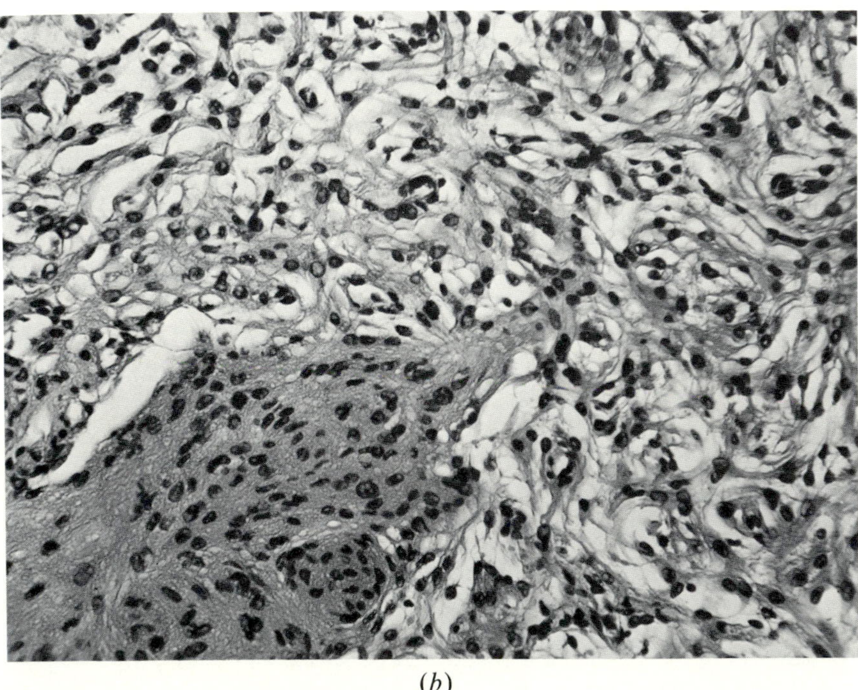

(*b*)

FIGURE 141
A case of frozen section diagnosis of fibrillary astrocytoma with meningioma diagnosed at the second operation. (*a*) Frozen biopsy showing stellate cells in syncytial arrangement. (*b*) Second specimen tissue (*left lower corner*) is more compact and shows meningothelial whorls. (Consultation material from Dr. L. Price, Bishop Clarkson Hospital, Omaha, Nebraska.)

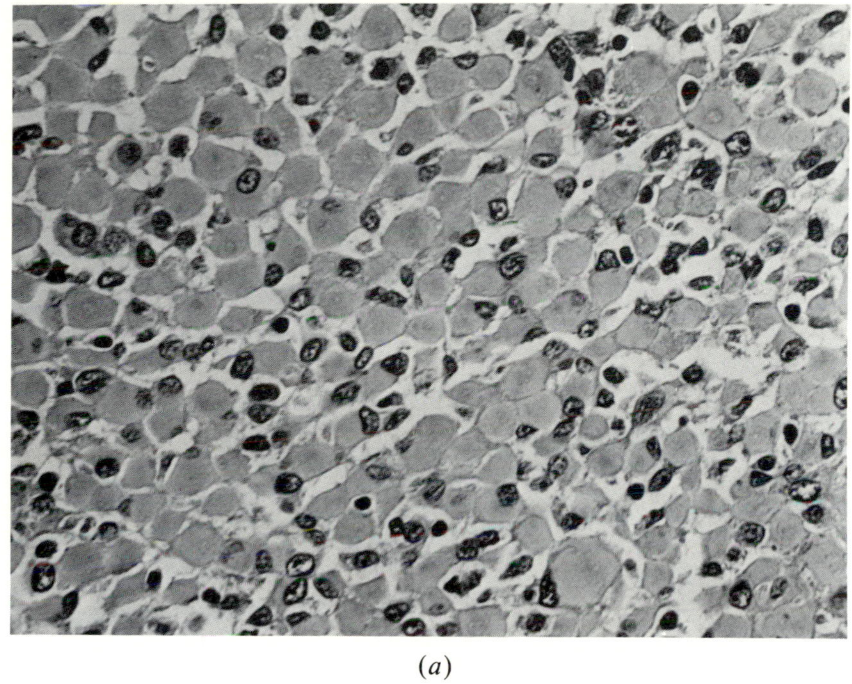

(*a*)

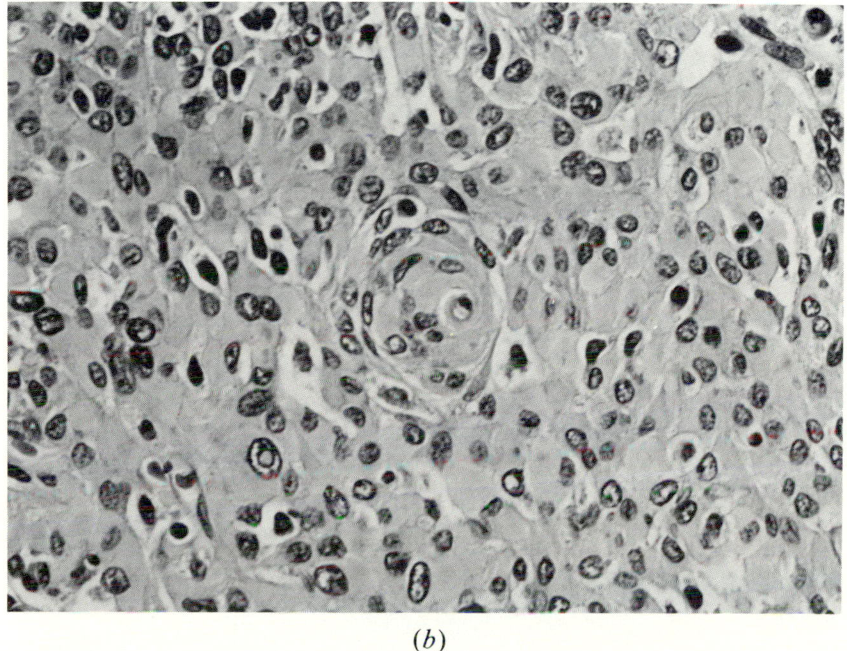

(*b*)

FIGURE 142
Plump epithelioid meningothelial cells imitating gemistocytic astrocytes. Convexity meningioma in 26-year-old man. (*a*) Entire area consists of plump eosinophilic cells with eccentric nuclei. (*b*) Whorling in center and vacuolated nuclei show the true nature of this meningioma.

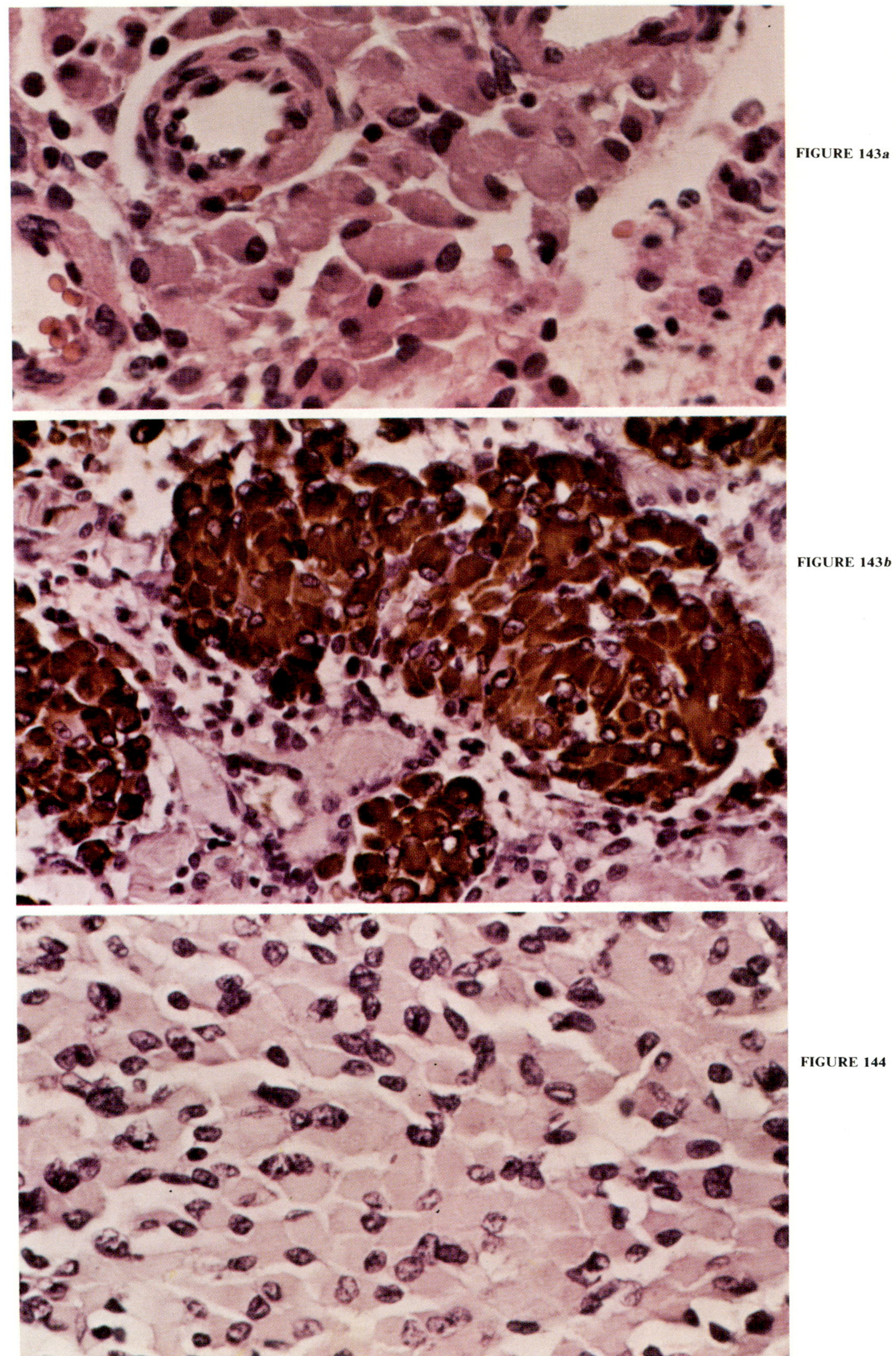

FIGURE 143*a*

FIGURE 143*b*

FIGURE 144

FIGURES 143 and 144
Comparison between gemistocytic astrocytoma and meningioma with gemistocytelike cells, using GFAP stain.

FIGURE 143
(*a*) Gemistocytic astrocytoma. H&E stain. (*b*) Same tumor stained for glial fibrillary acidic protein with the immunoperoxidase method. The tumor cells stain positively (*brown*).

FIGURE 144
Immunoperoxidase method for GFAP gives entirely negative result on gemistocytelike cells of meningioma.

---

described by Györi.[98] Others had their source in the breast. In a case reported by Fenyes and Kepes,[101] mammary carcinoma embolized into a meningioma without establishing a metastasis, but actual metastatic masses from breast cancer have been described by Bernstein,[102] Lapresle *et al.*,[90] Buge *et al.*,[103] Anlyan *et al.*,[104] Theologides,[105] and DiBonito and Bianchi.[106] Hockley's[107] case was unusual in that the breast carcinoma metastasized to a spinal meningioma.

Renal cell carcinoma was observed to create metastatic foci in meningiomas by Zülch,[108] Störtebecker,[109] and Osterberg.[94] Other less common primaries reported were gallbladder,[110] prostate,[111] and uterine cervix.[112] Rubinstein[113] referred to three cases of carcinoma metastases in meningiomas from his material, but did not specify the primary sources. Recent reports by Chambers *et al.*[114] include as primary sites prostate, breast, and lung, respectively, whereas Smith *et al*[115] described a malignant carcinoid tumor that has metastasized to a meningioma.

Figure 158 shows a heretofore unreported metastatic squamous cell carcinoma from the esophagus in a meningioma (case of Dr. N. Schumann, Kansas City). Figure 159 illustrates another previously unreported occurrence of a malignant lymphoma, with primary in the testicle, metastasizing to a meningioma.

It was mentioned earlier that cellular whorls are not the exclusive property of meningiomas, as they are occasionally seen in other primary and metastatic brain tumors. There exists one rare tumor, however—in the lung, of all places—that closely imitates meningiomas, not only by light microscopy, but even when examined with the electron microscope. These small collections of cells are known as minute pulmonary chemodectomas.[115]

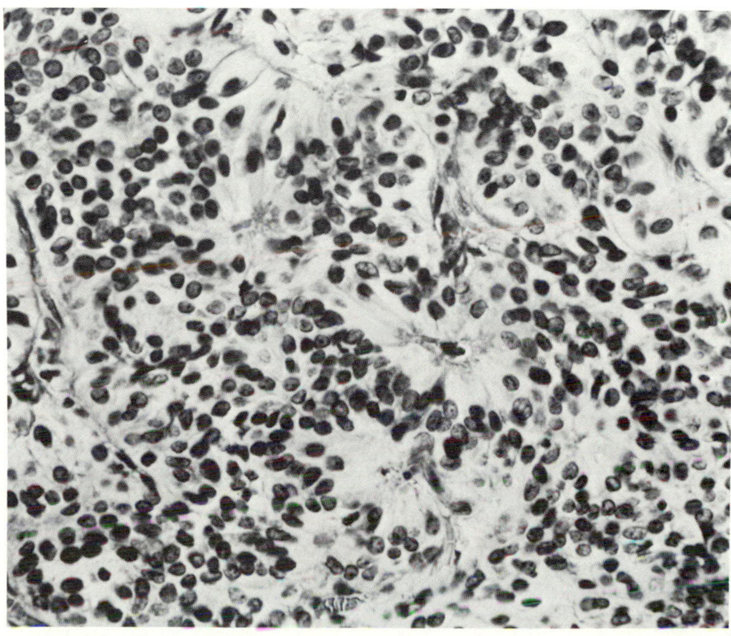

FIGURE 145
Meningioma from parapharyngeal area with pattern imitating that of cellular ependymoma.

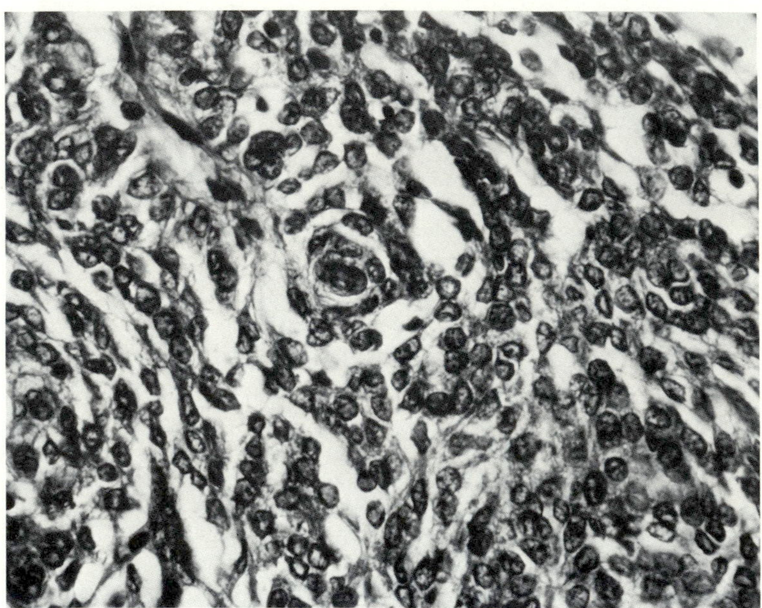

FIGURE 146
Cellular whorls in other areas of same tumor (Courtesy Dr. B. W. Scheithauer.)

The light microscopic features of this poorly understood lesion, which might actually be related to arachnoidal cells, are shown in Figure 160a,b.

MENINGIOANGIOMATOSIS

Benign meningiomas do not, as a rule, infiltrate the cerebral cortex (*vide supra*) and, in fact, deep penetration of the cerebral cortex by tumor cells is one of the histologic features commonly cited as denoting malignant biologic behavior of a given meningioma. There is, however, a rare condition in which a portion of the cerebral cortex is diffusely involved with, an ingrowth of both meningothelial cells and blood vessels, with a variable ratio of the two. These lesions do not behave in a malignant fashion; indeed, they are probably more of a hamartomatous than of a truly neoplastic nature.

This entity was termed meningioangiomatosis by Worster-Drought *et al.*,[117] who were the first to observe this lesion in a 25-year-old man who also suffered from neurofibromatosis. When the patient died, he was found to have, in addition to multiple intracranial and intraspinal neurilemmomas and meningiomas, several slightly depressed patches in the frontal and parietal cortices. Histologically, thick-walled leptomeningeal blood vessels penetrated the cortex in these areas, some of which were accompanied by meningothelial cells. The glial cells of the invaded area also took part in the proliferative process. Some of the multinucleated and gemistocytic astrocytes in the involved areas reminded the investigators of glial cells seen in tuberous sclerosis.

Subsequently reports of this condition have appeared, as in the original case of Worster-Drought *et al.* in association with von Recklinghausen's neurofibromatosis (Rubinstein[118]; Russell and Rubinstein[119]). But not all patients harboring this condition necessarily suffer from neurofibromatosis, or at least no stigmata of von Recklinghausen's disease were encountered in the cases of Davis,[120] Rhodes and Davis,[121] Clasen,[122] or in another recent case submitted to us by Dr. B. W. Scheithauer.

Not surprisingly, in view of the cortical involvement by the process, several of these patients, although not all, had a history of focal epileptic seizures. When first seen for their complaints referable to their cortical lesions, these patients were usually in their 2nd or 3rd decade of life. The first few reported patients' lesions were detected at autopsy, but in the more cases the lesions were discovered by craniotomy, usually after radiological finding of cortical mineralization (Fig. 161). Frontal and temporal gyri were often the most conspicuously involved areas.

The case submitted by Clasen,[122] in which the lesion was surgically excised from the temporal

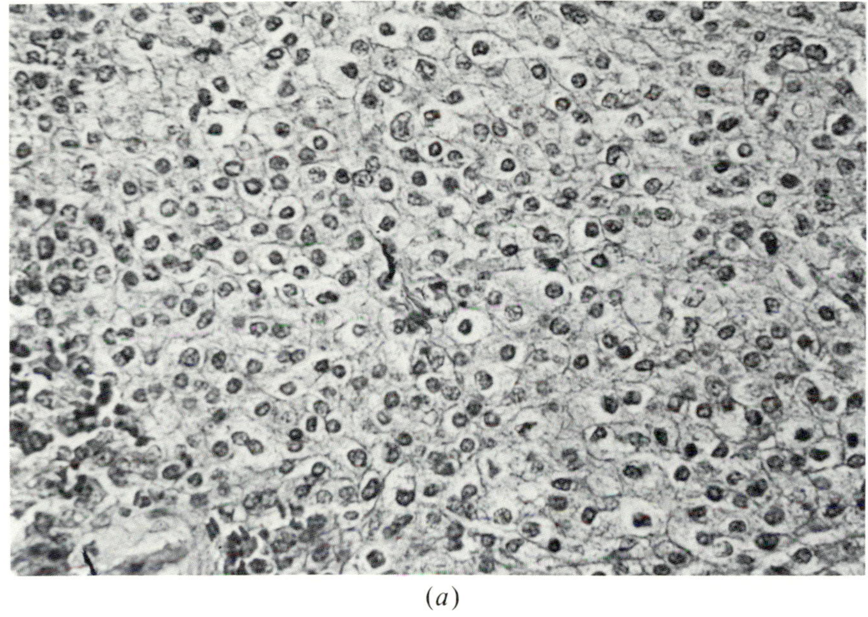

(*a*)

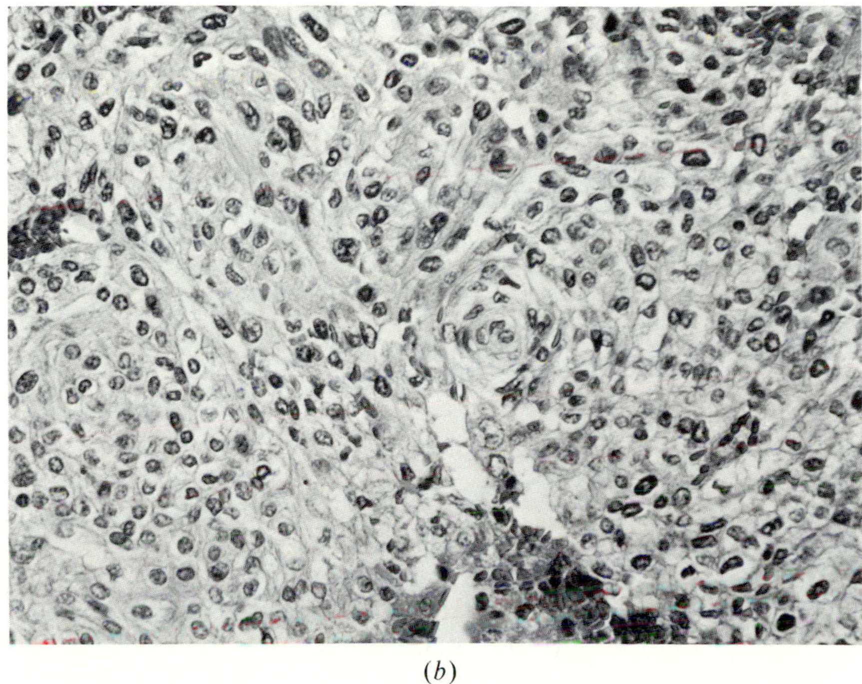

(*b*)

FIGURE 147
Oligodendrogliomalike pattern in meningioma. (*a*) This area with honeycomb or fried egg pattern closely resembles oligodendroglioma. (*b*) Deeper areas of same tumor reveal characteristic meningothelial pattern.

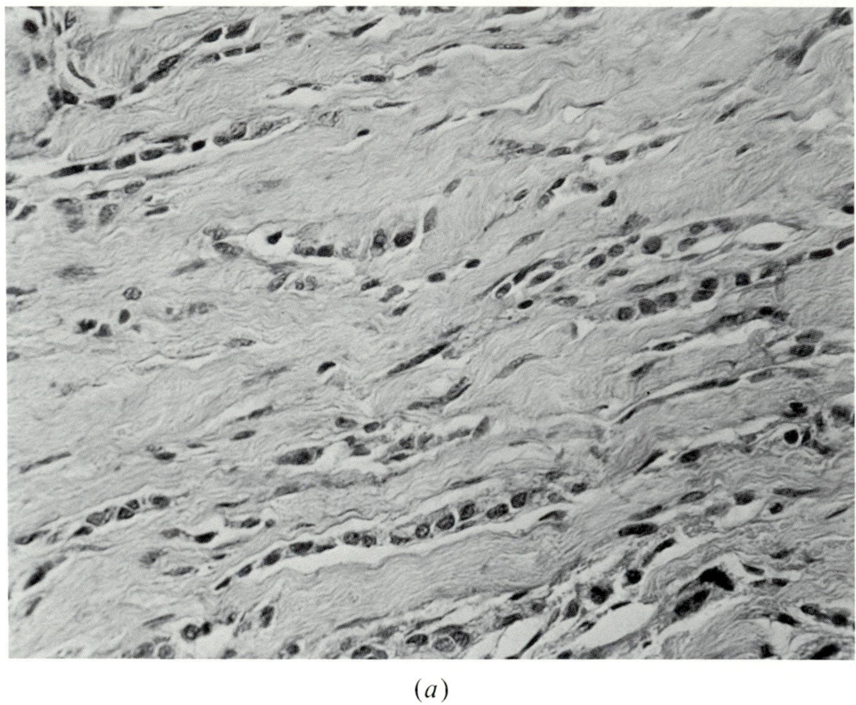

(*a*)

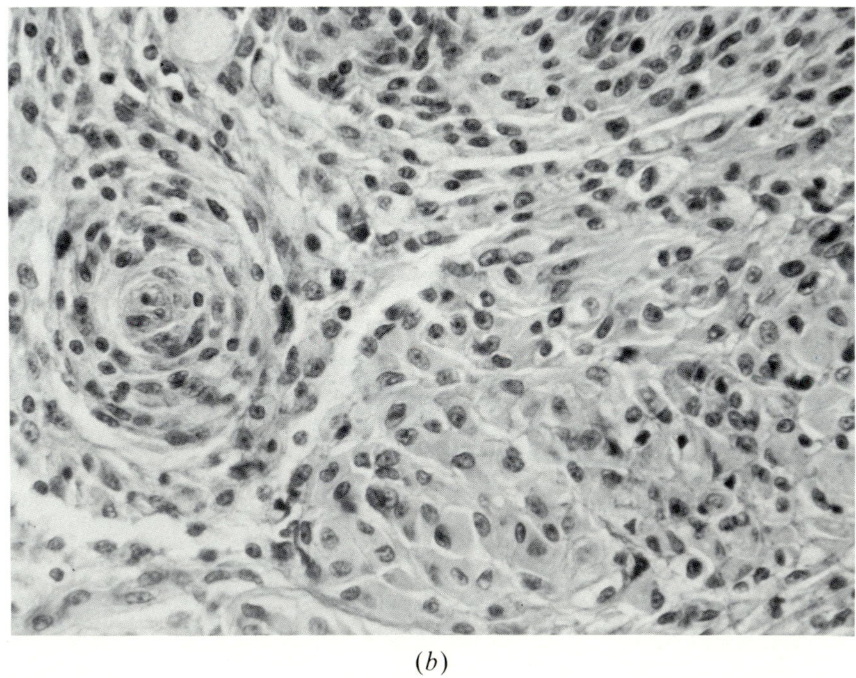

(*b*)

FIGURE 148
Imitation of metastatic scirrhous carcinoma by meningioma. (*a*) Single filing of tumor cells between layers of dura resembles pattern of invasive carcinoma from breast. (*b*) Deeper areas of same tumor show it to be a meningioma.

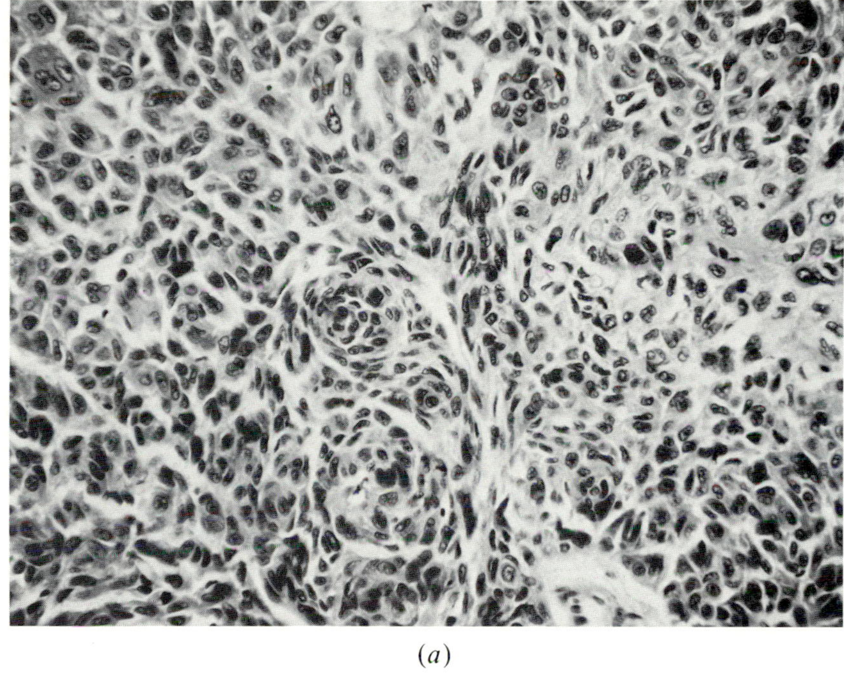

(*a*)

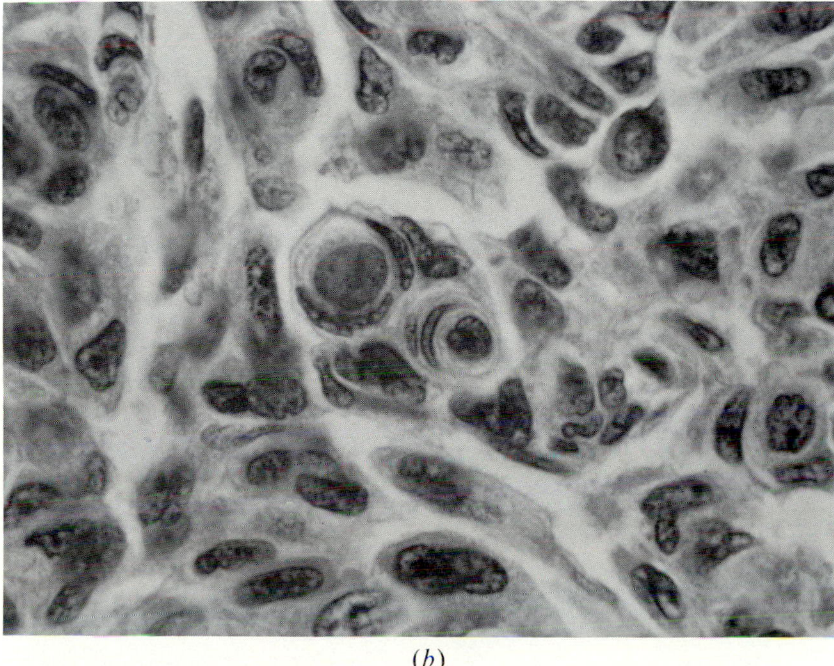

(*b*)

FIGURE 149
Poorly differentiated squamous cell carcinoma of larynx with metastases to brain. H&E. (*a*) ×160. (*b*) ×460. (From Kepes, J. J.: Cellular whorls in brain tumors other than meningiomas. *Cancer 37: 2232–2237, 1976.* Reproduced with permission.)

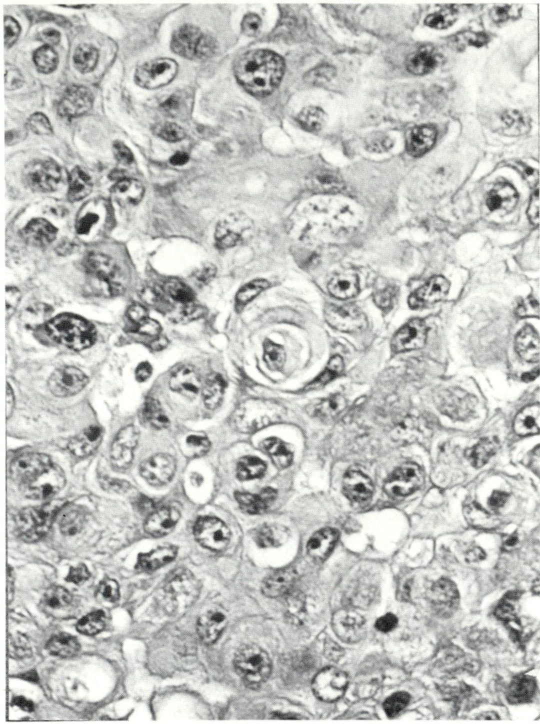

FIGURE 150. Cellular whorl in metastatic carcinoma from breast. (From Kepes, J. J.: Cellular whorls in brain tumors other than meningiomas. *Cancer 37: 2232–2237, 1976.* Reproduced with permission.)

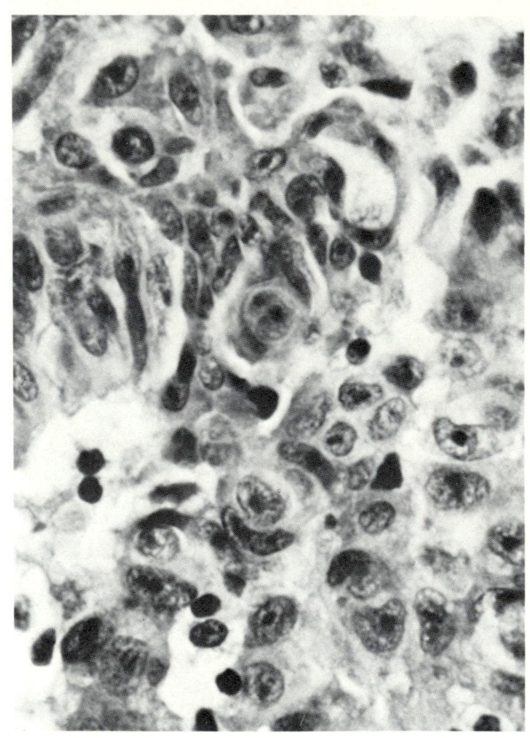

FIGURE 151. Metastatic melanoma in cerebellum. Tumor cells form whorls.

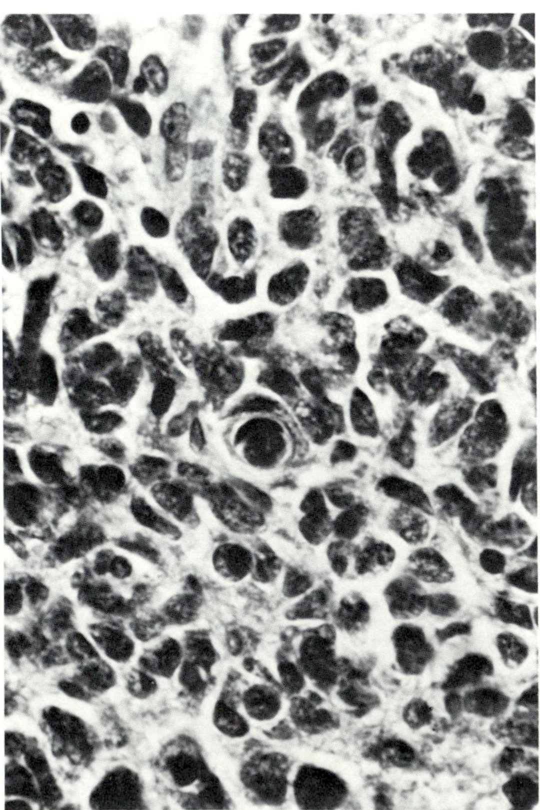

FIGURE 152. From a desmoplastic medulloblastoma of the cerebellum. Homer Wright rosette (*lower center*); whorling of cells (*center*).

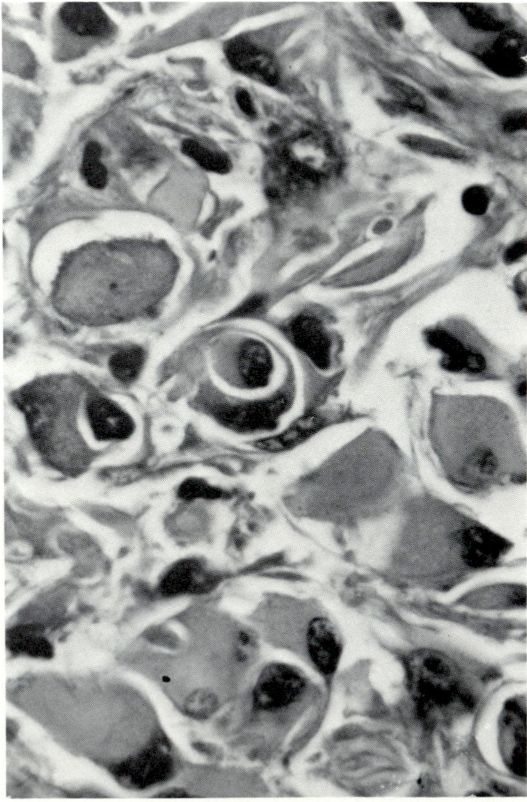

FIGURE 153. Cellular whorls in large cell glioblastoma of frontal lobe. (From Kepes, J. J.: Cellular whorls in brain tumors other than meningiomas. *Cancer 37: 2232–2237, 1976.* Reproduced with permission.)

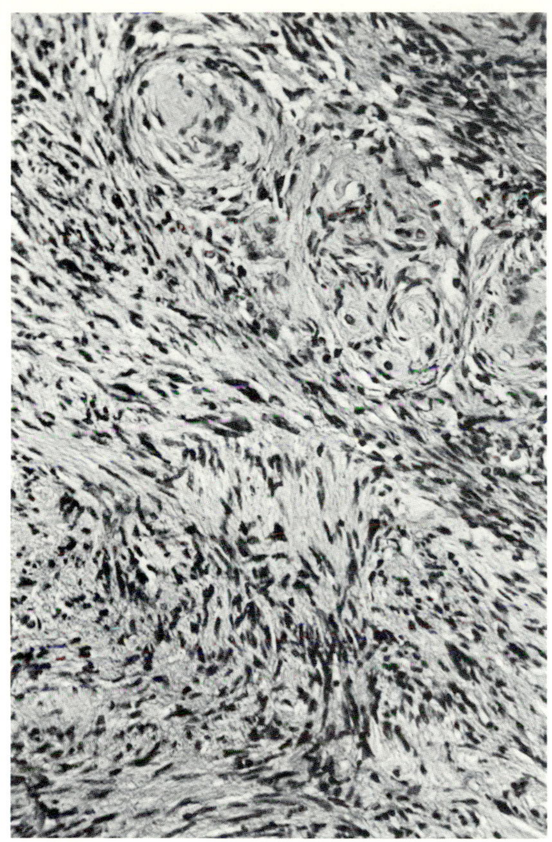

FIGURE 154
Schwannoma attached to dorsal nerve root of L_4 segment. *Lower half*, typical architecture for this neoplasm; *top half*, cellular whorls.

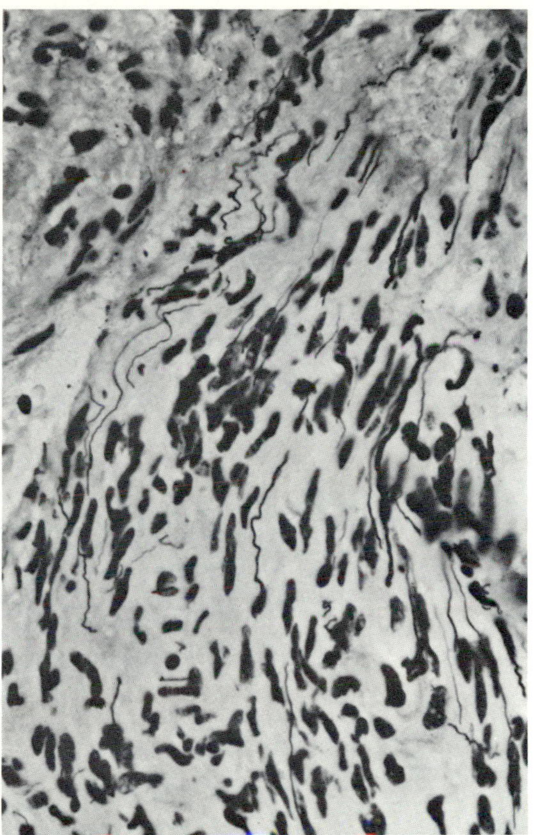

FIGURE 155
Same tumor shown in Fig. 154. Many axons are present between spindle-shaped tumor cells. (Bodian's silver impregnation.)

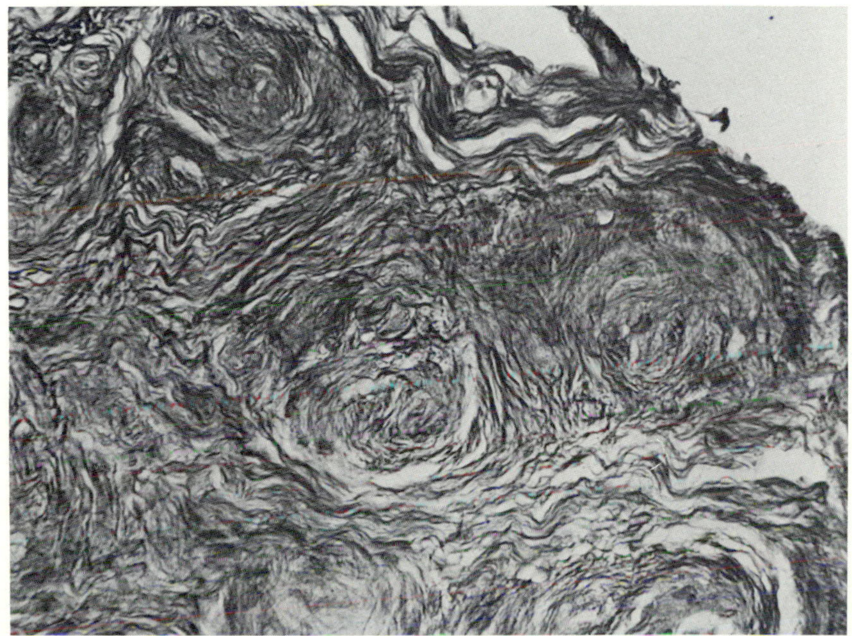

FIGURE 156
Same tumor shown in Figs. 154 and 155. Both the spindly areas and the whorls are rich in reticulin fibers. Wilder's reticulin stain.

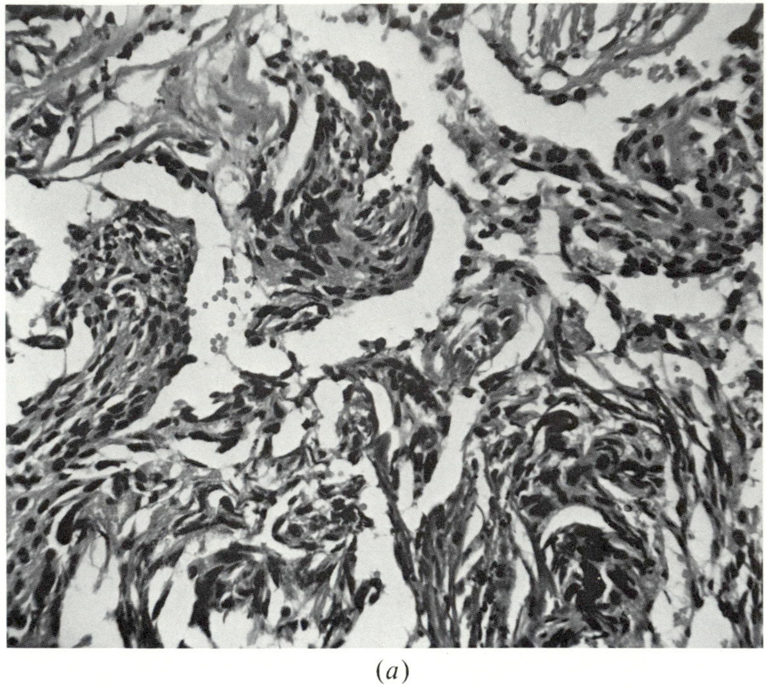

(*a*)

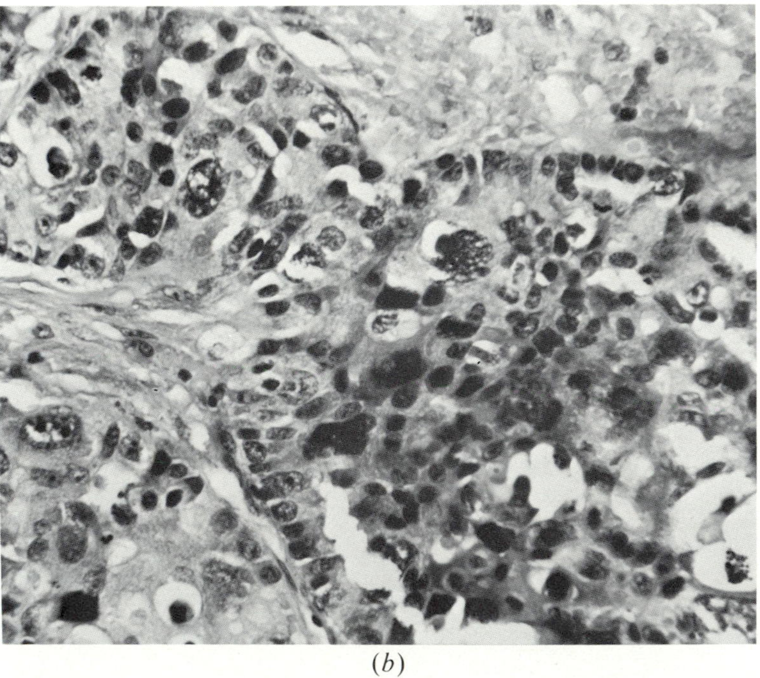

(*b*)

FIGURE 157
Thermal effect of cautery leading to diagnostic artifact. (*a*) Frozen section from cauterized area. Elongated nuclei and apparent whorl formation imitate pattern of meningioma. (*b*) Areas undistorted by cautery show true nature of tumor. Metastatic carcinoma (primary in lung).

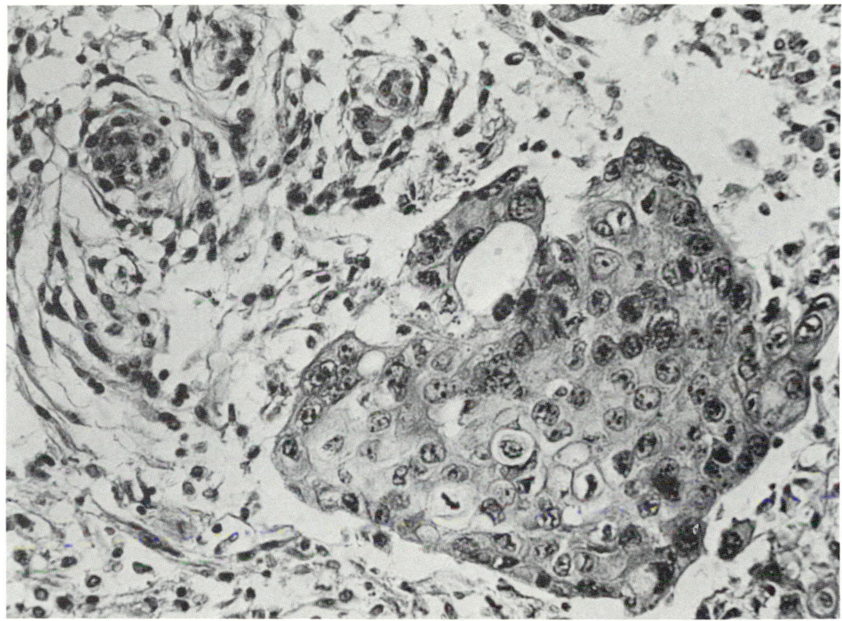

FIGURE 158
Squamous carcinoma of esophagus metastatic to meningothelial meningioma. (Case submitted by Dr. N. Schuman, Kansas City, Missouri.)

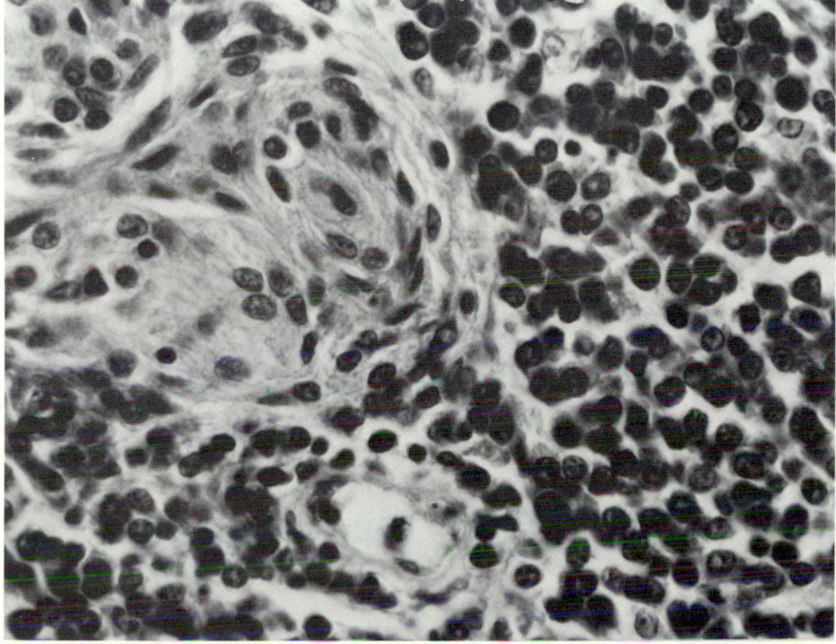

FIGURE 159
Malignant lymphoma metastatic to meningioma (primary tumor was in testis).

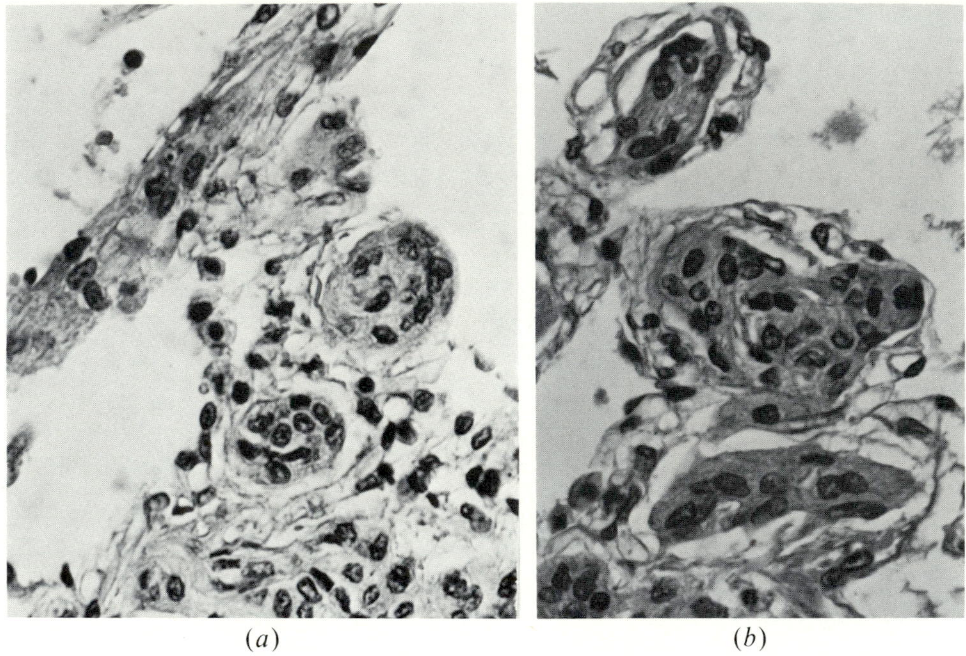

FIGURE 160
So-called pulmonary chemodectoma. Cellular whorls very similar to those seen in meningiomas are found in this lesion. (*a*) Low power. ×200. (*b*) Higher power. ×300.

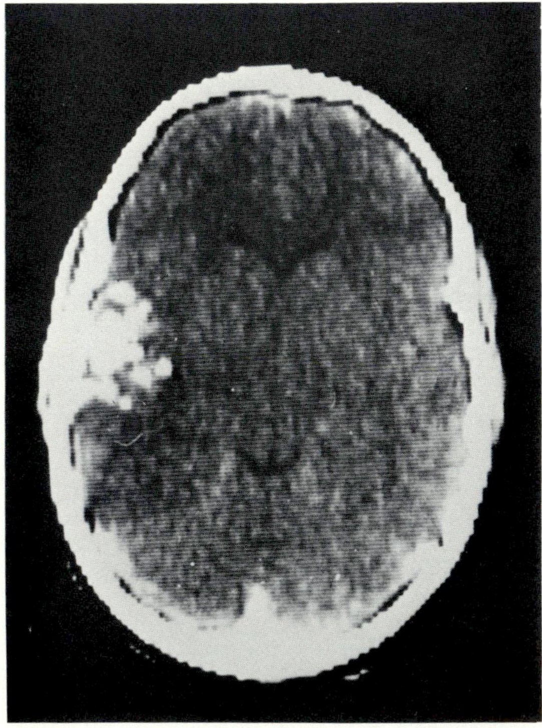

FIGURE 161
CT scan of 10-year-old girl with meningioangiomatosis. The opercular area of the right temporal cortex (*left*) shows greatly increased densities consistent with mineralization.

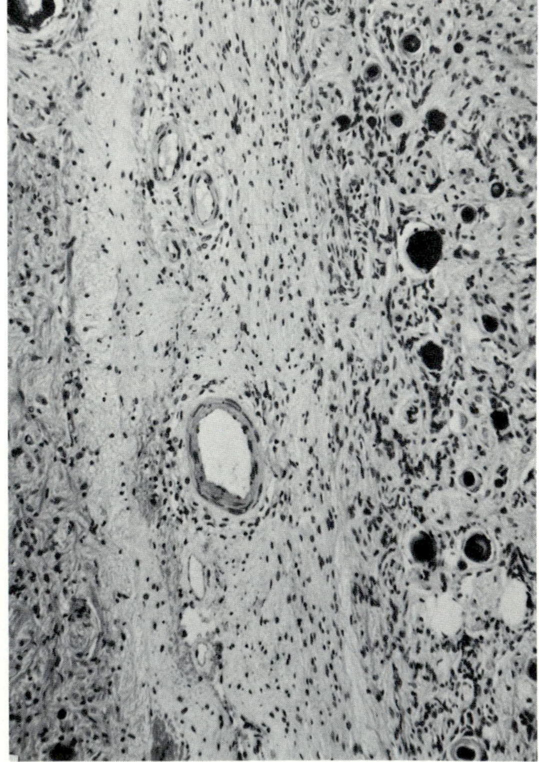

FIGURE 162
Same case shown in Figure 161. A sulcus between two neighboring gyri is obliterated by meningothelial cells and fibroblasts. The cortices also contain meningothelial elements with numerous psammoma bodies. H&E. ×90. (Figures 162–166 are photomicrographs from case submitted by Dr. R. A. Clasen.)

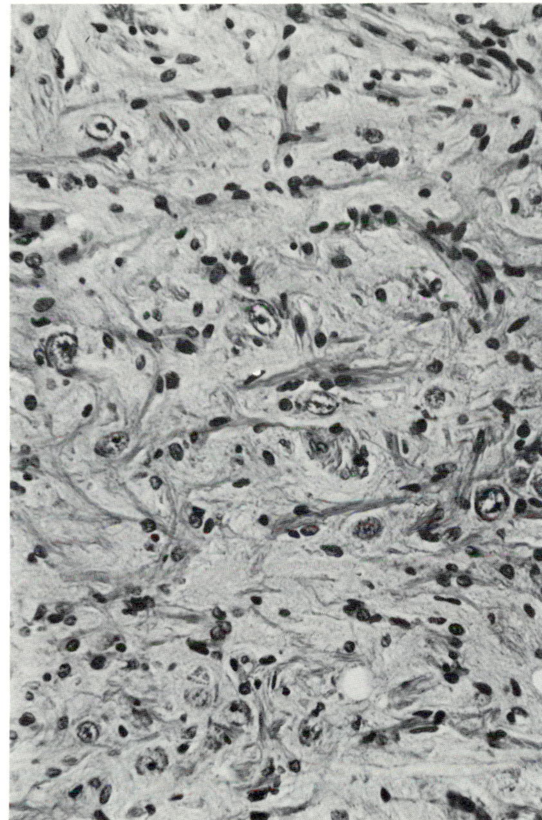

FIGURE 163
A network of thick-walled capillaries permeates the cortex in this area with neurons and glial cells trapped between vascular channels. H&E. ×200.

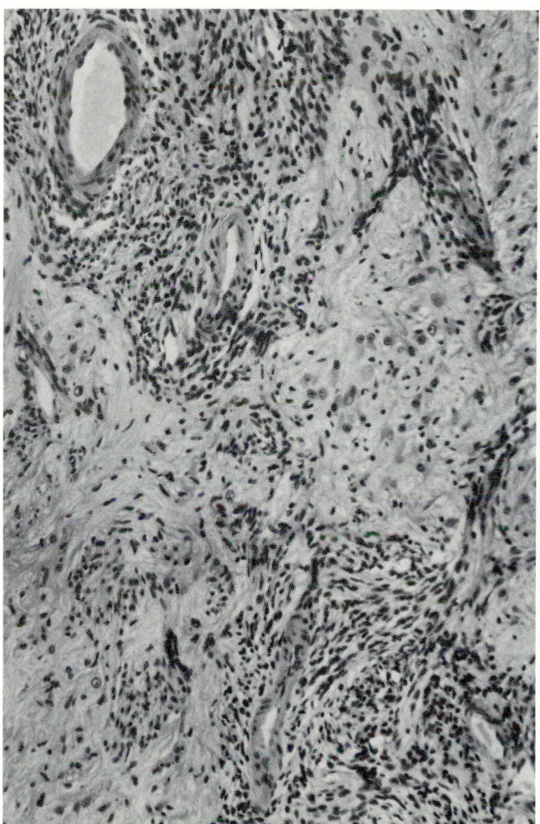

FIGURE 164
Blood vessels penetrating the cortex are accompanied by periadventitial clusters of meningothelial cells. H&E. ×120.

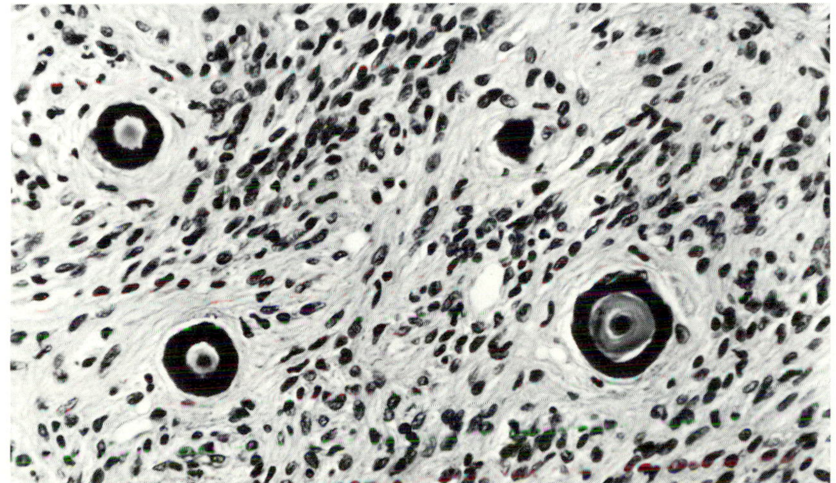

FIGURE 165
Some of the larger meningothelial clusters have cellular whorls and psammoma bodies. H&E. ×200.

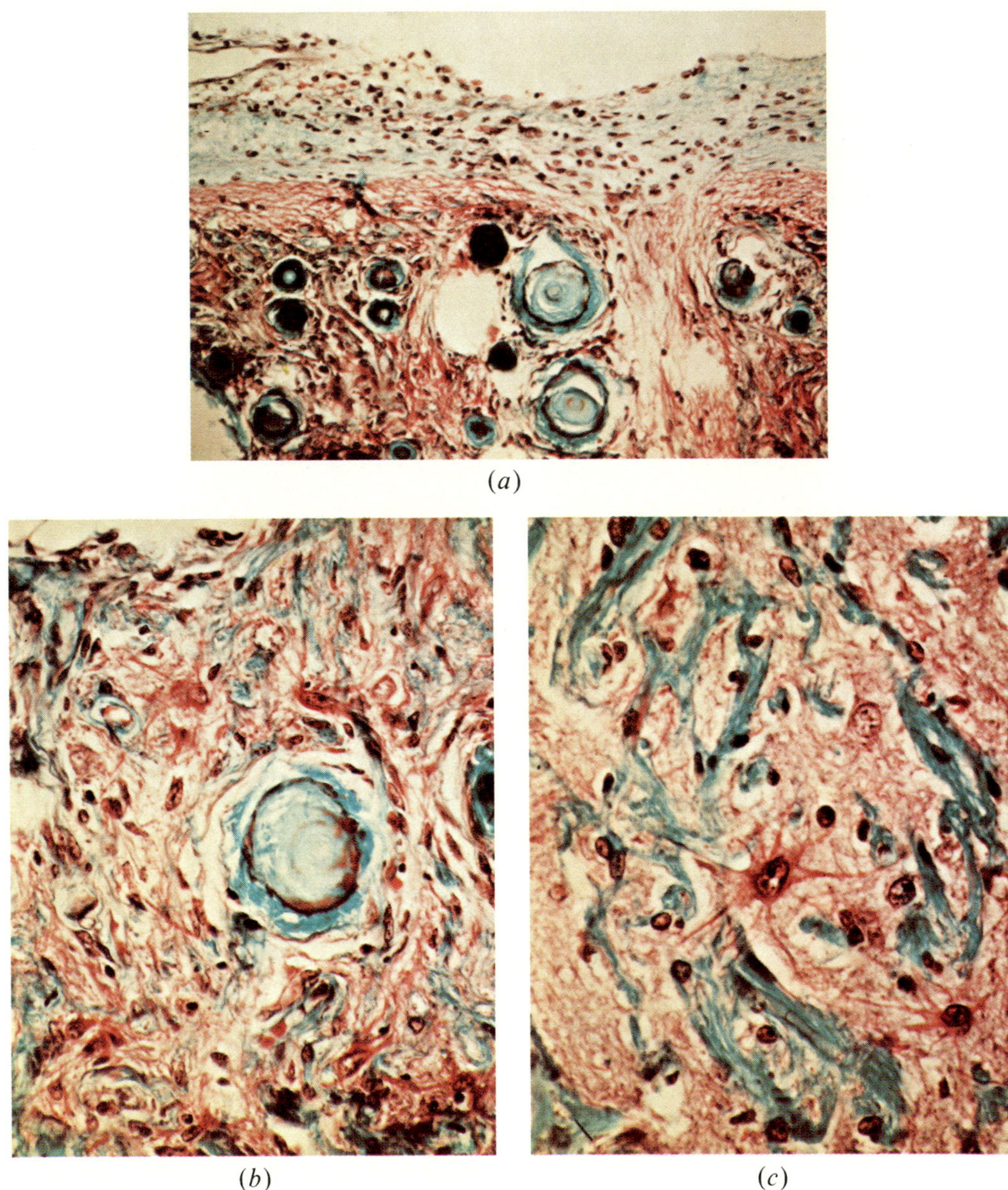

(*a*)

(*b*) (*c*)

FIGURE 166
Differential staining permits identification of meningeal and glial elements: meninges and collagenized whorls, *green*; astrocytes and glial fibers, *red*. Gomori's trichrome stain. (*a*) ×120. (*b*) ×200. (*c*) ×300.

lobe of a 10-year-old girl, shows the classic histological hallmarks of this entity. The sulcus between two neighboring gyri was completely obliterated by proliferating meningothelial cells, fibroblasts, and blood vessels (Fig. 162). The cerebral cortex has lost its original architecture because of the presence of proliferating blood vessels of diverse caliber (Fig. 163), accompanied in some areas by a sleeve of meningothelial cells. The latter formed fairly large intracortical clusters, with cellular whorls and psammoma bodies in some areas (Fig. 165). (In addition to ordinary psammoma bodies, Rhodes and Davis observed in their case larger clusters of mineralized material having the structure of fibroosseous nodules.) Neither the vascular nor the meningothelial components showed any histological or cytological hallmarks of malignancy. Astrocytic gliosis was prominent in the areas between blood vessels and meningothelial clusters. The two kinds of proliferations—meningovascular and glial—could be well distinguished by trichrome stain (Figs. 166a–c). It is not entirely clear whether the astrocytic proliferation is merely reactive in nature, that is, secondary to invasion of the cortex by meningovascular elements, or is part of the hamartomatous complex. The neurons in the involved areas also often show morphological abnormalities, one of the more striking changes having been encountered in the case of a 25-year-old patient submitted by Dr. Scheithauer, in which the neurons in the pyramidal layer of Ammon's horn, an area involved by meningoangiomatosis, showed almost without exception advanced changes of Alzheimer's neurofibrillary degeneration.

HISTOLOGICAL CLASSIFICATION OF MENINGIOMAS

As was pointed out by Russell and Rubinstein,[119] many classifications of meningiomas have been proposed in the past.[65,123–126] Russell[47] adopted Courville's classification of 1945,[127] later used by Russell and Rubinstein as well.[119] The main categories of this classification are (1) syncytial, (2) transitional, (3) fibroblastic, (4) angioblastic, and (5) malignant, the last category being separately dealt with in their book. Rather than propose still another classification, the purpose of our work is to acquaint the reader with the numerous variants of meningiomas, the main objective being that such variants should be recognized as those of meningiomas when encountered under the microscope. Where appropriate, e.g., hemangiopericytic tumors, papillary meningiomas, the biological connotations of some histological variants have been commented on.

As a most worthy effort is being made by WHO to create a worldwide standardized classification of neoplasms of various organ systems, it behooves us to present its classification of *Tumours of Meningeal and Related Tissues*,[128] included in WHO's general classification of brain tumors, outlined as follows:

A. Meningioma
   1. Meningiotheliomatous (endotheliomatous, syncytial, arachnotheliomatous)
   2. Fibrous (fibroblastic)
   3. Transitional (mixed)
   4. Psammomatous
   5. Angiomatous
   6. Hemangioblastic
   7. Hemangiopericytic
   8. Papillary
   9. Anaplastic (malignant) meningioma
B. Meningeal sarcomas
   1. Fibrosarcoma
   2. Polymorphic cell sarcoma
   3. Primary meningeal sarcomatosis
C. Xanthomatous tumors
   1. Fibroxanthoma
   2. Xanthosarcoma (malignant fibroxanthoma)
D. Primary melanotic tumors
   1. Melanoma
   2. Meningeal melanomatosis
E. Others

This classification will probably prove useful in many respects. Naturally, a review of the material presented by us in this section of the book will quickly indicate that some overlap is found among categories of the WHO classification. For example, there is a very smooth transition between meningiomas with few and those with many psammoma bodies. Just how many psammoma bodies should be present to warrant the use of the category psammomatous is open to question. Papillary formations can be found in both meningothelial and in hemangiopericytic meningiomas, so this category provides an overlap between at least two other categories. Also, anaplastic (malignant) features may be found in papillary meningiomas as well as in hemangiopericytic forms.

References

1. Roy, S., Chopra, P., Brahm Prakash, B., and Tandon, P.N.: Chondrosarcoma of the meninges. *Acta Neuropathol. (Berl.) 22: 272–274, 1972.*
2. Alvira, M.M., and McLaurin, R.L.: Asymptomatic subdural chondrosarcoma. Case report. *J. Neurosurg. 48: 825–828, 1978.*
3. Lichtenstein, L., and Bernstein, D.: Unusual benign and malignant chondroid tumors of the bone: A survey of some mesenchymal cartilage tumors and malignant chondroblastic tumors including a few multicentric ones as well as many atypical benign chondroblastomas and chondromyxoid fibromas. *Cancer 12: 1142–1157, 1959.*
4. Dahlin, D.C., and Henderson, E.D.: Mesenchymal chondrosarcoma: Further observations on a new entity. *Cancer 15: 410–417, 1962.*
5. Raskind, R., and Grant, S.: Primary mesenchymal chondrosarcoma of the cerebrum: Report of a chondroma and a mesenchymal chondrosarcoma. *J. Neurol. Neurosurg. Psychiatry 33: 469–475, 1970.*
6. Wu, W.Q., and Lapi, A.: Primary non-skeletal intracranial cartilaginous neoplasms. Report of a chondroma and a mesenchymal chondrosarcoma. *J. Neurol. Neurosurg. Psychiatry 33: 469–475, 1970.*

7. Guccion, J.G., Font, R.L., Enzinger, F.M., and Zimmerman, L.E.: Extra-skeletal mesenchymal chondrosarcoma.
Arch. Pathol. Lab. Med. 95: 335–340, 1973.
8. Scheithauer, B.W., and Rubinstein, L.J.: Meningeal mesenchymal chondrosarcoma. Report of 8 cases with review of the literature.
Cancer 42: 2744–2752, 1978.
9. Rengachary, S.S., and Kepes, J.J.: Spinal epidural metastatic "mesenchymal" chondrosarcoma. Case report.
J. Neurosurg. 30: 71–73, 1969.
9a. Lam, R.M.Y., Malik, G.M., and Chasen, J.L.: Osteosarcoma of the meninges. Clinical, light, and ultrastructural observations of a case.
Am. J. Surg. Pathol. 5: 203–208, 1981.
10. Cushing, H., and Eisenhardt, L.: *Meningiomas. Their Classification, Regional Behaviour, Life History, and Surgical End Results.* Sringfield, Ill., Charles C Thomas, 1938, pp. 44–45.
11. Rochat, G.F.: Grosshirnangiom bei der Lindauschen Erkrankung.
Klin. Monatsbl. Augenheilkd. 86: 23–27, 1931.
12. Hoff, J.T., and Ray, B.S.: Cerebral hemangioblastoma occurring in a patient with von Hippel-Lindau disease: Case report.
J. Neurosurg. 28: 365–368, 1968.
13. Perks, W.H., Cross, J.N., Sivapragasam, S., and Johnson, P.: Supartentorial haemangioblastoma with polycythemia.
J. Neurol. Neurosurg. Psychiatry 39: 218–220, 1976.
14. Bachmann, K., Markwalder, R., and Seiler, R.W.: Supratentorial haemangioblastoma. Case report.
Acta Neurochir. (Wien) 44: 173–177, 1978.
15. Lee, K.R., Kishore, P.R.S. Wulfsberg, E., and Kepes, J.J.: Supratentorial leptomeningeal hemangioblastoma.
Neurology (Minneap.) 28: 727–730, 1978.
16. Bailey, P., Cushing, H., and Eisenhardt, L.: Angioblastic meningioma.
Arch. Pathol. Lab. Med. 6: 453–490, 1928.
17. Cushing, H., and Eisenhardt, L.: *Meningiomas. Their classification, regional Behaviour, Life History and Surgical End Results.* Springfield, Ill., Charles C Thomas, 1938, pp. 43–44.
18. Begg, C.F., and Garret, R.: Hemangiopericytoma occurring in the meninges.
Cancer 7: 602–606, 1954.
19. Kruse, F., Jr.: Hemangiopericytoma of the meninges (angioblastic meningioma of Cushing and Eisenhardt). Clinicopathologic aspects and follow-up studies in 8 cases.
Neurology (NY) 11: 771–777, 1961.
20. Popoff, N.A., Malinin, T.I., and Rosomoff, H.C.: Fine structure of intracranial hemangiopericytoma and angiomatous meningioma.
Cancer 34: 1187–1197, 1974.
21. Peña, C.E.: Intracranial hemangiopericytoma. Ultrastructural evidence of its leiomyoblastic differentiation.
Acta Neuropathol. (Berl.) 33: 279–284, 1975.
22. Choux, R., Chrestian, M.A., Tripier, M.F., Gambarelli, D., Hassoun, J., and Toga, M.: Hémangiopéricytome cérébral. Étude ultrastructurale d'un cas.
J. Neurol. Sci. 28: 361–371, 1976.
23. Goellner, J.R., Laws, E.R., Soule, E.H., and Okazaki, H.: Hemangiopericytoma of the meninges. Mayo Clinic experience.
Am. J. Clin. Pathol. 70: 375–380, 1978.
24. Jellinger, K., and Slowik, F.: Histologic subtypes and prognostic problems in meningiomas.
J. Neurol. 208: 279–298, 1975.
25. Rubinstein, L.J.: *Tumors of the Central Nervous System.* Washington, D.C., Armed Forces Institute of Pathology, 1972, fasc. 6, pp. 180–182.
26. Horten, B.D., Urich, H., Rubinstein, L.J., and Montague, S.R.: The angioblastic meningioma: A reappraisal of a nosological problem.
J. Neurol. Sci. 31: 387–410, 1977.
27. Bergstrand, H., and Olivecrona, H.: Angioblastic meningiomas.
Am. J. Cancer 24: 522–530, 1935.
28. Pitkethly, D.T., Hardman, J.M., Kempe, L.G., and Earle, K.M.: Angioblastic meningiomas.Clinicopathologic study of 81 cases.
J. Neurosurg. 32: 539–544, 1970.
29. Muller, J., and Mealey, J., Jr.: The use of tissue culture in differentiation between angioblastic meningioma and hemangiopericytoma.
J. Neurosurg. 34: 341–348, 1971.
30. Ludwin, S.K., Rubinstein, L.J., and Russell, D.S.: Papillary meningioma: a malignant variant of meningioma.
Cancer 36: 1363–1373, 1975.
31. Jellinger, K., and Denk, H.: Blood group isoantigens in angioblastic meningiomas and hemangioblastomas of the central nervous system.
Virchows Arch. [Pathol. Anat.] 364: 137–144, 1974.
32. Mirra, S.S., and Miles, M.L.: Unusual pericytic proliferation in a meningotheliomatous meningioma: An ultrastructural study. (Abstract.)
J. Neuropathol. Exp. Neurol. 39: 376, 1980.
33. Challa, V.R.: Personal communication, 1979.
33a. Challa, V.R., Moody, D.U., Marshall, R.B., and Velley, D.L., Jr.: The vascular component in meningiomas associated with severe cerebral edema.
Neurosurgery 7: 363–368, 1980.
34. Kepes, J.J., MacGee, E.E., Vergara, G., and Sil, R.: Malignant meningioma with extensive pulmonary metastases.
J. Kans. Med. Soc. 72: 312–316, 1971.
35. Petito, C.K., and Porro, R.S.: Angioblastic meningioma with hepatic metastasis.
J. Neurol. Neurosurg. Psychiatry 34: 541–545, 1971.
36. Lowden, R.G., and Taylor, H.B.: Angioblastic meningioma with metastasis to the breast.
Arch. Pathol. Lab. Med. 98: 373–375, 1974.
37. Skullerud, K., and Löken, A.C.: The prognosis of meningiomas.
Acta Neuropathol. (Berl.) 29: 337–344, 1974.
38. Sirang, H., Scharrer, E., and Wohlfahrstädter, H.: Epidurales Hämangioperizytom.
Acta Neurochir. (Wien) 33: 113–121, 1976.
39. Pitlyk, P.J., Dockerty, M.B., and Miller, R.H.: Hemangiopericytoma of the spinal cord. Report of three cases.
Neurology (Minneapolis) 15: 649–653, 1965.
40. Fathie, K.: Hemangiopericytoma of the thoracic spine. Case report.
J. Neurosurg. 32: 371–374, 1970.
41. Harris, D.J., Fornasier, V.L., and Livingston, K.E.: Hemangiopericytoma of the spinal canal. Report of three cases.
J. Neurosurg. 49: 914–920, 1978.
42. Bertrand, I., Guillaume, J., and Olteanu, I.: Étude histologique de 130 meningiomes.

Rev. Neurol. (Paris) 80: 81–99, 1948.
43. Cushing, H., and Eisenhardt, L.: *Meningiomas. Their Classification, Regional Behaviour, Life History and Surgical End Results.* Springfield, Ill., Charles C Thomas, 1938, pp. 692–719.
44. Hamblet, J.B.: Arachnoidal fibroblastoma (meningioma) with metastases to liver. *Arch. Pathol. 37: 216–218, 1944.*
45. Christensen, E., Kiaer, W., and Winblad, S.: Meningeal tumours with extracerebral metastases. *Br. J. Cancer 3: 485–493, 1949.*
46. Ringsted, J.: Meningeal tumors with extracranial metastases. *Acta Pathol. Microbiol. Scand. [B] 43: 9–20, 1958.*
47. Russell, D.S.: Meningeal tumours (a review). *J. Clin. Pathol. 3: 191–211, 1950.*
48. Russell, D.S., and Rubinstein, L.J.: *Pathology of Tumours of the Nervous System* London, Edward Arnold, 1959, p. 53.
49. Miller, A.A., and Ramsden, F.: Malignant meningioma with extracranial metastases and seeding of the subarachnoid space and ventricles. *Pathol. Res. Pract. 7: 167–175, 1972.*
50. Ludwin, S.K., and Conley, F.K.: Malignant meningioma metastasizing through the cerebrospinal pathways. *J. Neurol. Neurosurg. Psychiatry 38: 136–142, 1975.*
51. Gonzalez-Vitale, J.C., Slavin, R.E., and McQueen, J.D.: Radiation-induced intracranial malignant fibrous histiocytoma. *Cancer 37: 2960–2963, 1976.*
52. Lam, R.M-Y., and Colah, S.A.: Atypical fibrous histiocytoma with myxoid stroma. A rare lesion arising from dura mater of the brain. *Cancer 43: 237–245, 1979.*
53. Kyriakos, M., and Kempson, R.L.: Inflammatory fibrous histiocytoma. *Cancer 37: 1584–1606, 1976.*
54. Ferrer, I., and Aceves, J.: Cambios xantomatosos y contenido de melanina en tumores meningeos. Xanthomatous changes and melanin content in meningeal tumors. *Morfol. Normal Pathol. [B] 2: 531–539, 1978.*
55. Limas, C., and Tio, F.O.: Meningeal melanocytoma ("melanotic meningioma"). Its melanocytic origin as revealed by electron microscopy. *Cancer 30: 1286–1294, 1972.*
56. Steinberg, J.M., Gillespie, J.J., MacKay, B., Benjamin, R.S., and Leavens, M.E.: Meningeal melanocytoma with invasion of the thoracic spinal cord. Case report. *J. Neurosurg. 48: 818–824, 1978.*
57. Scott, M., Ferrara, V.L., and Peale, A.R.: Multiple melanotic meningiomas of the cervical cord. Case report. *J. Neurosurg. 36: 555–559, 1971.*
58. Ray, B.S., and Foot, N.C.: Primary melanotic tumors of the meninges: Resemblance to meningiomas. Report of two cases in which operation was performed. *Arch. Neurol. Psychiatry 44: 104–117, 1940.*
59. Abbott, M., Killeffer, F.A., and Crandall, P.H.: Melanotic meningioma. Case report. *J. Neurosurg. 29: 283–286, 1968.*
60. Keegan, H.R., and Mullan, S.: Pigmented meningiomas: An unusual variant. Report of a case with review of the literature. *J. Neurosurg. 19: 696–698, 1962.*
61. Bakody, J.T., Hazard, J.B., and Gardner, W.J.: Pigmented tumor of the central nervous system. *Cleve. Clin. Q. 17: 89–101, 1950.*
62. Turnbull, I.M., and Tom, M.I.: Pigmented meningioma. *J. Neurosurg. 20: 76–80, 1963.*
63. Russell, D.S., and Rubinstein, L.F.: *Pathology of Tumours of the Nervous System*, 4th ed. Baltimore, William & Wilkins, 1977, pp. 79–80.
64. Goldman, J.E., Horoupian, D.S., and Johnson, A.B.: Granulofilamentous inclusions in a meningioma. *Cancer 46: 156–161, 1980.*
65. Cushing, H., and Eisenhardt, L.: *Meningiomas. Their Classification, Regional Behaviour, Life History and Surgical End Results.* Springfield, Ill., Charles C Thomas, 1938, p. 175.
66. Kepes, J.: Observations on the formation of psammoma bodies and pseudopsammoma bodies in meningiomas. *J. Neuropathol. Exp. Neurol. 20: 255–262, 1961.*
67. Kepes, J.J.: The fine structure of hyaline inclusions (pseudopsammoma bodies) in meningiomas. *J. Neuropathol. Exp. Neurol. 36: 282–289, 1975.*
68. Buerger, L., and Scarpelli, D.G.: Intracellular duct formation in human breast cancer. *In Proceedings, Fifth International Congress for Electron Microscopy.* New York, Academic Press, 1962, Vol. 2, p. 12.
69. Wang, N.S.: Electron microscopy in the diagnosis of pleural mesotheliomas. *Cancer 31: 1046–1054, 1974.*
70. Berard, M., Tripier, F., Choux, R., Chrétien, A., Hassoun, J., and Toga, M.: Étude ultrastructurale des corps hyalins d'un méningeome pseudoepithelial. *Acta Neuropathol. (Berl) 42: 59–62, 1978.*
71. Moraci, A., and Cioffi, F.: La méningiome kystique. Aboutissement de la "forme humide" de Masson. *Neurochirurgie 22: 701–710, 1976.*
72. Masson, P.: *Tumeurs Humaines. Histologie Diagnostic et Ethniques*, 2nd ed. Paris, Maloîne, 1968, p. 980.
73. Cushing, H., and Eisenhardt, L.: *Meningiomas. Their Classification, Regional Behaviour, Life History and Surgical End Results.* Springfield, Ill., Charles C Thomas, 1938, pp. 26, 577–578.
74. Lake, P., Heiden, J.S., and Minckler, J.: Cystic meningioma. Case report. *J. Neurosurg. 38: 638–641, 1973.*
75. Henry, J.M., Schwartz, F.T., Sartawi, M.A., and Fox, J.G.: Cystic meningiomas simulating astrocytomas. Report of three cases. *J. Neurosurg. 40: 647–650, 1974.*
76. David, M., Guillaumat, L., and Askénasy, H.: Méningiome intraventriculaire. *Rev. Neurol. (Paris) 67: 504–514, 1937.*
77. Olivecrona, H.: The parasagittal meningiomas. *J. Neurosurg. 4: 327–341, 1947.*
78. Russell, D.S., and Rubinstein, L.J.: *Pathology of Tumours of the Nervous System*, 4th ed. Baltimore, Williams & Wilkins, 1977, p. 73.
79. Nauta, H.J.W., Tucker, W.S., Horsey, W.J., Bilbao, J.M., and Gonsalves, C.: Xanthochromic cysts associated with meningioma. *J. Neurol. Neurosurg. Psychiatry 42: 529–535, 1979.*
80. Rengachary, S., Batnitzky, S., Kepes, J.J., Morantz, R.A., O'Boynick, P., and Watanabe, I.: Cystic lesions associated with intracranial meningiomas. *Neurosurgery 4: 107–114, 1979.*
81. Banerjee, A.K., and Blackwood, W.: A subfrontal tumour with the features of plasmocytoma and meningioma. *Acta Neuropathol. (Berl.) 18: 84–88, 1971.*

82. Russell, D.S., and Rubinstein, L.J.: *Pathology of Tumours of the Nervous System*, 4th ed. Baltimore, Williams & Wilkins, 1977, pp. 80–81.
83. Horten, B.C., Urich, H., and Stefoski, D.: Meningiomas with conspicuous plasma cell–lymphocytic components. A report of five cases. *Cancer 43: 258–264, 1979.*
84. Stam, F.C., van Alphen, H.A.M., and Boorsma, D.M.: Meningioma with conspicuous plasma cell components. A histopathological and immmunohistochemical study. *Acta Neuropathol. (Berl.) 49: 241–243, 1980.*
85. West, S.G., Pittman, D.L., and Coggin, J.T.: Intracranial plasma cell granuloma. *Cancer 46: 330–335, 1980.*
86. Henderson, J.W., and Campbell, R.J.: Primary intraorbital meningioma with intraocular extension. *Mayo Clin. Proc. 52: 504–508, 1977.*
87. Fabiani, A., Trebini, F., Favero, M., Peres, B., and Palmucci, L.: The significance of atypical mitoses in malignant meningiomas. *Acta Neuropathol. (Berl.) 38: 229–231, 1977.*
88. Kepes, J., and Kernohan, J.W.: Meningiomas: Problems of differential diagnosis. *Cancer 12: 364–370, 1959.*
89. Kepes, J.J.: Differential diagnostic problems of brain tumors. *In Pathology of the Nervous System*, J. Minckler (ed.) New York, McGraw-Hill, 1971, pp. 2219–2238, Vol. II.
89a. Rubinstein, L.J.: Tumors of the central nervous system. *In Atlas of Tumor Pathology*. Washington, D.C., Armed Forces Institute of Pathology, 1972, fasc. 6, pp. 188–189.
90. Lapresle, J., Netsky, M.G., and Zimmerman, H.M.: The pathology of meningiomas. A study of 121 cases. *Am. J. Pathol. 28: 757–791 (Fig. 30), 1952.*
90a. Horoupian, D.S., Lax, F., and Suzuki, K.: Extracerebral leptomeningeal astrocytoma mimicking a meningioma. *Arch. Pathol. Lab. Med. 103: 676–679, 1979.*
91. Burger, P.C., and Vogel, F.S.: Surgical pathology of the nervous system and its coverings. John Wiley and Sons, New York, p. 93, 1976.
92. Kepes, J.J.: Cellular whorls in brain tumors other than meningiomas. *Cancer 37: 2232–2237, 1976.*
92a. Feigin, I.: Mixed mesenchymal tumors: Meningioma and nerve sheath tumor. *J. Neuropathol. Exp. Neurol. 37: 459–470, 1978.*
93. Fried, B.M.: Metastatic inoculation of meningioma by cancer cells from a bronchiogenic carcinoma. *Am. J. Pathol. 6: 47–52, 1930.*
94. Osterberg, D.H.: Metastases of carcinoma to meningioma. *J. Neurosurg. 14: 337–343, 1957.*
95. Best, P.V.: Metastatic carcinoma in a meningioma. *J. Neurosurg. 20: 892–894, 1963.*
96. Wilson, C.B., Jenevein, E.P., Jr., and Bryant, L.R.: Carcinoma of the lung metastatic to falx meningioma. Case report. *J. Neurosurg. 27: 161–165, 1967.*
97. Wilintz, A.H., and Mastri, A.: Metastasis of carcinoma of lung to sphenoidal ridge meningioma. Case report. *NY State J. Med. 70: 2592–2598, 1970.*
98. Györi, E.: Metastatic carcinoma in meningioma. *South. Med. J. 69: 514–517, 1976.*
99. Weems, T.D., and Garcia, J.H.: Intracranial meningioma containing metastatic foci. *South. Med. J. 70: 503–505, 1977.*
100. Hope, D.T., and Symon, L.: Metastasis of carcinoma to meningioma. *Acta Neurochir. (Wien) 40: 307–313, 1978.*
101. Fenyes, G., and Kepes, J.: Über das gemeinsame Vorkommen von Meningeomen und Geschwülsten anderen Typs im Gehirn. *Zentralbl. Neurochir. 16: 251–260, 19.*
102. Bernstein, S.A.: Über Karzinommetastase in einem Duraendotheliom. *Zentralbl. Allg. Pathol. 58: 163–166, 1933.*
103. Buge, A., Escourolle, R., Martin, M. Poirier, J., and Devoise, C.: Métastases cérébro-méningees d'un epitheliome du sein. Meningiomatose multiple. Intrication des deux processus. *Rev. Neurol. (Paris) 114: 308–312, 1966.*
104. Anlyan, F.H., Heinzen, B.R., and Carras, R.: Metastasis of tumor to second different tumor: Collision tumors. *JAMA 212: 2124, 1970.*
105. Theologides, A.: Tumor to tumor metastasis. *JAMA 219: 384, 1972.*
106. Di Bonito, L., and Bianchi, C.: Métastase d'un cancer mammaire dans un méningiome. *Sem. Hop. Paris 55: 171–172, 1979.*
107. Hockley, A.D.: Metastatic carcinoma in a spinal meningioma. *J. Neurol. Neurosurg. Psychiatry 38: 695–697, 1975.*
108. Zülch, K.J.: Biologie und Pathologie der Hirngeschwülste *In Handbuch der Neurochirurgie*, H. Olivecrona and W. Tönnis (eds.). Berlin-Göttingen-Heidelberg, Springer-Verlag, 1956, Vol. III, p. 589.
109. Störtebecker, T.P.: Metastatic hypernephroma of the brain from a neurosurgical point of view. A report of 19 cases. *J. Neurosurg. 8: 185–197, 1951.*
110. Peison, W.B., and Feigin, I.: Suprasellar meningioma containing metastatic carcinoma. Report of a case. *J. Neurosurg. 18: 688–689, 1961.*
111. Döring, L.: Metastasis of carcinoma of prostate to meningioma. *Virchows Arch. [Pathol. Anat.] 366: 87–91, 1975.*
112. Wu, W.Q., and Hiszczynskyj, R.: Metastasis of carcinoma of cervix to convexity meningioma. *Surg. Neurol. 8: 327–329, 1977.*
113. Rubinstein, L.J.: *Tumors of the Central Nervous System*, series 2. Washington, D.C. Armed Forces Institute of Pathology, 1972, Vol. 6, p. 321.
114. Chambers, P.W., Davis, R.L., Blanding, J.D., and Buck, F.S.: Metastases to primary intracranial meningiomas and neurilemmomas. *Arch. Pathol. Lab. Med. 104: 350–354, 1980.*
115. Smith, T.W., Wang, S.-Y., and Schoene, W.C.: Malignant carcinoid tumor metastatic to a meningioma. *Cancer 47: 1872–1877, 1981.*
116. Kuhn, C., and Askin, F.B.: The fine structure of so-called minute pulmonary chemodectomas. *Hum. Pathol. 6: 681–691, 1975.*
117. Worster-Drought, C., Carnegie Dickson, W.E., and McMenemey, W.H.: Multiple meningeal and perineural tumours with analogous changes in the glia and ependyma (neurofibroblastomatosis). *Brain 60: 85–117, 1937.*
118. Rubinstein, L.J.: *Tumors of the Central Nervous System*, Series 2. *Atlas of Tumor Pathology*. Washington, D.C., Armed Forces Institute of Pathology, 1972, Vol. 6, pp. 305–306.

119. Russell, D.S., and Rubinstein, L.J.: *Pathology of Tumours of the Nervous System*, 4th ed. Baltimore, Williams & Wilkins, 1977, p. 52.
120. Davis, R.L.: Case #4. Diagnostic Slide Seminar. American Association of Neuropathologists, San Juan, Puerto Rico, 1971.
121. Rhodes, R.H., and Davis, R.L.: An unusual fibro-osseous component in intracranial lesions. *Hum. Pathol. 9: 309–319, 1978.*
122. Clasen, R.A.: Case #6. Diagnostic Slide Seminar. American Association of Neuropathologists, Vancouver, B.C., Canada, 1981.
123. Bailey, P., and Bucy, P.C.: The origin and nature of meningeal tumors. *Am. J. Cancer 15: 15–54, 1931.*
124. Globus, J.H.: Meningiomas: Their origin, divergence in structure, and relationship to contiguous tissues in the light of the phylogenesis and ontogenesis of the meninges, with a suggestion of a simplified classification of meningeal neoplasms. *Res. Publ. Assoc. Nerv. Ment. Dis. 16: 210–265, 1937.*
125. del Rio-Hortega, P.: Nomenclatura y classificacion de los tumores del sistema nervioso. *Arch. Argent. Neurol. 24: 7–28, 1941.*
126. Kernohan, J.W., and Sayre, G.P.: *Tumors of the Central Nervous System*, series 2. *Atlas of Tumor Pathology.* Washington, D.C., Armed Forces Institute of Pathology, 1952, Vol. 35, pp. 97–117.
127. Courville, C.B.: *Pathology of the Central Nervous System.* [A study based on a survey of Lesions found in a thirty thousand autopsies.] Mountain View, Calif., Pacific Press, 1945, pp. 369–372.
128. World Health Organization. *Histological Typing of Tumours of the Central Nervous System*, K.J. Zülch (ed.). Geneva, WHO, p. 21, 1979.

CHAPTER 26

Electron Microscopy

Transmission Electron Microscopy

At the time of this writing, the study of meningiomas through the electron microscope is a little over 20 years old. Prior to that time, fine structure of the non-neoplastic meninges, including the arachnoid membrane of rats, had already been examined by Pease and Schultz,[1] a study to be amplified some years later by Waggener and Beggs[2] in their ultrastructural observations of the meninges of rats and guinea pigs.

Leventhal[3] was the first to present electron microscopic features of brain tumors at the Ninth Congress of Neurological Surgeons in 1959. He included meningiomas in his study, suggesting that meningothelial and fibroblastic cells could be distinguished in these neoplasms. This and other early works dealing with meningiomas centered on the more conventional meningeal and fibroblastic forms, as hemangiopericytomatous tumors of the meninges are relatively rare. Luse[4] studied a great variety of CNS tumors with the electron microscope, and she too included meningiomas in her work. These were of the meningotheliomatous form. That author was the first to call attention to the interdigitation of plasma membranes between neighboring meningioma cells, a pattern that causes the blurring of cell margins when viewed under the light microscope, and as a result is responsible for the syncytial appearance of some meningiomas. Luse went a step beyond this and recognized the importance of this particular electron microscopic finding in diagnosing a tumor as being a meningioma, even though the light microscopic features of such neoplasm may fall short of being pathognomonic. She illustrated this with the case of a poorly differentiated malignant tumor that by light microscopy resembled a fibrosarcoma, but that nevertheless had characteristic dovetailing of plasma membranes under the electron microscope, making the diagnosis of a meningioma possible. Luse's paper also included the first illustration of tonofibrils in the cytoplasm of meningioma cells.

Kepes[5,6] was the first to dedicate a study entirely to the submicroscopic structure of meningiomas. He examined 14 surgically removed meningiomas, 12 of which were meningotheliomatous and two fibroblastic by light microscopy. No significant difference was found between the cells of these two groups when viewed by the electron microscope. The presence of complex interdigitations of plasma membranes described the previous year by Luse was confirmed in all 14 cases. The cytoplasmic tonofilaments were given special emphasis; it was pointed out that they are the same structures that Romhanyi,[7] on the basis of his polarizing microscopic analysis of meningiomas, predicted would one day be found by ultrastructural studies. The work of Kepes included electron microscopic observations on the formation of psammoma bodies in meningiomas. It was shown that what appears as a homogeneous, hyalinized whorl, prior to calcification, in reality consists of a mixture of degenerating cytoplasmic organelles, amorphous intercellular material, and sometimes collagen fibers. This was also the first study to show that pockets of collagen in the tumor may be entirely surrounded by typical meningothelial cells, thereby strongly suggesting that the latter cells are capable of collagen production. The close apposition of young collagen fibers to the outer surface of the cell membranes, with the latter being focally indistinct, was also used in arguing for the fibroblastic potential of meningothelial cells. This effacement of the cell membrane in the vicinity of young collagenous and protocollagenous fibers, has also been observed by Koizumi,[8] Rascol,[9] and Choux *et al.*[10]

It was thus suggested by Kepes that not only do

meningothelial and fibroblastic meningioma cells have the same ultrastructural characteristics, but that cells that are certainly meningothelial under the light microscope are capable to assume the nature of connective tissue cells by virtue of producing collagen.

This unitarian view of the basic character of meningothelial and fibroblastic meningioma cells was in opposition to the original observations of Leventhal,[3] and came under strong attack from Raimondi *et al.*,[11] Gonatas and Besen,[12] and Koinov *et al.*,[13] all of whom felt that they could demonstrate a significant basic difference between fibroblasts and meningothelial cells in various types of meningiomas. The unitarian concept, however, was upheld and further strengthened by the observations of Gusek[14] in his study of 14 meningiomas, and by Napolitano *et al.*,[15] Koizumi,[8] Ishida *et al.*,[16] Rascol,[9] Rascol *et al.*,[17] Nyström,[18] Castaigne *et al.*,[19] Cervós-Navarro,[20] Cervós-Navarro and Vazquez,[21] Woyke *et al.*,[22] and Humeau *et al.*[23,24] in their respective studies.

While Luse and Kepes described dovetailing of plasma membranes in meningiomas, Gusek[14] was the first to observe desmosomes between neighboring meningioma cells. He has also observed the same type of intercellular junctions in the nonneoplastic arachnoid. Raimondi *et al.*[11] in the same year (independently) and Napolitano *et al.*[15] also nicely depicted desmosomes in meningiomas. Tani *et al.*[25] rendered careful analysis of specialized junctional complexes in meningiomas and found that they comprise, in addition to desmosomes, gap-(nexus) and tight (zonula occludens) junctions. In a subsequent paper, Tani *et al.*[26] specifically examined gap junctions of meningiomas with freeze-fracture studies. It has been suggested that gap junctions are widely implicated in intercellular communication between neighboring cells and that they permit ionic and metabolic coupling. In general, such junctions are more readily found in benign than in malignant tumor tissues. It is therefore perhaps not surprising that large numbers of them should be found in meningiomas.

Sipe[27] gave a very detailed electron-microscopic analysis of such gap junctions as observed in meningiomas maintained in organ culture. Copeland *et al.*[28] pointed to the presence of hemidesmosomelike intercellular specializations in meningiomas.

The nuclei of meningiomas often appear vacuolated or containing inclusion bodies by light microscopy (Fig. 25). Such intranuclear inclusions in meningiomas were first described by Wolf and Orton,[29] later confirmed by Russell *et al.*,[30] and were found in tissue cultures of meningiomas by Bland and Russell.[31] These same workers also differentiated between intranuclear inclusions and vacuoles. Inclusions were thought to be suggestive of viral activity, whereas vacuoles appeared optically empty and occurred in older cultures. Later Fischmann and Russell[32] found that the inclusions did not contain nucleic acid, and therefore concluded that the evidence did not support a viral nature of these inclusions.

Gusek[14] was the first to recognize under the electron microscope that the intranuclear inclusions contained cytoplasmic organelles, and therefore represented invaginations of cytoplasm into nuclei of meningioma cells. Gusek thought that, in contrast, intranuclear vacuoles were glycogen droplets, a view not confirmed by others.[22,33]

The most precise and detailed electron microscopic study of intranuclear inclusions and vacuoles in meningiomas was undertaken by Robertson.[33] He demonstrated how cytoplasmic organelles trapped within an intranuclear inclusion at times undergo degeneration. Nuclear vacuoles turned out to be loose areas in a chromatin-free region of the nucleus. Whereas cytoplasmic inclusions are surrounded by a membrane, vacuoles have no wall of their own. In addition to inclusions and vacuoles, Robertson also described less common intranuclear dense bodies. There is another constituent sometimes found in nuclei of meningioma cells. Cervos-Navarro and Vazquez[21] were the first to describe intranuclear sphaeridions in meningiomas, that is, collections of filamentous material.

While Gusek[14] found centrioles in some of the tumor cells in his meningioma material, Cervós-Navarro and Vazquez[33] were the first to observe cilia in 10 out of 14 endotheliomatous and in two out of three fibroblastic meningiomas. These authors found no cilia in angiomatous meningiomas but later Peña[35] demonstrated their presence in a hemangiopericytomatous meningeal tumor.

The existence of pinocytosis in meningiomas was emphasized by Cervós-Navarro and Vazquez.[21] These workers were also able to demonstrate some amorphous basement membrane material between meningothelial cells, as well as the occasional presence of mast cells in meningiomas.

Meningiomas do not possess a barrier between the lumen of their blood vessels and the tumor parenchyma, in contradistinction to the blood-brain barrier found within the CNS. A detailed ultrastructural study of blood vessels in meningiomas by Long[35] demonstrated that the absence of such a barrier is attributable to three factors: 1) widely open endothelial junctions, 2) marked pinocytosis in endothelial cytoplasm, and 3) fenestrated endothelial cells. Long[35] showed that protein-rich blood plasma material can easily escape through the open junctions of endothelial cells and become part of the extracellular space in the tumor. There is a striking similarity between this material, as illustrated in his article, and the granular basement membranelike substance often seen between neighboring meningioma cells, particularly but not exclusively in the hemangiopericytomatous forms. However, the same material has been shown in meningioma cultures in the absence of blood vessels by Horten *et al.*[37] Ermel[38] found a similar substance filling the lacunar system of meningiomas, and he believed that cells of a meningioma by rearranging themselves around such material may in time become newly formed blood vessels. This form of angiogenesis in meningiomas has not been confirmed by others, however.

With regard to calcification of psamomma bodies, Kepes[39] suggested that in addition to a whorling arrangement of tumor cells, they are secreting some type of PAS-positive material, which later may attract calcium. Nyström[40] believed he could demonstrate this material by electron microscope. Other authors[12,41] also devoted studies to the formation of psamomma bodies. An important contribution was provided by Lipper *et al.*,[42] who have followed the steps of calcium deposition in early psammomma bodies in cell cultures of meningiomas. They found that similarly to other types of calcifications under normal and pathologic conditions in the human body[43] matrix vesicles derived from the cytoplasm of a meningothelial cell in some instances preceded the deposition of calcium apatite crystals, although according to their studies, such crystals were found mostly outside the matrix vesicles. They also postulated that in addition to this mechanism, PAS-positive material, likely to represent glycoproteins and degenerating cellular organelles, may play a role in attracting calcium salts to the developing psamomma body.

That meningiomas which appear quite malignant under the light microscope might still retain their typical ultrastructural features was, as mentioned earlier, first realized by Luse.[4] This aspect of malignant meningiomas was reaffirmed through the findings of Ishida *et al.*[16] and Nyström,[18] in one case of Mena and Garcia,[44] and in the case of Pietruszka *et al.*[45]

As indicated earlier, Cushing and Eisenhardt[46] found what they called hyaline inclusions in a meningioma removed by the first author in 1913. These highly refractile, glassy-appearing inclusion bodies were described as being distinct from psamomma bodies. Light and histochemical features of such inclusions were analyzed in detail by Kepes.[39] (See Figs. 106–112). Kepes[47] was also first to describe the electron-microscopic appearance of these structures, which have since become well-known. In essence, these inclusions were found to occupy intracellular lumina, similar to structures previously described in breast carcinoma cells and in mesotheliomas, among others. These lumina are lined by microvilli, whereas the inclusions themselves consist of a granular proteinaceous material and masses of larger osmiophilic granules. Berard *et al.*[68] made further contributions to this matter in that they have shown that in addition to simple hyaline inclusions with fine granular material, a more complex form also exists that contains lamellar bodies, quite possibly—even likely—derived from the microvilli which eventually disintegrate and their membranous wall becomes part of the contents of the inclusion. It was pointed out that in the larger intracellular cavities, microvilli are no longer easily found in the lining. These workers also concluded that hyaline inclusions are likely to remain intracellular in every phase of their development. A glycolipid component was identified in the inclusion bodies by Font and Croxatto.[49]

Important observations regarding the submicroscopic structure of xanthomatous meningiomas were made by Ferrer and Aceves.[50] Rather than always having to invoke the presence of macrophages to account for xanthomatous elements in meningiomas, these investigators showed lipidic transformation of otherwise typical meningothelial cells themselves.

Electron microscopic studies of melanin-containing meningeal tumors were first undertaken by Limas and Tio,[51] who believed that these tumors are in essence melanocytomas of the meninges, and not true meningiomas. This view was also shared by Ferrer and Aceves[50] on the basis of the study of one of their melanocytic meningeal tumors.

Finally, with reference to still another type of intracellular material that could be studied under the electron microscope, Goldman *et al.*[52] described a new variant of granulofilamentous intracytoplasmic inclusion bodies (Fig. 105a,b), which when studied by electron microscopy, turned out to be composed of granular masses attached to tonofilaments, in turn connected to desmosomes.

Whether hemangiopericytic tumors of the meninges are related to meningiomas or are a separate breed by themselves, simply duplicating hemangiopericytomas elsewhere in the body, is a problem that has been extensively debated by light microscopists. With the advent of electron microscopy the debate spilled over into this territory, again with arguments both pro and con voiced in the debate. Ramsey[53] was the first to describe the submicroscopic features of an intracranial hemangiopericytoma in a 19-year-old man with recurrent frontal masses. She found that the tumor was composed of crowded cells with few processes, and the vessels in the tumor were surrounded by expanses of extracellular granular material, broader than the typical basement membrane associated with capillaries of the normal brain. Ramsey also found throughout the tumor septa made up of extremely fine fibrillary component and flocculent substance "rather like that of a basement membrane." Unlike the case of normal pericytes individually surrounded by basement membrane, there was no such membrane found between many adjacent individual tumor cells. The intricate interdigitation of plasma membranes, so characteristic of meningiomas, was not a prominent feature in this tumor. Popoff *et al.*[54] reported similar findings and stressed that unlike ordinary meningiomas, the intracranial hemangiopericytoma they studied had only weak desmosomes and half-desmosomes. There were fine filaments in the cytoplasm of tumor cells 60 to 80 Å thick, sometimes occurring in fascicles. These investigators believed that intracranial hemangiopericytomas are not meningiomas and should not be called by that name, as Cushing and Eisenhardt did when they listed this tumor as the type IV, variation 1 of meningiomas. Peña[35] examined a meningeal tumor of the hemangiopericytic type and found intracytoplasmic fusiform dense bodies as well as plaquelike bodies attached to the inner surface of the plasma membrane in the tumor cells. He thought these features represented leiomyomatous differentiation, consistent with the pericytic derivation of the tumor cells but contrary to meningothelial origin. Choux *et al.*[55] made essentially the same observations, stressing that in a typical case of intracranial hemangiopericytoma, they found no real desmosomes between cells, only zonulae adherentes, as well as filaments of 60–80 Å with some condensations. No interdigitation was seen between cells. Where the tumor cells were very close to each other, there was no basement membrane between them. Elsewhere, there were clusters of basement membrane material. There were many blood vessels present, often fenestrated. Goellner *et al.*,[56] in their cases of meningeal hemangiopericytomas, found nonspecific intracytoplasmic fibers in the tumor cells. No hemidesmosomes, pinocytosis, or myofilaments with dense bodies were encountered by these authors. They believed that the important features setting this type of tumor apart from meningiomas is the presence of 60 to 80-Å wide filaments with focal condensations in the cytoplasm, whereas meningiomas have filaments 80–100 Å wide. They claimed that conversely meningiomas lacked basement membranes, but show desmosomes and their thicker filaments have no condensations.

Horten *et al.*[37] took issue with all the above. They were not contesting the fact that meningeal tumors of hemangiopericytic character are histologically and biologically distinct entities. Nevertheless, they were able to show what they felt were transitions to meningothelial as well as fibroblastic meningiomas, both at the light and electron microscopic level. As to the latter, they felt that condensations of cytofilaments were not pathognomonic for hemangiopericytomas, because they were able to show such clumping of filaments in a transitional meningioma as well. They also found in hemangiopericytomatous tumors occasional cells containing abundant filaments 90–100 Å in diameter. Finally, although they agreed that in the tumor itself the cells were apposed to each other with only rare intervening cytoplasmic extensions and infrequent junctions consisting only of focal thickening of adjacent plasma membranes, nevertheless, when they grew such hemangiopericytic tumors on a Millipore filter, elaborate interdigitating cytoplasmic extensions did develop between cells. As to the granular floccular basement membrane-type material between tumor cells, they too have observed this in hemangiopericytomatous tumors, but then such accumulations are not uncommon between cells of meningothelial and fibroblastic meningiomas either.

As indicated in Chapter 25, Challa[57] and Mirra[58] independently observed the striking proliferation of pericytes within meningothelial meningiomas. The two cell populations were closely intermingled in Mirra's case (Fig. 203). The very loose and edematous type of meningioma, containing accumulations of both intra- and extracellular fluid first described by Masson as the humid form or *forme humide* was studied by Choux *et al.*[10] They found much lipid material related to lysosomal structures in the tumor cells

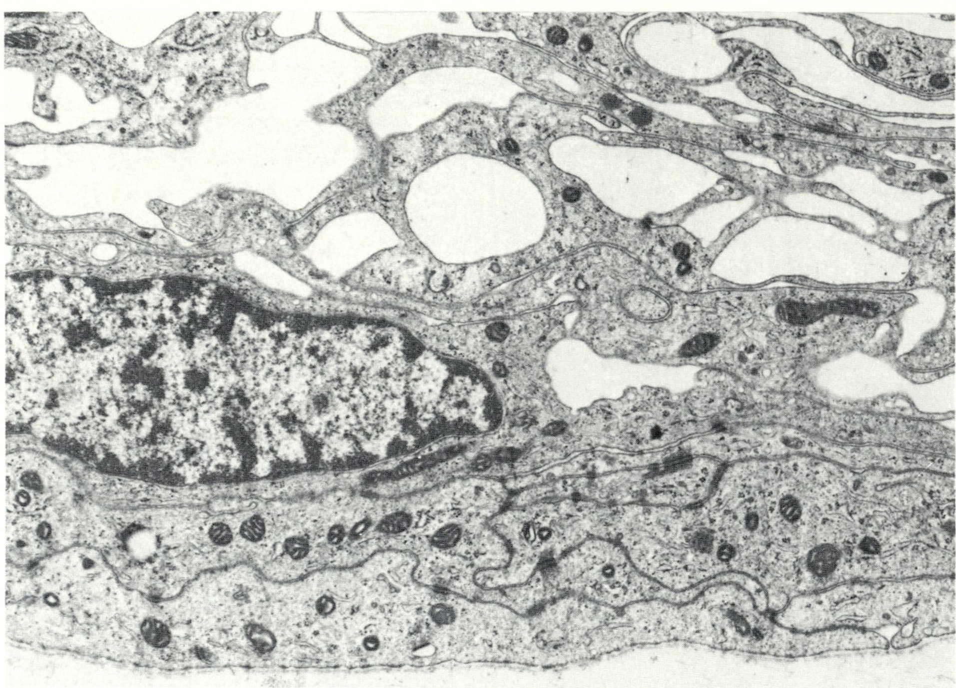

FIGURE 167
Normal arachnoid membrane biopsied during surgery. Several layers of flat, elongated cells are seen. *Top*, Cells are either closely appositioned to each other or have distended, cisternlike intercellular spaces between them. *Lowest five layers*, Cells are much more closely packed and exhibit more desmosomes than do the cells at the top. *Bottom*, a thin basal lamina separates the lower-most cells from the subarachnoid space. ×10,000. (Courtesy Dr. I. Watanabe.)

and in the extracellular spaces there were filaments of the proto- and precollagenous type, mixed in some areas with fibrin.

From the illustrations of Kleinman *et al.*,[59] it would appear that a very spongy microcystic pattern may develop in meningiomas by virtue of dilatation of the extracellular spaces only. This would indicate, then, that although light microscopically they look alike, there are two forms of humid meningiomas: one with enlarged extracellular spaces only, and the other, as described by Choux et al.[10] and also found in our own material (Figs. 204 and 205) containing fluid-filled distended spaces both intra- and extracellularly. Eimoto and Hashimoto,[60] who earlier observed similar cases, wondered if the distention of extracellular spaces may not represent pia-arachnoid differentiation within a meningioma.

OUR PRESENT OBSERVATIONS

In electron-microscopic studies of meningiomas of our own material accumulated since our original studies, we found many examples that we believe can be included here to illustrate our own findings as well as those of the literature.

The many close similarities between the submicroscopic structure of the normal arachnoid and that of meningiomas become evident if these two are compared. Figure 167 shows the ultrastructure of human arachnoid membrane removed during a neurosurgical operation in a patient who did not have a meningioma. A rather intricate interdigitation of neighboring cells may be observed, with some cells, particularly in the lower aspects of the arachnoid, lying closely apposed to each other. They are interconnected through many desmosomes and other intercellular junctions, whereas in the upper part of this membrane, the cells are not nearly as closely packed, and focal cistern-like spaces are seen between cells. Figure 168, representing a detail from a meningothelial meningioma, shows the interdigitation of cell membranes and desmosomal junctions, very like the ones seen in the normal arachnoid. Here, too, cells are either closely apposed to each other or permit the development of dilated cisternlike spaces. It is easy to

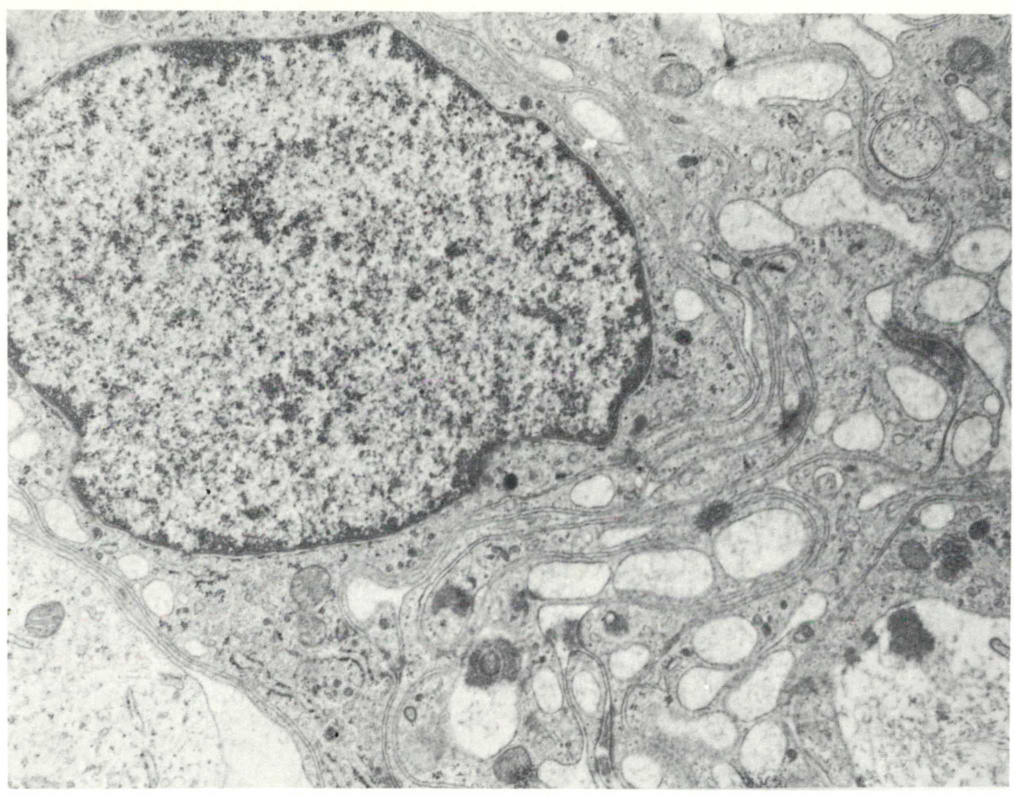

FIGURE 168
Detail from a meningothelial meningioma. Interrelationships of cells (close apposition with desmosomes in some areas, distended, cisternlike extracellular spaces in others), closely mimick the structure of the normal arachnoid as shown in Fig. 161. ×11,000.

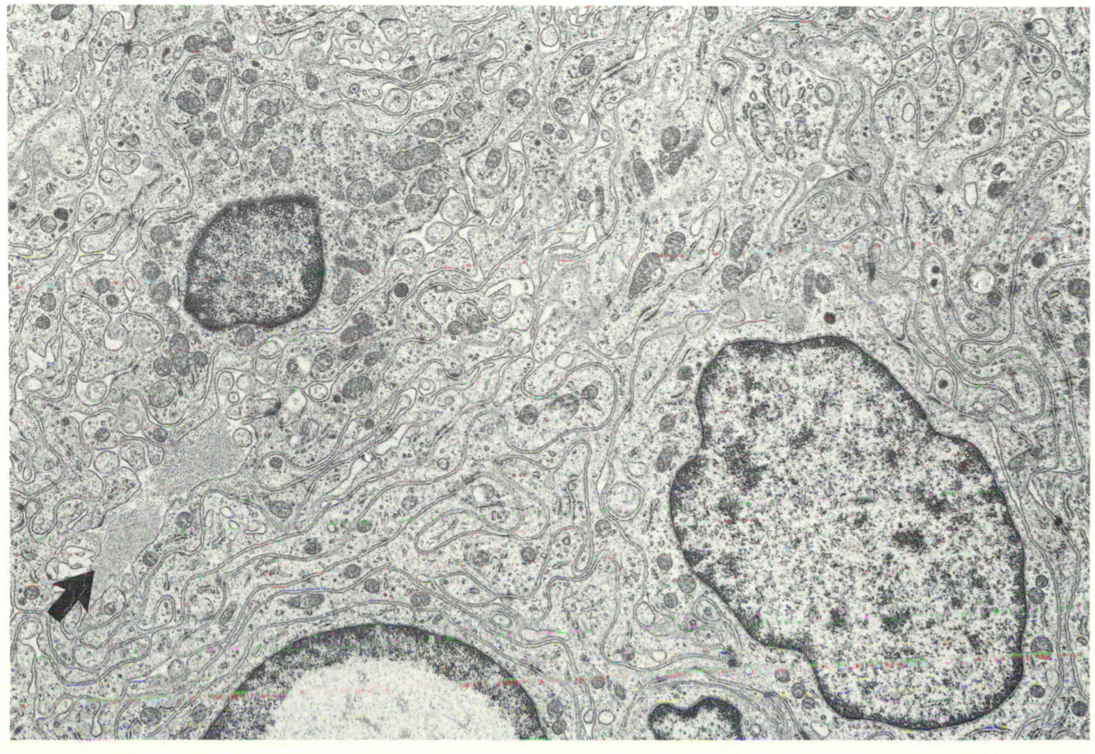

FIGURE 169
Syncytial meningioma. The intricate interdigitation of cell membranes creates a jig-saw puzzlelike appearance. Multiple desmosomes are seen, as well as granular material between neighboring cells (*left lower corner*, *arrow*). ×13,000.

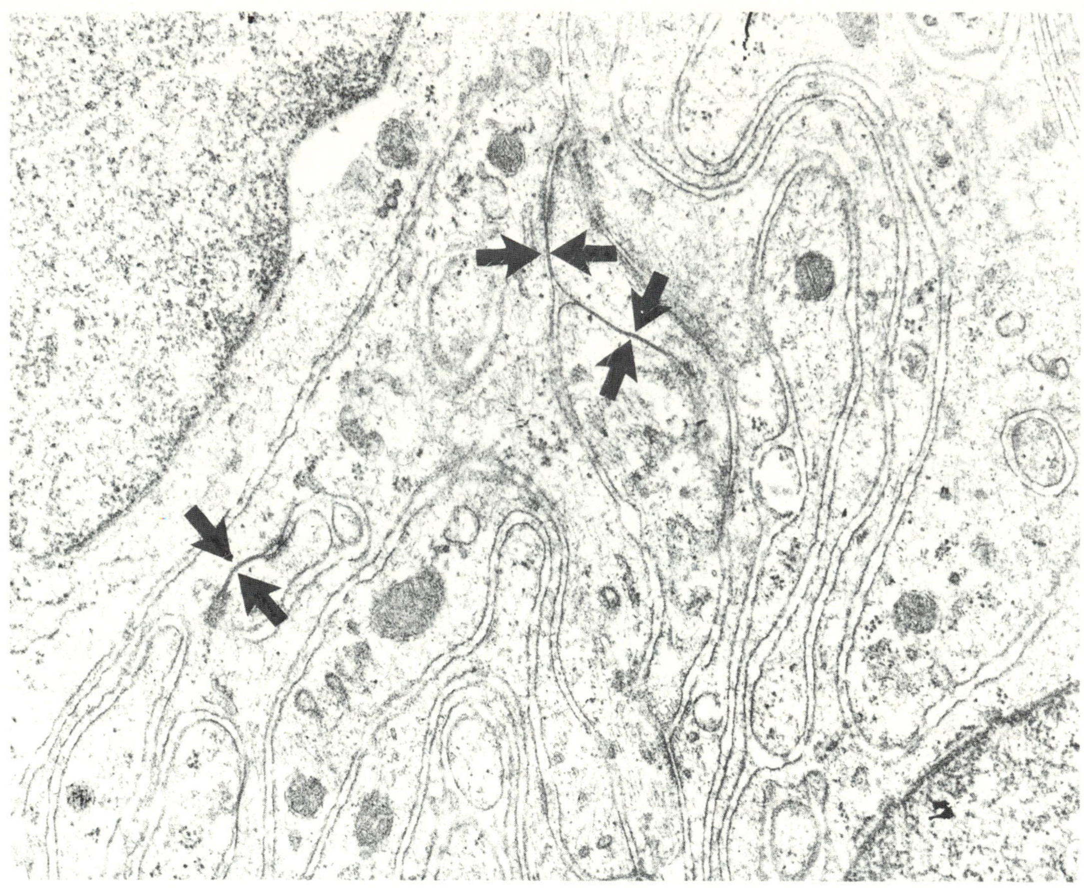

FIGURE 170
Higher-power view of interdigitating cell membranes with various types of plasma membrane differentiation. Three tight junctions are indicated (*arrows*). ×48,000.

see how cell borders become completely blurred under the light microscope when one observes the mazelike intricate interdigitations of cell membranes creating a veritable jigsaw puzzle in some meningiomas, as shown in Figure 169. Tight junctions, including desmosomes, gap junctions and zonulae adherentes mark the connections between these cells (Fig. 170). The formation of cellular whorls can also be followed under the electron microscope, with a tumor cell in some instances forming the center of the whorl. It is just as possible to find a capillary assuming the role of the central structure of a cellular whorl (Fig. 171). Tonofilaments that sometimes reach considerable thickness in the cytoplasm are depicted in Figure 172, whereas the finer details of a desmosomal attachment between neighboring tumor cells are shown in Figure 173. We found cilia in some, but not all, of the meningiomas examined. Most of the time, as in Figure 174, rather than protruding from its surface, they were deeply ensheathed within the cytoplasm of the tumor cell. Scattered aggregates of extracellular osmiophilic granular–floccular material were observed in many of the meningiomas we examined, including meningothelial fibroblastic and hemangiopericytic types. Figure 175 shows this material accumulating in clumps and flecks between some neighboring tumor cells, whereas other cells maintain their close adherence to each other without the presence of such material between them. On higher power the relationship of this granular material to the cell membranes is seen. It appears that in places where the material is in close apposition to the outer surface of the cell membrane, there is frequently a plaquelike electron-dense condensation on the cytoplasmic side of the membrane (Figs. 176 and 177).

Figure 177 also shows the beginning of the for-

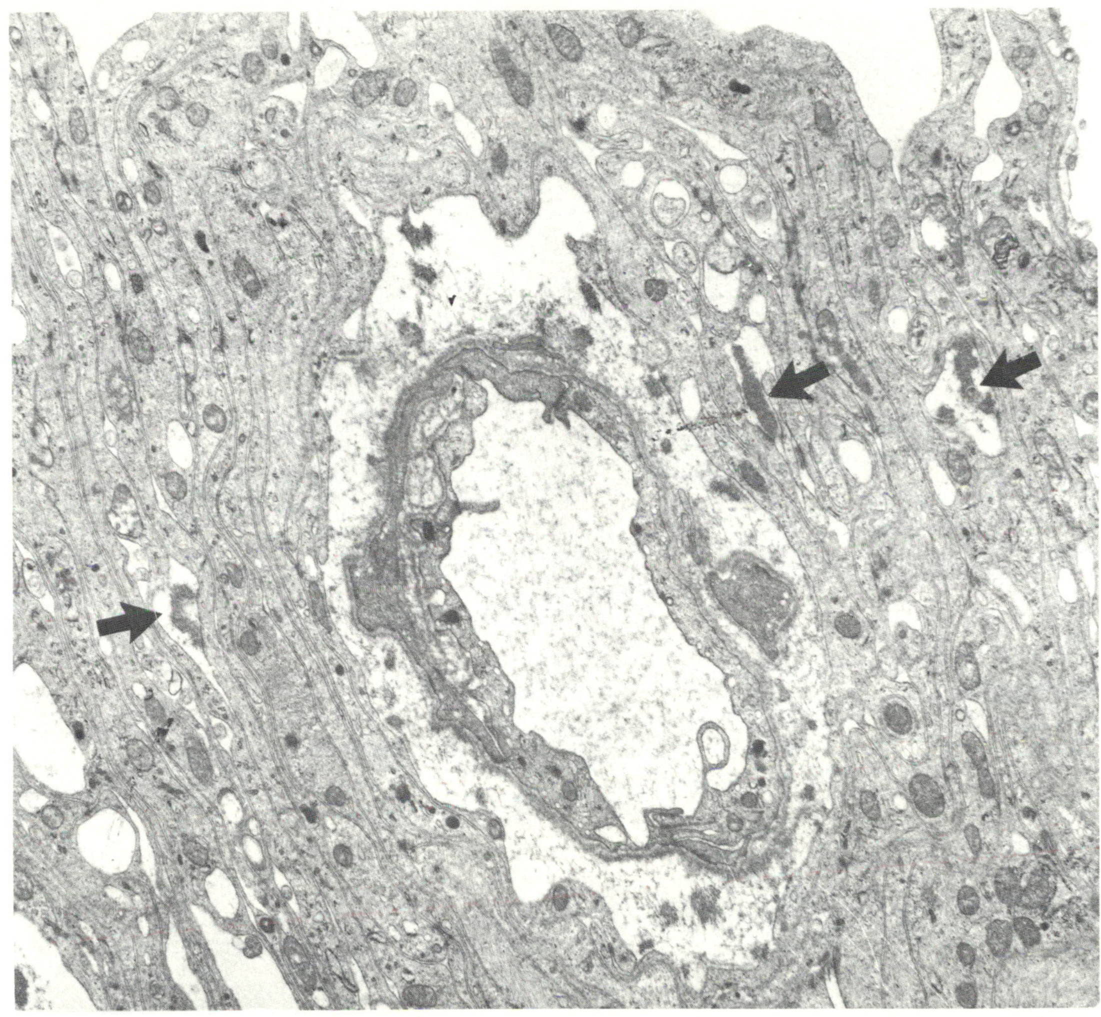

FIGURE 171
Concentric arrangement of meningothelial tumor cells around a small blood vessel. The innermost layer of tumor cells is separated from the basement membrane of the blood vessel by amorphous granular material, similar to that seen farther to the left and right between neighboring tumor cells (*arrows*). ×4,600.

mation of filamentous material in close relationship to the granular substance attached to the outer cell walls. In many instances neighboring tumor cells permitted the formation of fibrillary and granular material between them (Figs. 178 and 179). This area contains, in addition to granular substance, fine and coarse filaments corresponding to protocollagen and more mature collagen fibers. These three components (granular material, fine filaments, and collagen with well-developed cross-banding) are depicted in Figure 180, in which the apparent effacement between plasma membrane and these filamentous structures as observed by Kepes[6] and other authors in the past, is discernible. Whereas cells bordering these enclosures with granular material and collagen fibers do not always show morphological evidence of ongoing protein production, every once in awhile, as in Figure 181, this is strongly suggested by distended cisterns of rough endoplasmic reticulum within the tumor cells, a feature often seen in fibroblasts actively engaged in the synthesis of collagen fibers.

What appears by light microscopy as homogeneous hyaline material in the center of degenerating whorls, can be seen to contain a conglomerate

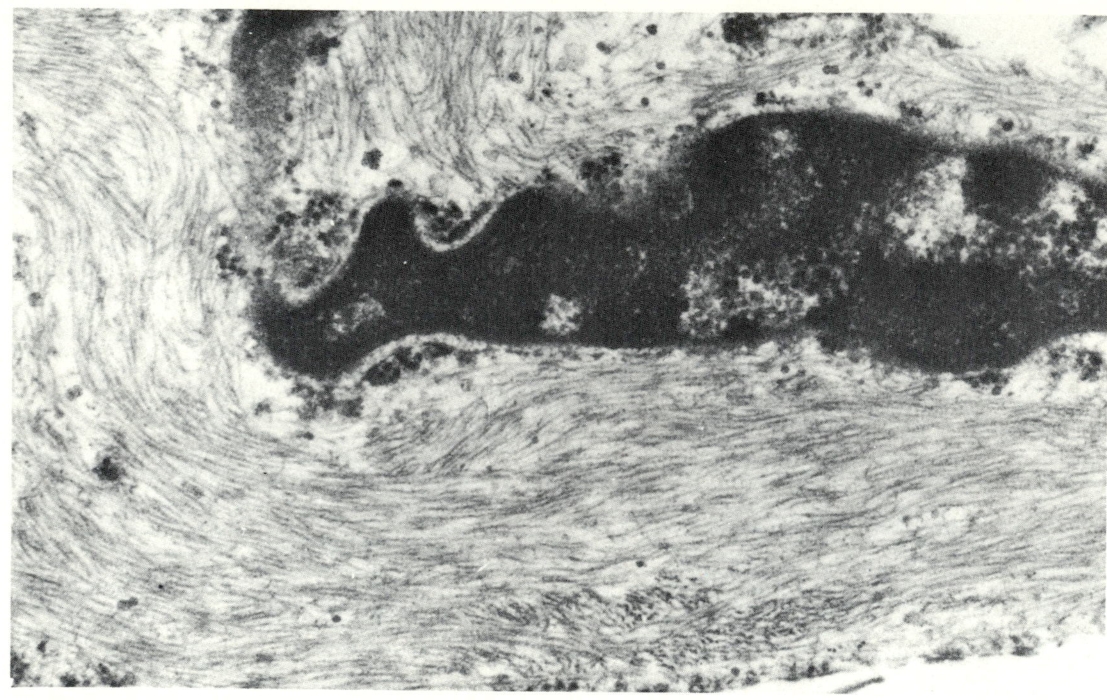

FIGURE 172
High-power view of tumor cell in a meningioma. The nucleus is elongated the nuclear membrane slightly undulating. Bundles of rather thick (80–100-Å) filaments are present in the cytoplasm. ×44,000.

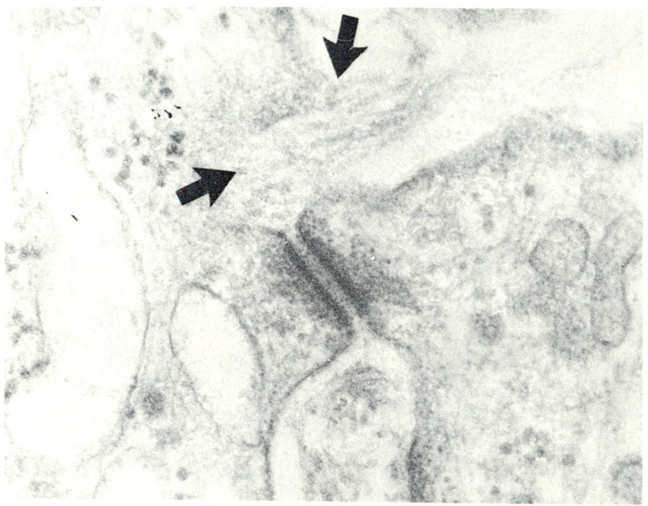

FIGURE 173
At a point of junction between two neighboring cells, a clearly defined desmosome is seen. Elsewhere the cell membrane is indistinct and (particularly at *upper half, arrow*) appears to blend with collagen fibers. ×52,000.

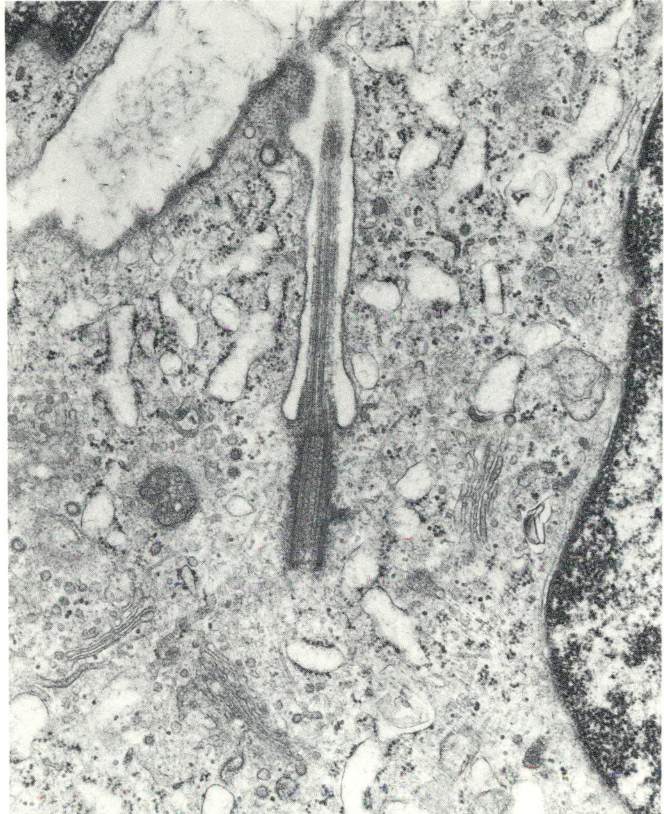

FIGURE 174
A fully developed cilium is shown in this meningothelial tumor cell. This organelle is entirely ensheathed, that is its tip is not protruding beyond the cell membrane. Profiles of endoplasmic reticulum and of Golgi apparatus are also seen. ×26,000.

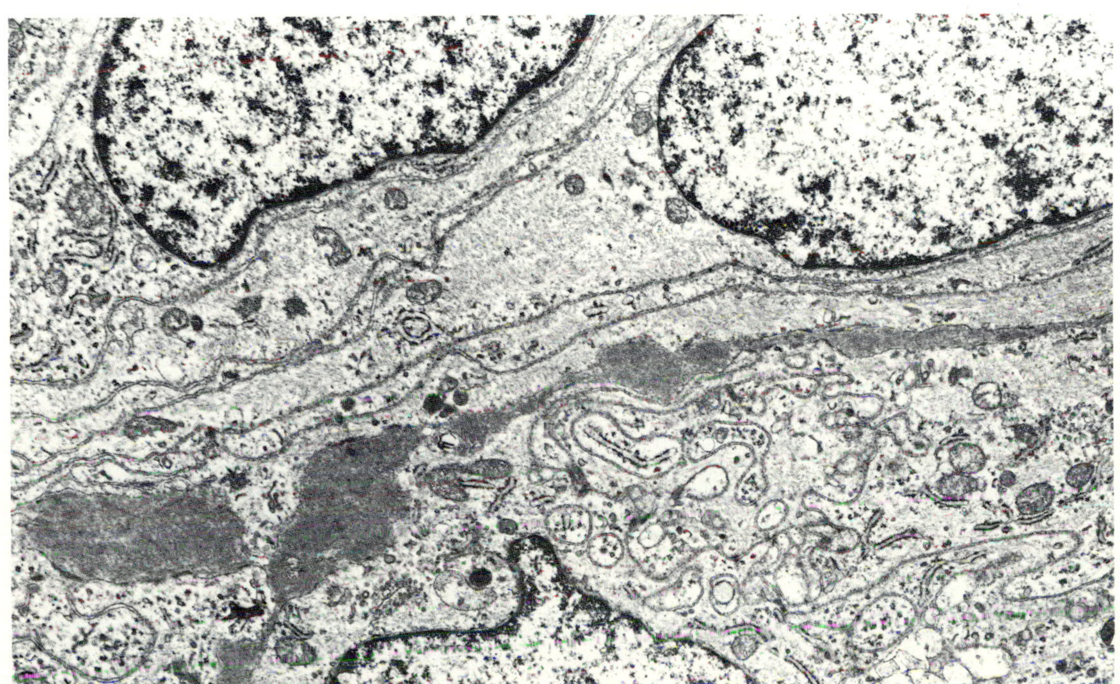

FIGURE 175
In this meningothelial meningioma some cells are closely appositioned with virtually no extracellular space separating them, but the irregular deposits (*center*) of granular-floccular material separate two neighboring cells from each other. ×12,000.

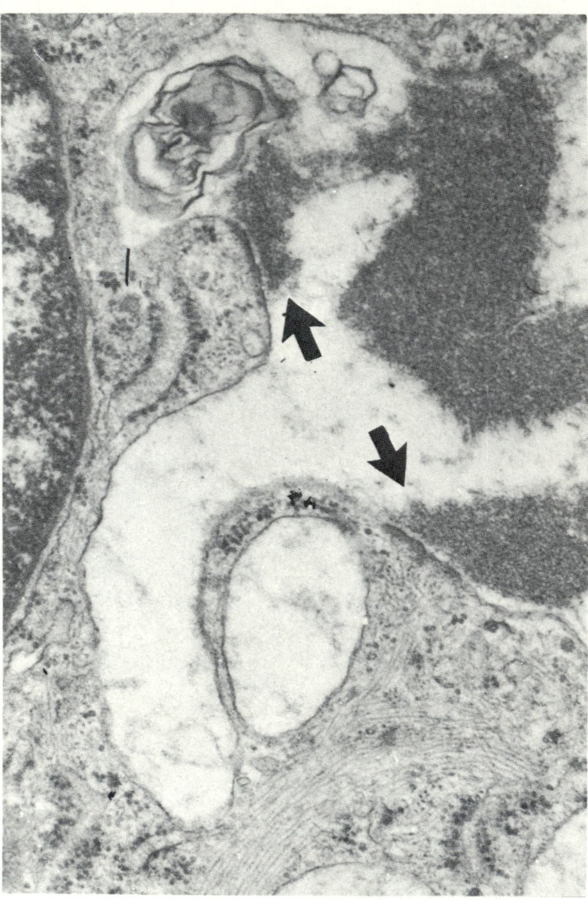

FIGURE 176
Extracellular granular material is in close proximity to the outer surface of the cell membrane in two areas (*arrows*), both marked with plaquelike thickening on the cytoplasmic side of the cell membrane. ×36,000.

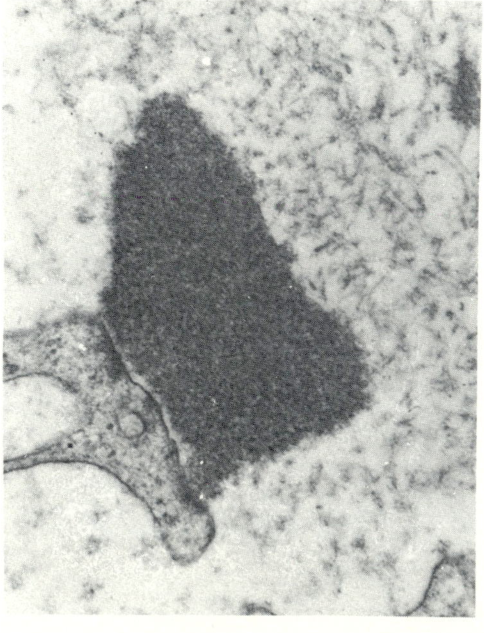

FIGURE 177
Another area of attachment between extracellular granular material and cell membrane. To the right side of the granular deposit, and in continuity with it, material of more fibrillary character is seen corresponding to protocollagen fibers. ×38,000.

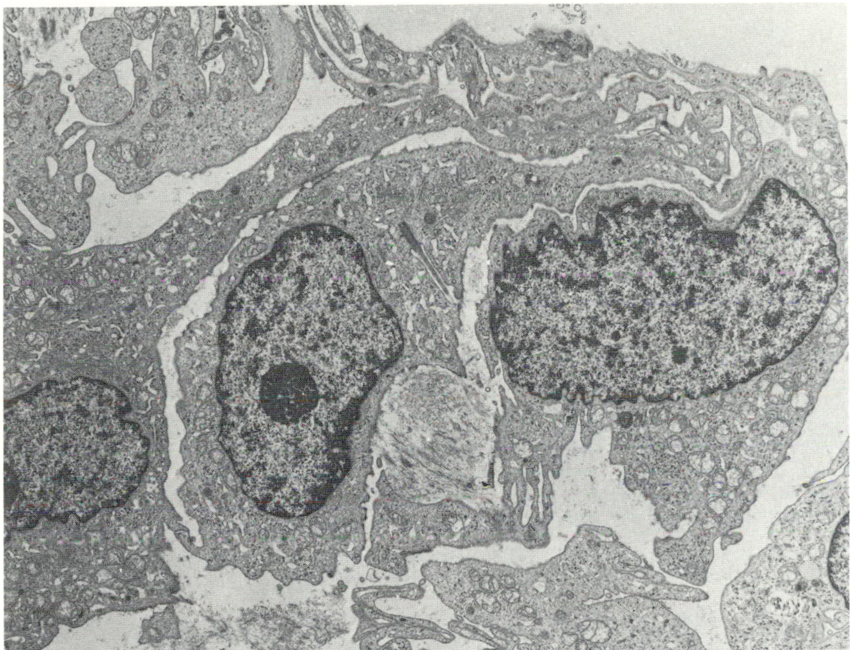

FIGURE 178
Low-power electron micrographic view of two neighboring meningioma cells with a small pocket of extracellular space enclosed by them. ×6,000.

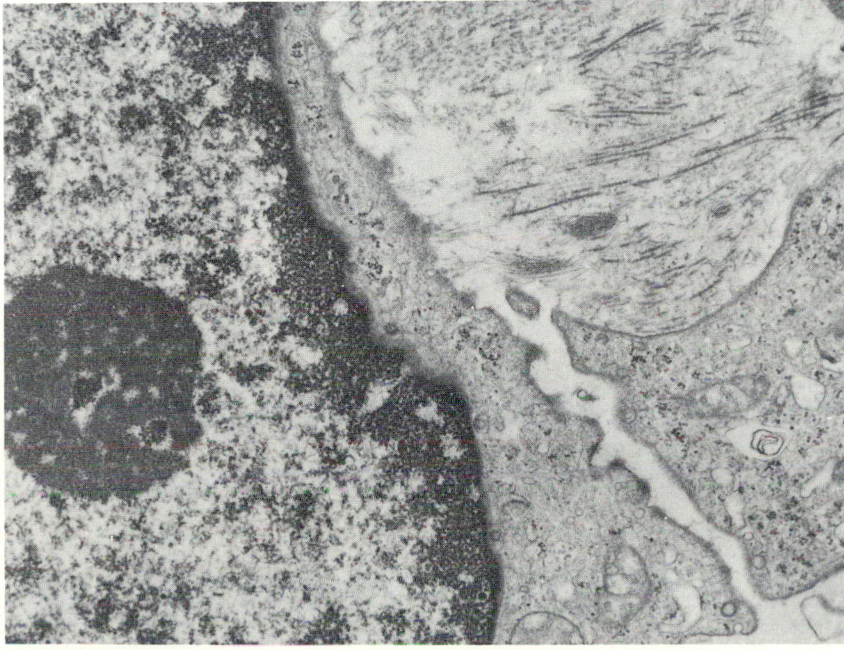

FIGURE 179
Higher-power of Figure 12 shows that the enclosure contains fibers of varying diameters. The thinner ones (left, *enclosure*) appear to be continuous with the plasma membrane of the tumor cell. ×19,000.

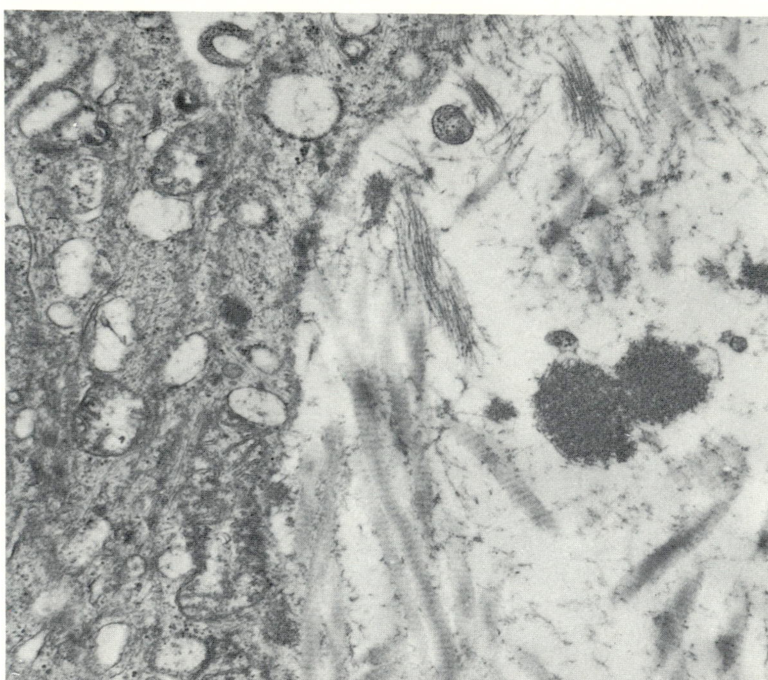

FIGURE 180
High-power view of another enclosure with granular material, protocollagen, and well-developed collagen fibers with 640 Å cross-banding. The plasma membrane is focally indistinct and in the upper portion of the picture seems to blend with perpendicularly arranged, fine extracellular fibers. ×32,000.

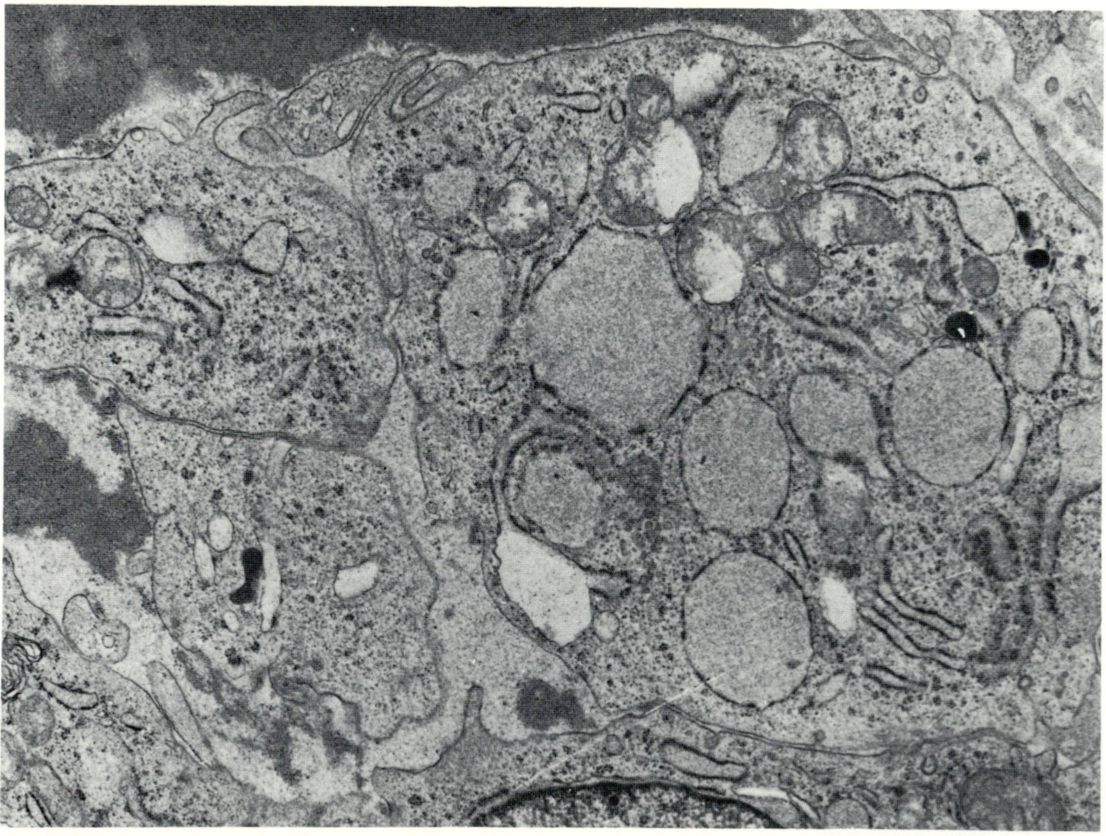

FIGURE 181
In another meningioma, the cells surrounding the spaces with granular material have some characteristics of active fibroblasts with distended rough endoplasmic reticulum. ×15,000.

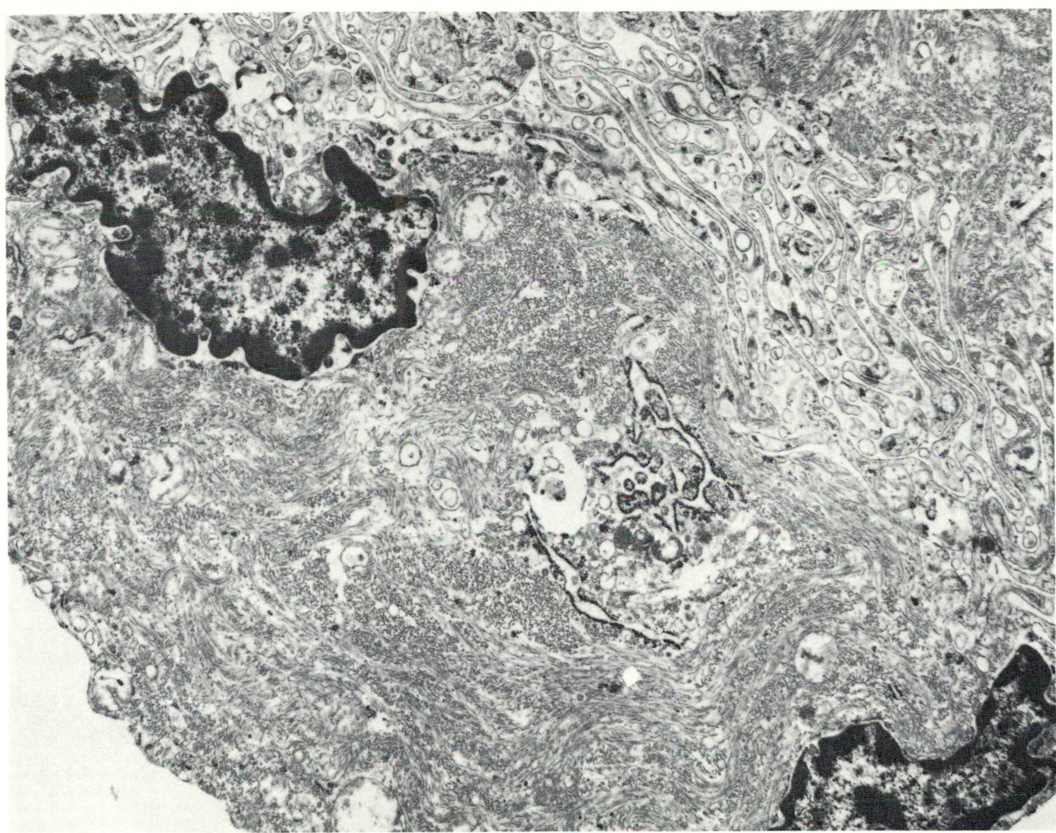

FIGURE 182
A low-power view of a cellular whorl with a hyalinized center. The latter area, which appeared homogeneous by light microscopy, contains fibrillary material as well as broken up fragments of ergastoplasm. ×12,500.

of filamentous and fibrillary material as well as fragments of cytoplasmic organelles. In Figure 182, these are represented by broken up remnants of rough endoplasmic reticulum, no longer surrounded by a cell membrane. The intermingling of fibrillary material and what appear to be previous lysosomal components, as well as degenerating mitochondria, are shown in Figure 183. Lipper,[42] who has studied psammoma body formation in tissue cultures of meningiomas, kindly contributed Figure 184, which shows the appearance of calcium apatite crystals in close relationship to membrane bound vesicles considered to represent matrix vesicles that are derived from the body of neighboring meningothelial tumor cells.

The origin of intranuclear cytoplasmic inclusions can be well followed in Figures 185 and 186, the former with a peninsulalike invagination of the cytoplasm into the nucleus, the latter with total intranuclear encasement still showing cytoplasmic organelles, which permit the viewer to identify the inclusion as being derived from the cytoplasm. By contrast, simple nuclear vacuoles (Fig. 187) have no delineating membrane and consist merely of fine floccular material with no further identifying marks. Cytoplasmic inclusions and intranuclear vacuoles may coexist within the same nucleus, as shown in Figure 188, whereas dense osmiophilic inclusions, as originally described by Robertson,[33] may also be seen in some nuclei (Fig. 189). Finally, intranuclear structures composed predominantly of filamentous material and corresponding to the sphaeridions, shown to occur in the meningiomas by Cervós-Navarro and Vazquez[21] are shown in Figure 190a,b.

Tumor cells in meningiomas are often seen engaged in active pinocytosis (Fig. 191). Every once in awhile, one encounters within meningiomas mast cells with their characteristic heparin granules, but with no apparent relationship to the main tumor cells (Fig. 192).

Hyaline inclusions, or pseudopsamomma bodies,

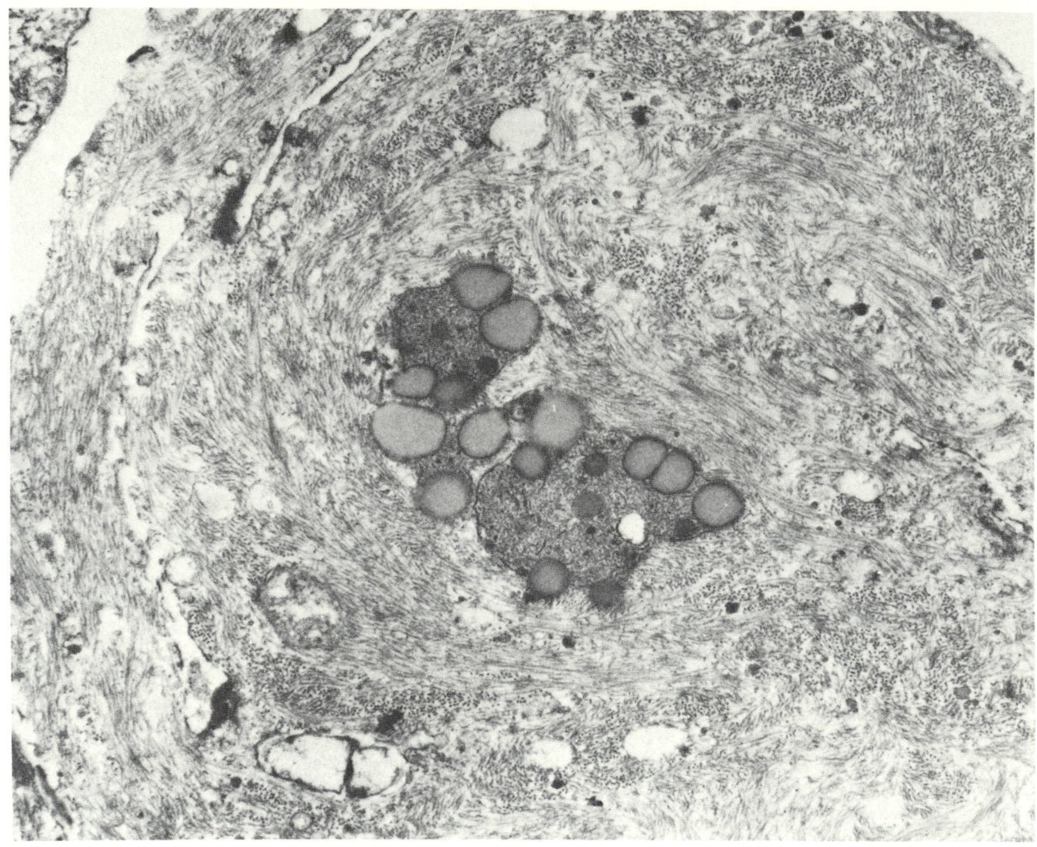

FIGURE 183
Distended, degenerated mitochondria are seen at periphery and osmiophilic round vesicles, probably remnants of lysosomal structures, are present in the center of this whorl. ×26,000.

the light-microscopic features of which have been discussed earlier (see Figs. 106–112) appear under the electron microscope as single or multiple intracellular inclusions (as many as eight inclusions in a single tumor cell are shown in Fig. 193). In simpler forms they are composed of granular moderately osmiophilic material, situated within an intracellular ductulelike cavity, which in turn is lined by microvilli (Fig. 194). The microvilli themselves appear to contain the same granular material as the one present within the lumen (Fig. 195) and in some instances a direct continuity between the intra- and extravillous portion of this material can be established (Fig. 196). Intracellular spaces containing this granular material are often surrounded in the nearby cytoplasm by dense aggregates of tonofilaments (Fig. 197). As Berard *et al.*[48] have observed, in what appears to be a more advanced stage of these inclusions, the microvilli lining the cavities eventually undergo fragmentation and become part of the contents of the cavity (Fig. 198) as circular profiles or multilamellar bodies mixed in with the original granular material of the hyaline inclusion.

Those of our tumors that showed the classical light-microscopic features of hemangiopericytomatous meningiomas, showed a submicroscopic structure described by earlier authors: closely packed tumor cells with few poorly developed cellular processes (Fig. 199). A granular basement membranelike material is present in many areas of the tumor, sometimes also between neighboring tumor cells, but at the same time there are many closely appositioned cells without such material intruding between the neighbors (Fig. 200). Interestingly, however, some attempts of whorl formation or at least nuclear molding may be detected between neighboring cells, as shown in Figure 200. In most instances no desmosomes or other tight junctions are observed between neighboring tumor cells (Fig. 201). Condensations of intracytoplasmic filaments giving rise to dense bodies, similar to

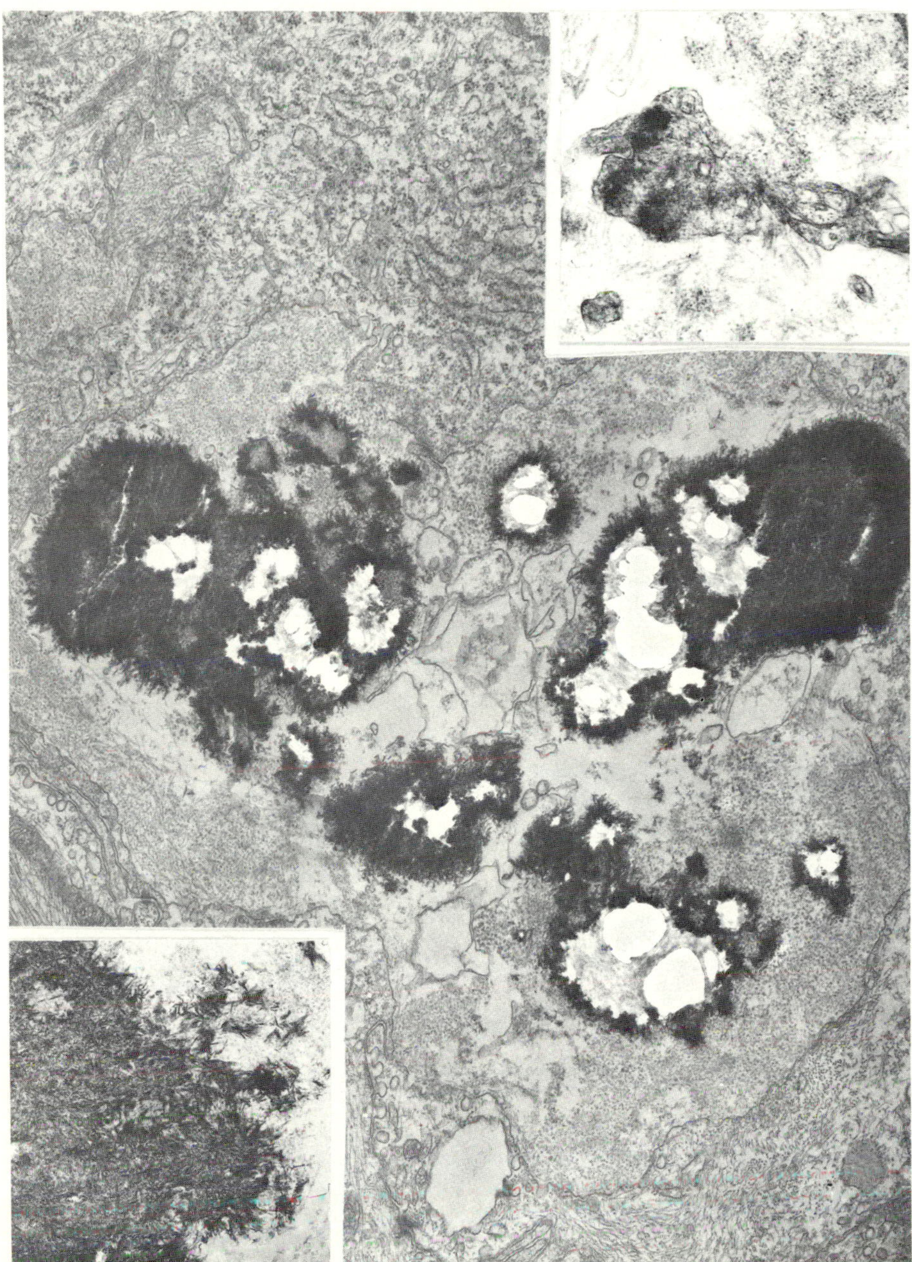

FIGURE 184
Psamomma body that formed in a tissue culture of meningioma cells. Central enclosure surrounded by tumor cells contains distended vesicles and deposition of calcium apatite crystals. ×13,200. *Upper right insert*, Club-shaped cytoplasmic process with apparent intracytoplasmic depositions of calcium. ×16,050. *Lower left insert*, Needlelike hydroxyapatite crystals. ×14,040. (Courtesy Dr. Lipper.)

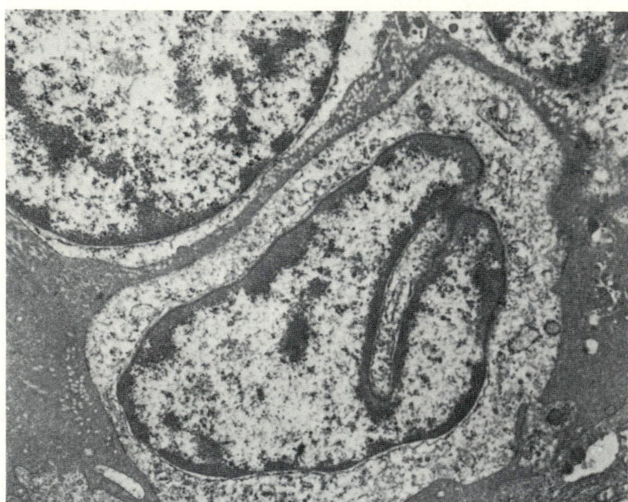

FIGURE 185
This figure shows the mechanism of the development of intracellular cytoplasmic inclusions. The cytoplasm is protruding into the nucleus in the form of a peninsula. The connections to the remaining cytoplasm, however, are still clear. ×8,000.

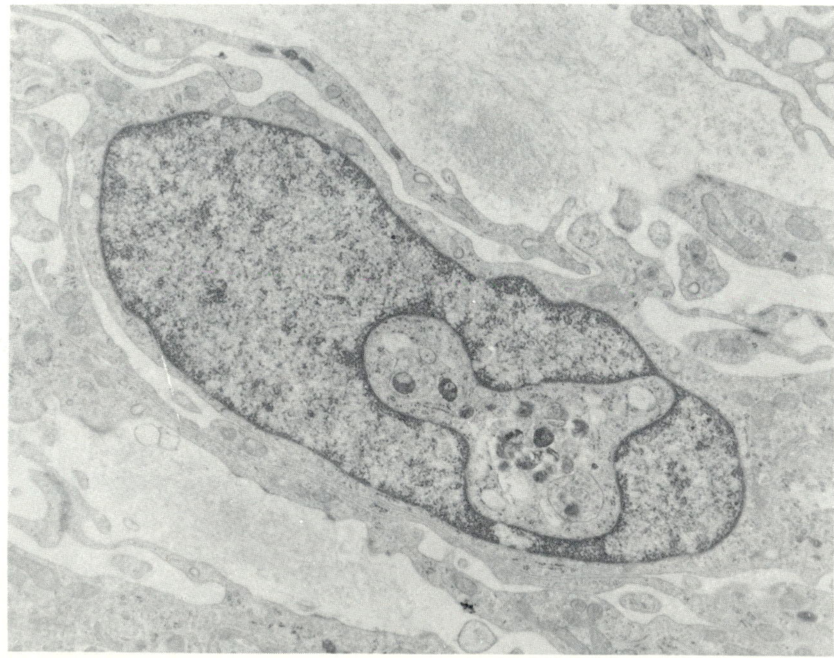

FIGURE 186
This intranuclear cytoplasmic inclusion appears to be totally isolated from the surrounding cell body. It contains various cytoplasmic organelles. ×11,000.

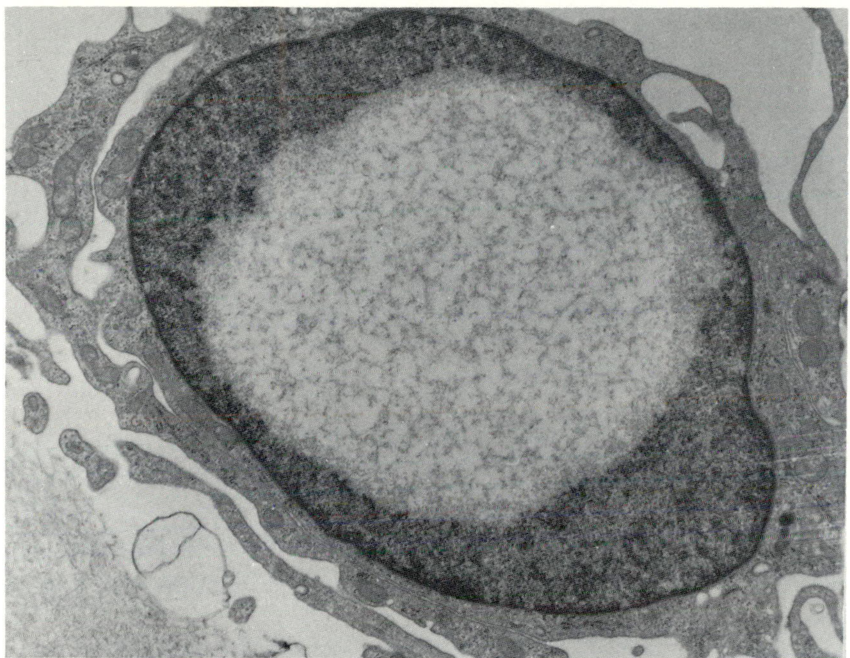

FIGURE 187
Intranuclear vacuole. This is an area of the nucleus not delineated by any particular membrane and contains loosely arranged floccular material. ×11,000.

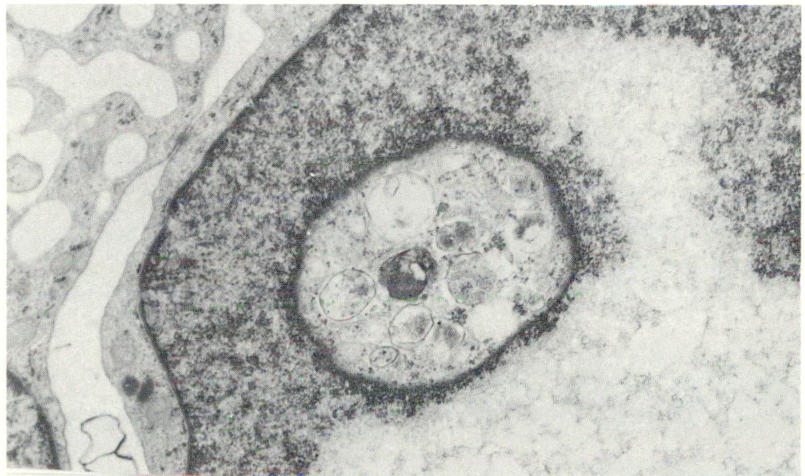

FIGURE 188
A cytoplasmic inclusion (*left*) and simple vacuole (*right*) are seen side by side in the same nucleus. ×42,000.

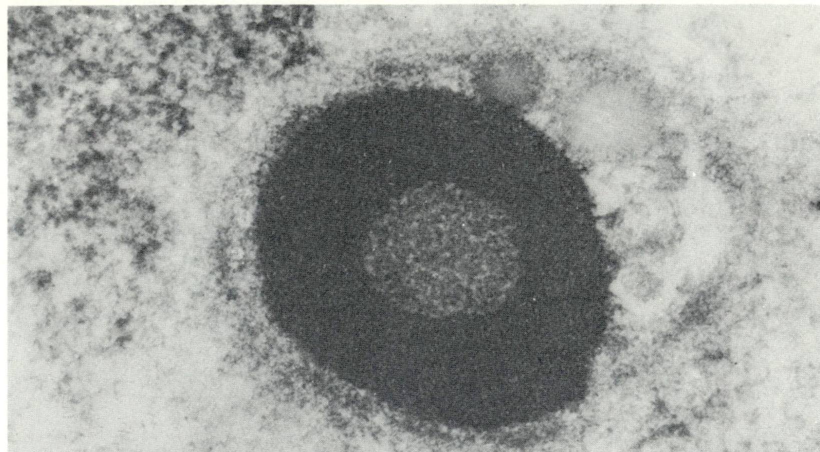

FIGURE 189
Still another intranuclear inclusion in the form of a dense, concentric body. ×52,000.

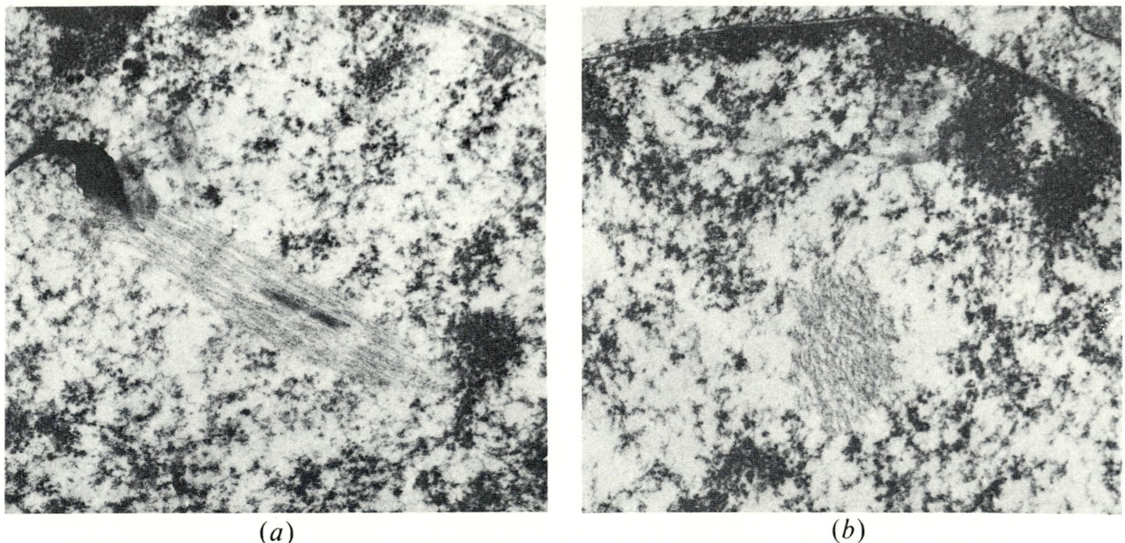

(*a*) (*b*)

FIGURE 190
Intranuclear filamentous inclusions (sphaeridions). (*a*) Longitudinal profiles. (*b*) Cross section of filaments. ×56,000.

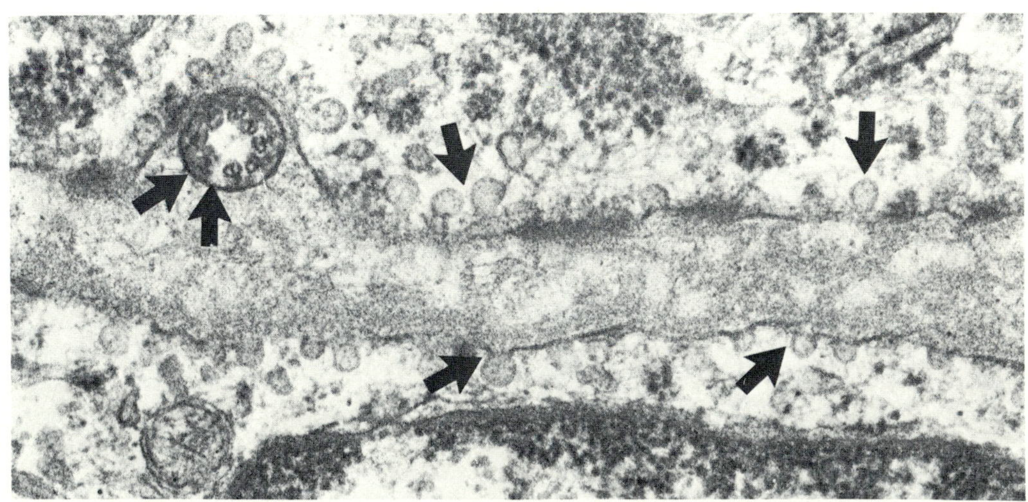

FIGURE 191
Cell borders of two neighboring meningothelial tumor cells showing large numbers of pinocytotic vesicles (*arrows*) at their respective interface with extracellular granular material. *Double arrow*, Cross section of a cilium. ×26,000.

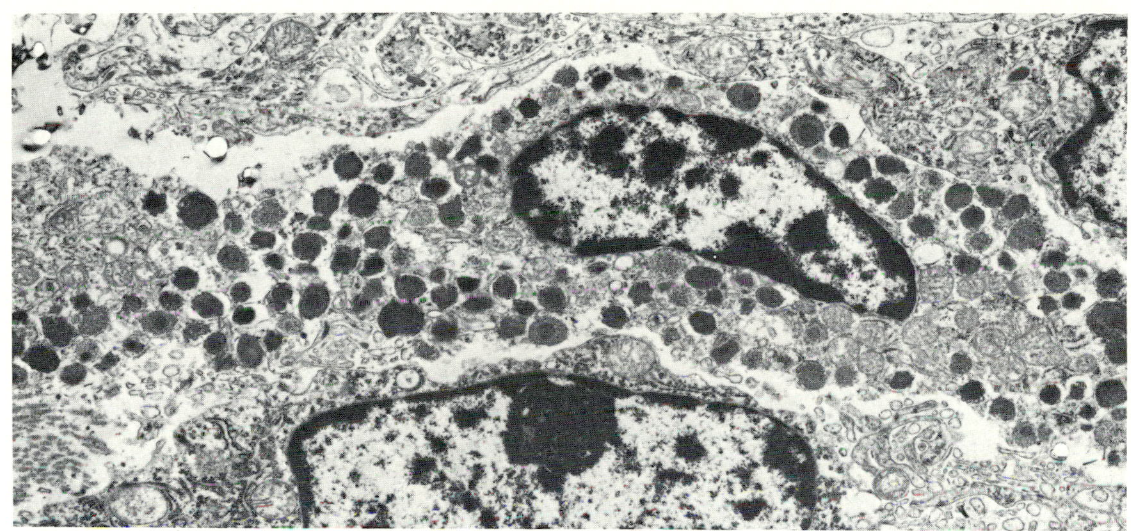

FIGURE 192
A slender mast cell with characteristic heparin granules has insinuated itself between two neighboring meningothelial tumor cells. ×9,000.

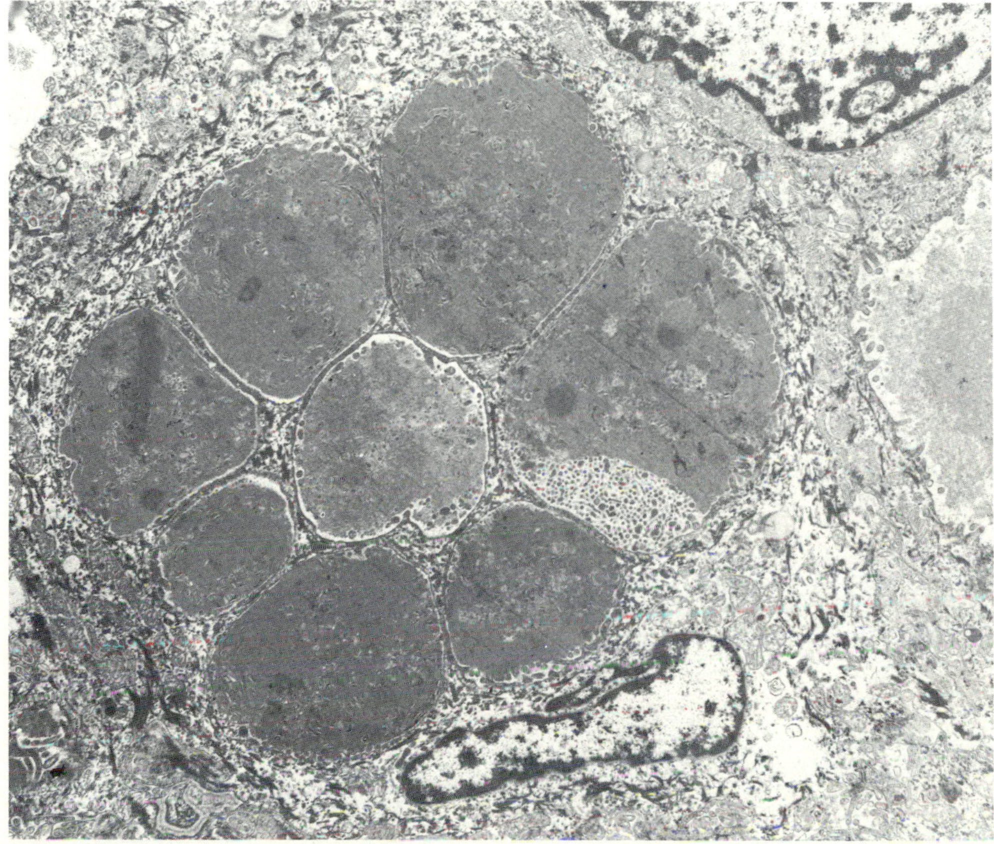

FIGURE 193
Hyaline inclusions (pseudopsamomma bodies) in a meningioma: Eight small intracellular inclusions are seen, with half of an inclusion in the neighboring cell (*right*). ×10,000.

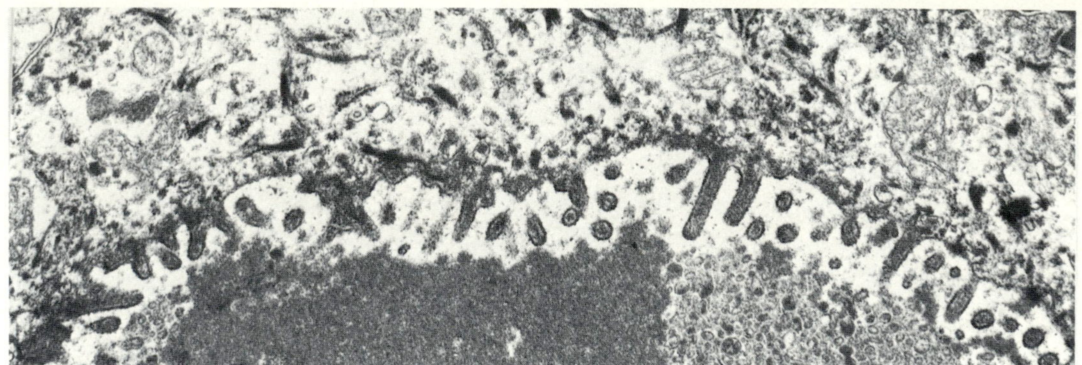

FIGURE 194
The cavities containing the inclusion bodies are lined by microvilli of varying lengths. ×22,000.

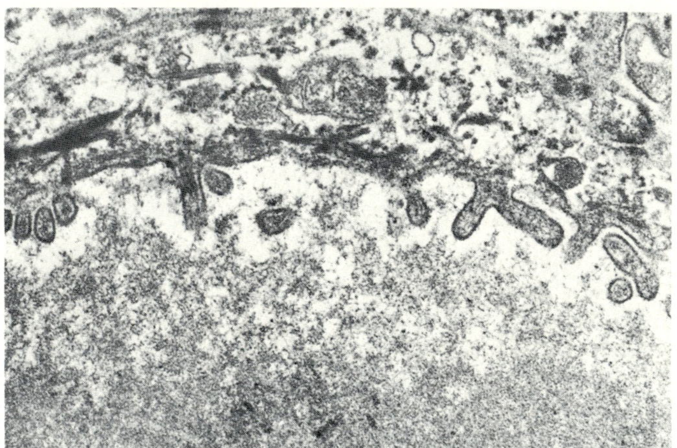

FIGURE 195
Microvilli contain the same type of granular material as the inclusion. ×36,000.

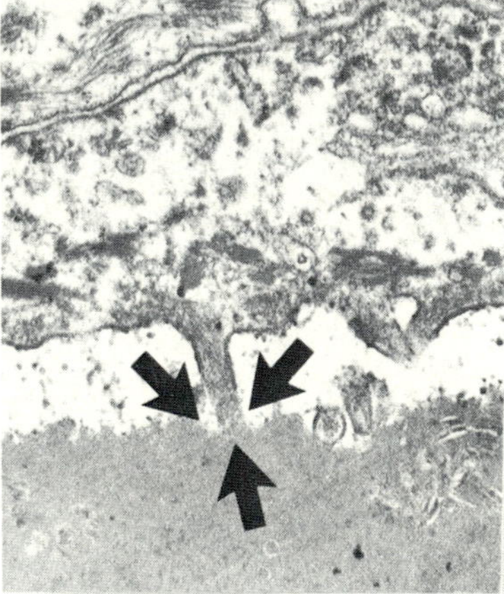

FIGURE 196
This illustrates the continuity between the contents of a microvillus and the substance of the inclusion (*arrows*). ×36,000.

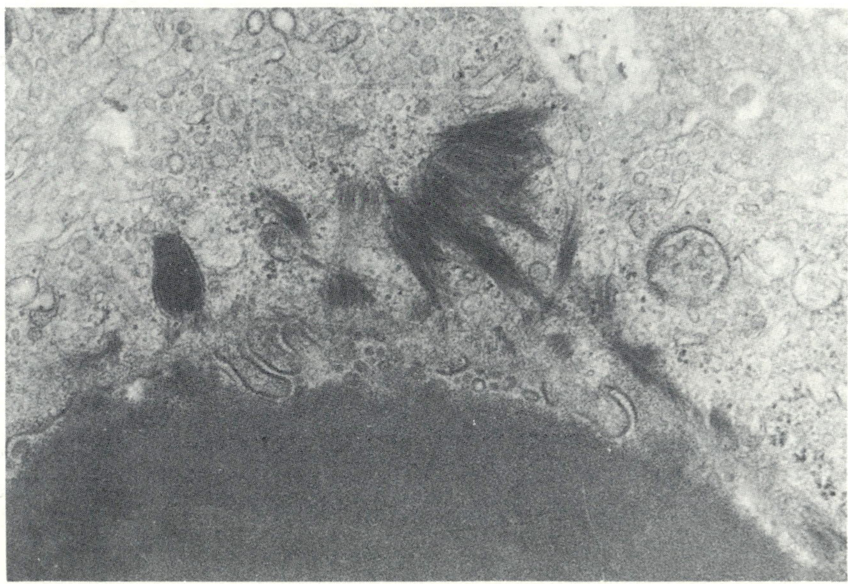

FIGURE 197
Dense aggregates of intracytoplasmic filaments are seen close to the wall of the lumen containing the inclusion. ×34,500.

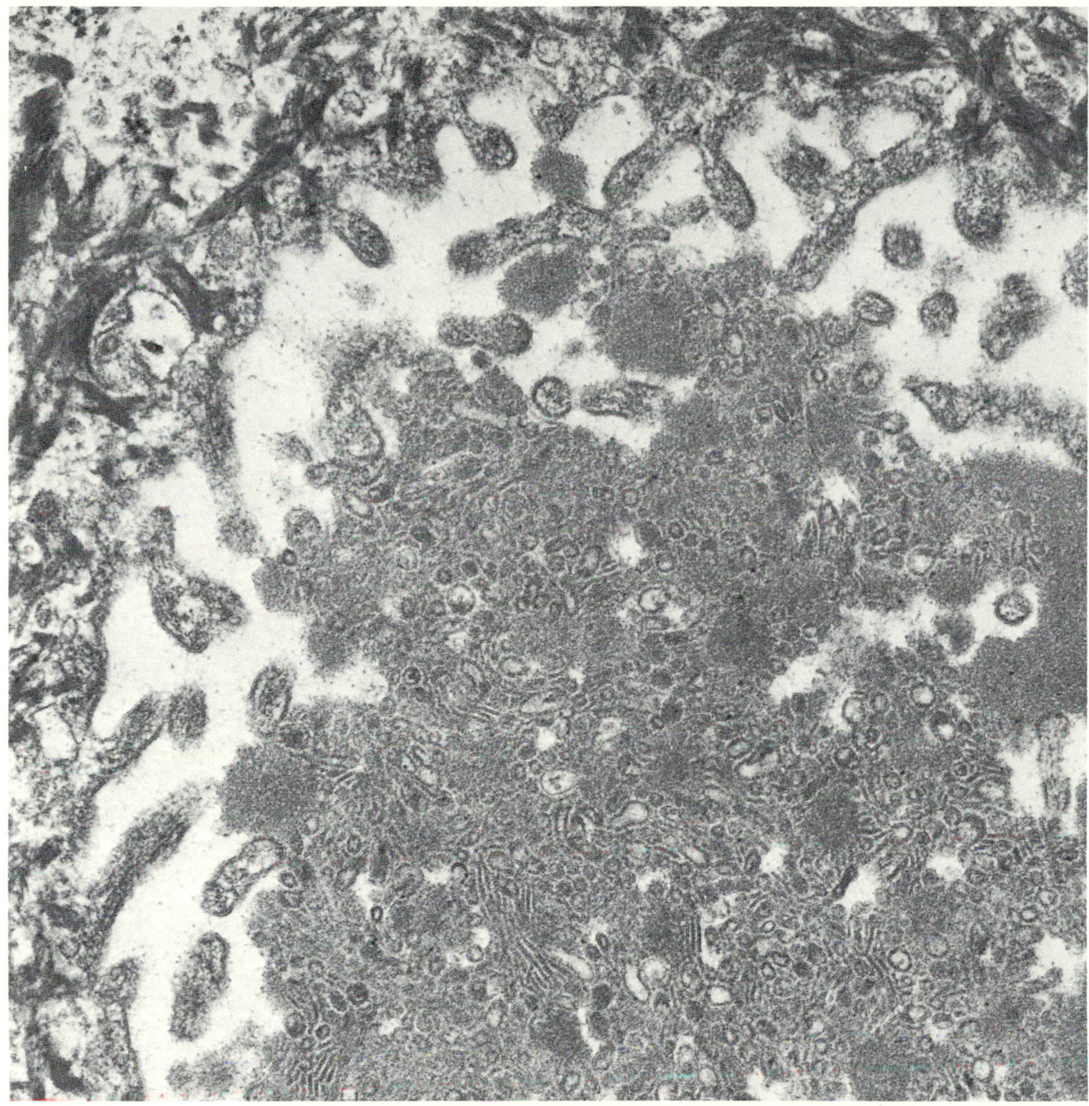

FIGURE 198
A more complex intracellular inclusion shows an admixture of broken-up microvilli and the original granular contents of a cavity. Circular profiles and multilamellar bodies can be observed in the central dense area. ×66,000.

those seen in smooth muscle cells, have been observed by Peña[35] (1975). The same investigator kindly contributed an illustration of this phenomenon for this volume (Fig. 202). The admixture of proliferating pericytes and ordinary meningothelial tumor cells in meningiomas were observed independently by Challa[57] and Mirra[58] (Fig. 76). Dr. Mirra contributed Figure 203, which illustrates the simultaneous presence of these two types of cells in the same tumor at the submicroscopic level. It seems that no transitional cells can be observed between the two constituents of this lesion, but even the parallel proliferative tendencies of these two cell types within the same neoplasm clearly have important theoretical implications.

Extensive accumulation of fluid, in both intra- and extracellular compartments can make diagnosis of a "humid" form of meningioma quite difficult by light microscopy. However, as seen in the case of Dr. Scheithauer of the Mayo Clinic (Figs. 137 and 138), even though some portions of the tumor contain large amounts of edema fluid,

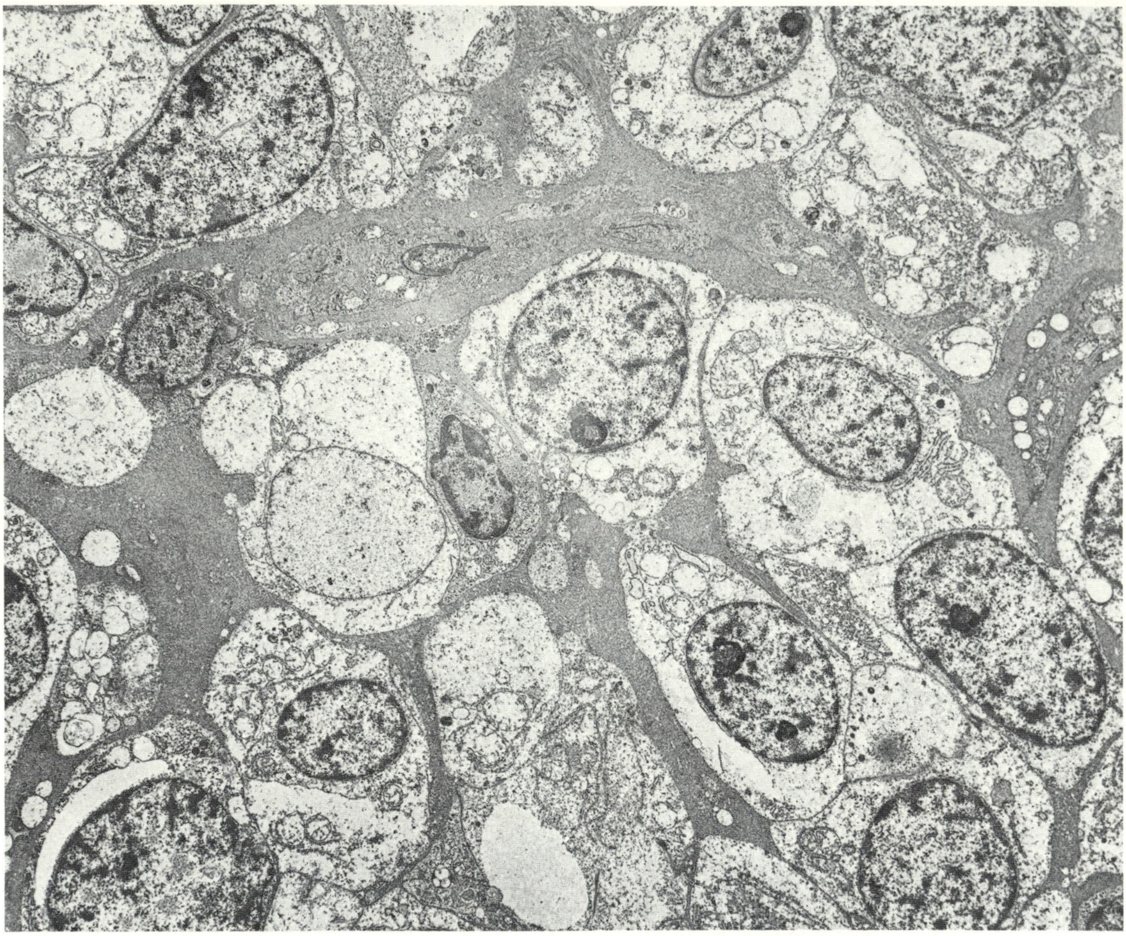

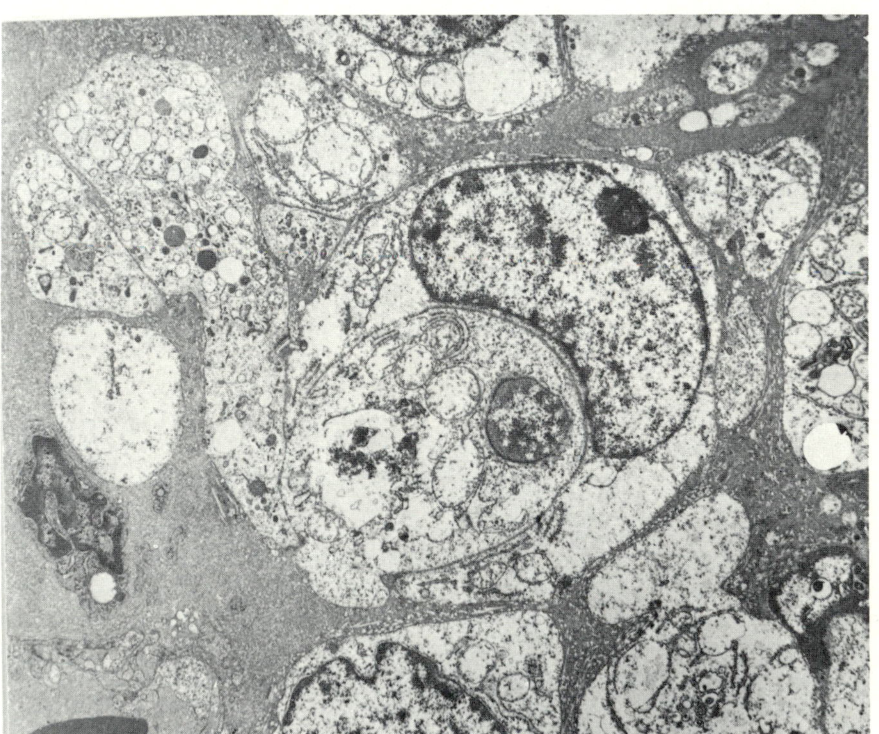

FIGURE 200
Another area of the same tumor shows two closely approximated cells forming what appears to be an abortive whorl. ×6,600.

FIGURE 199
From a hemangiopericytic tumor of the meninges. Cells have fairly large cytoplasms and are partially surrounded by granular basement membranelike material, which, however, does not extend everywhere between neighboring cells. Reduced from ×3,200.
←

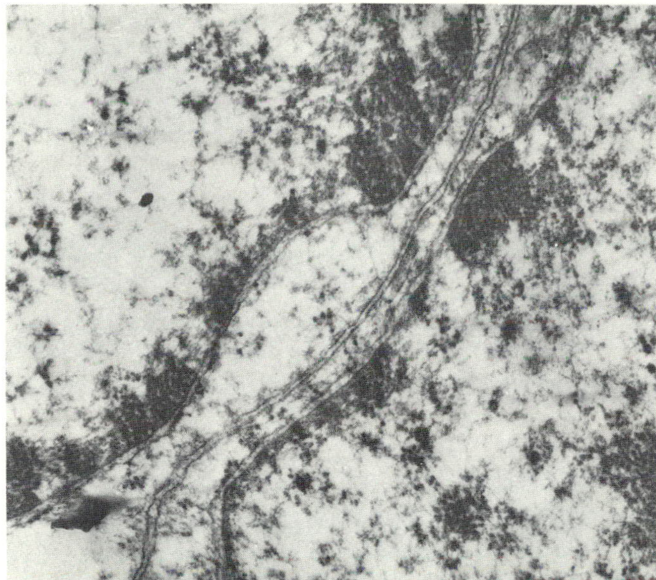

FIGURE 201
Cell walls of neighboring cells show no evidence of desmosomes or other forms of tight junctions in this area. ×20,000.

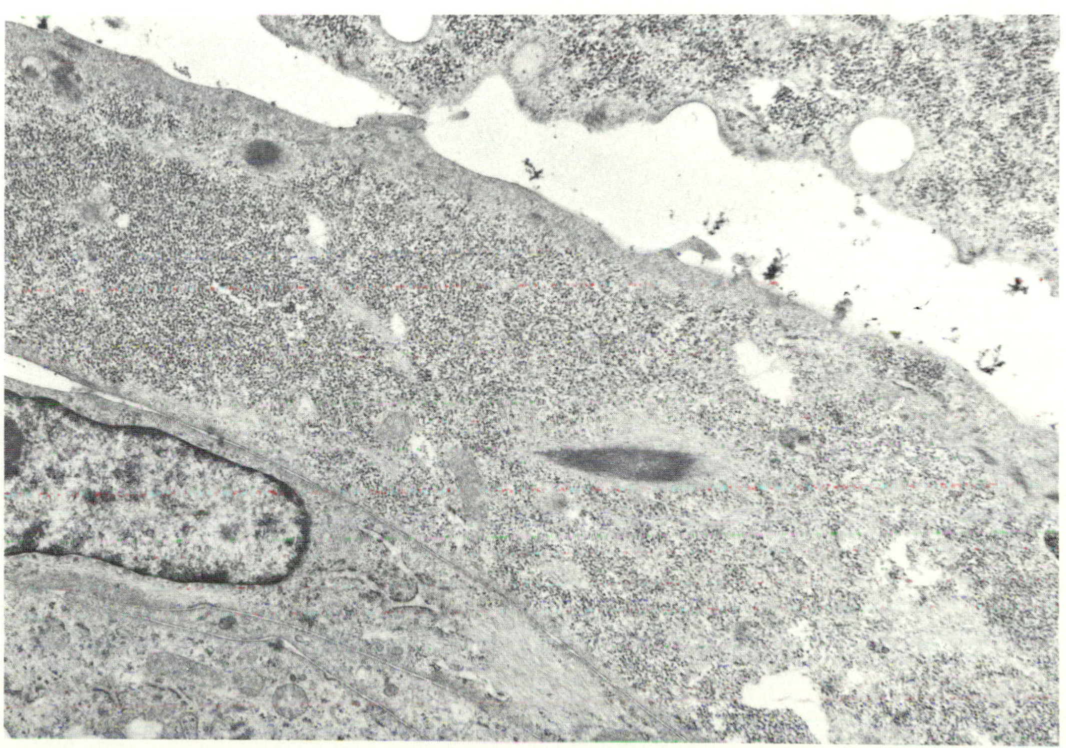

FIGURE 202
A tumor cell from a meningeal hemangiopericytic tumor shows condensation of cytoplasmic fibers in the center similar to that seen in smooth muscle cells. (Courtesy Dr. C. Pena.) ×12,000.

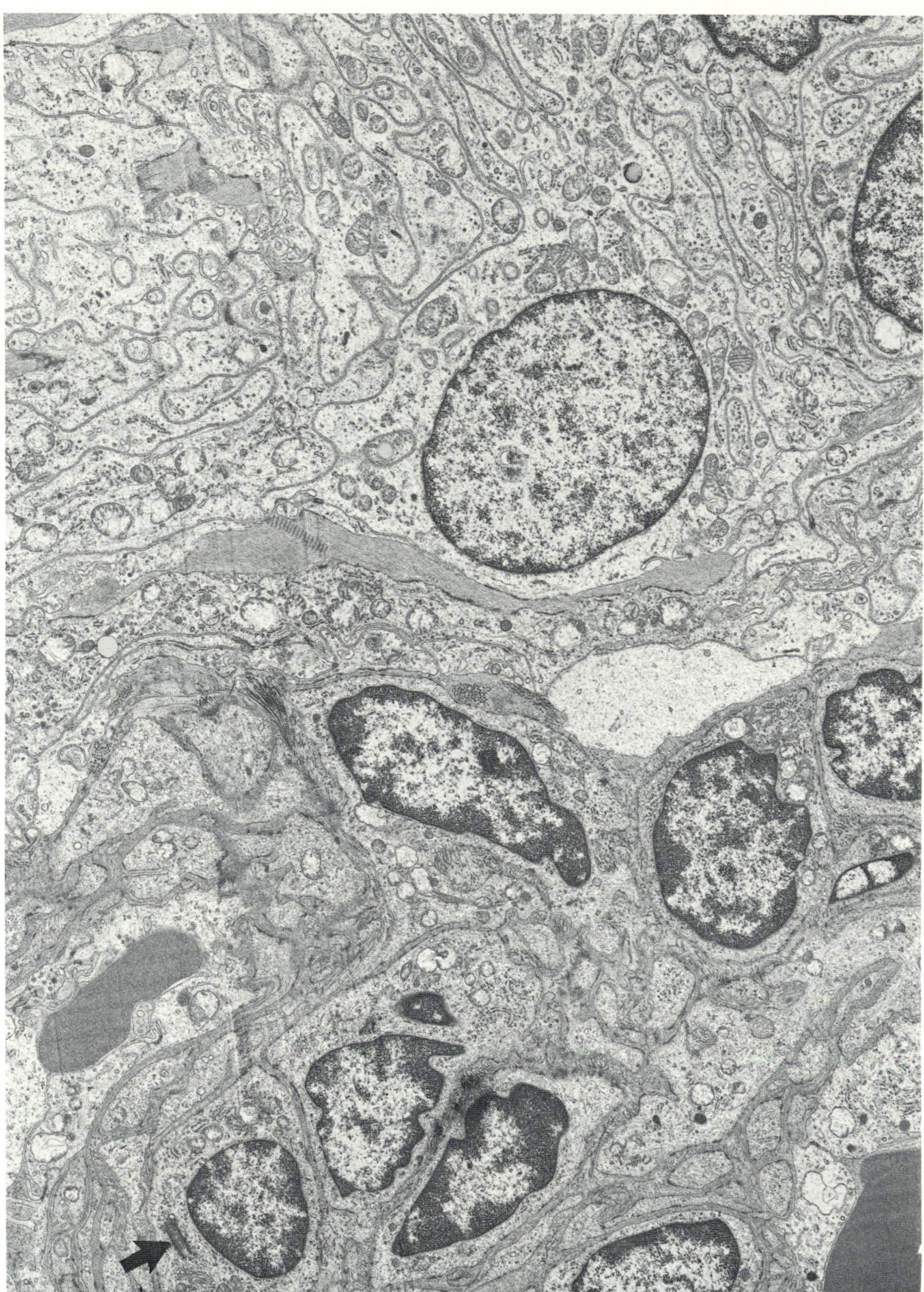

FIGURE 203
Meningothelial meningioma with proliferation of pericytic elements. Typical interdigitating cell membranes of the meningothelial tumor (*upper half*) in contrast to more closely packed pericytic elements surrounding a blood vessel (*right lower corner*). Nuclei of the pericytic elements are smaller than those of the meningothelial cells and have fewer processes. Basement membrane material, however, is seen between cells in both the lower and upper portion of the picture. *Arrow*, the shaft of a cilium in a pericytic cell. (Courtesy Dr. S. Mirra.) Reduced from ×9,000.

FIGURES 204 and 205
From an intradural humid meningioma of the region of the cauda equina. (For light microscopy, see Figs. 137–138.)

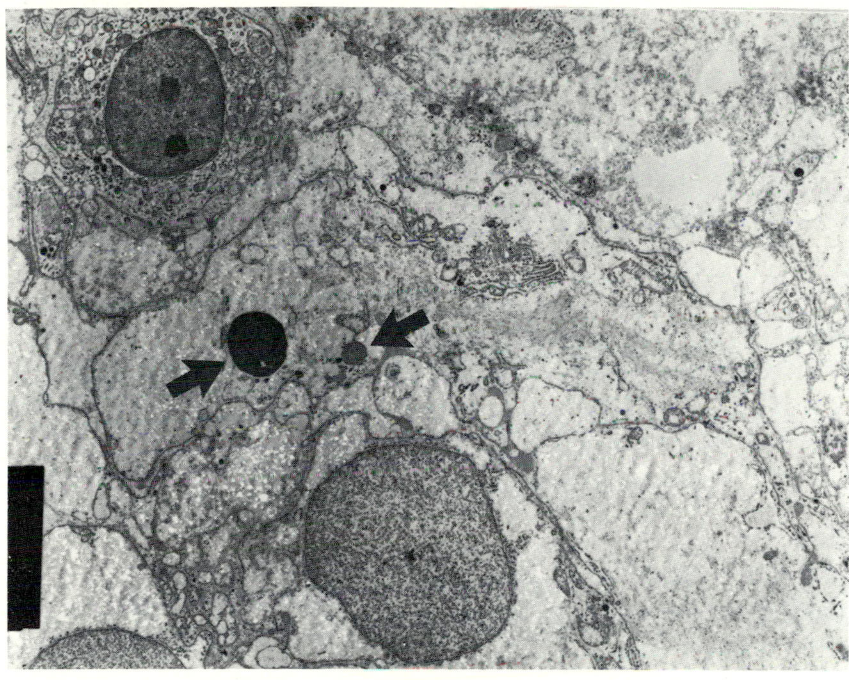

FIGURE 204
Both intra- and extracellular spaces are distended by what appears to be proteinaceous edema fluid plus osmiophilic lipid droplets (*arrow*). ×22,000.

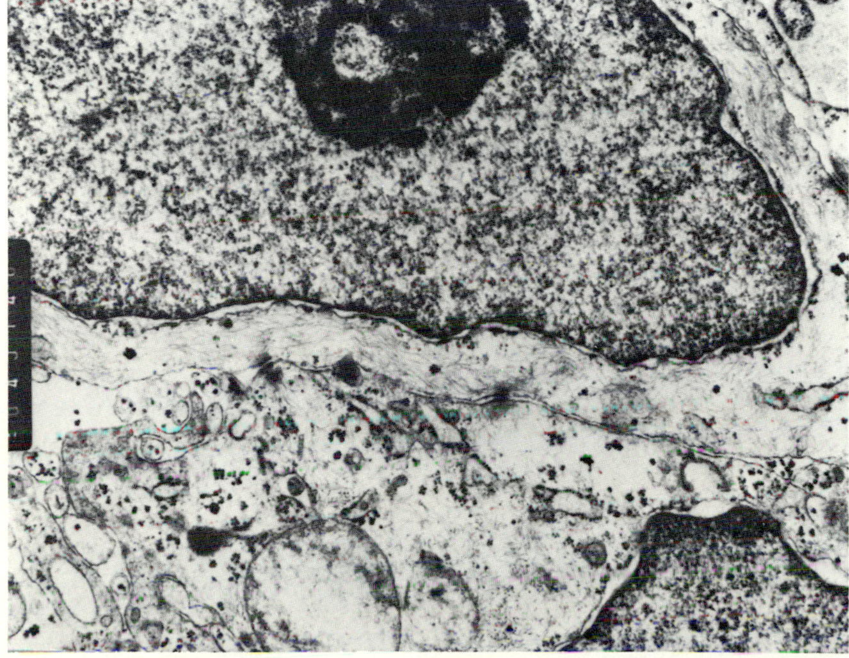

FIGURE 205
In a more condensed portion of the tumor, intracytoplasmic filaments aand desmosomes are well recognizable. ×36,000.

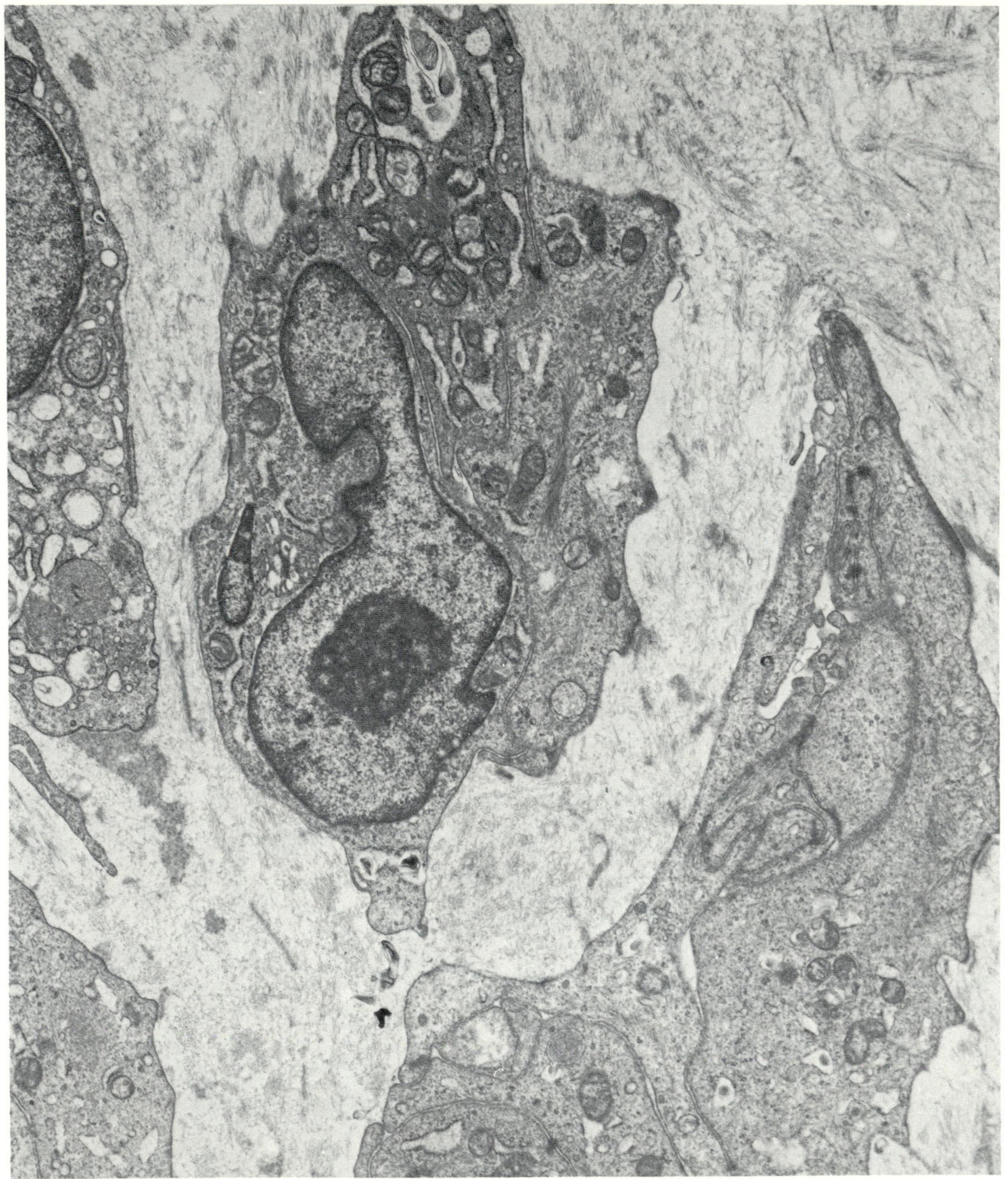

FIGURE 206
Electron micrographic view of cells from a malignant xanthofibromatous meningioma, depicted in Figures 94–100. Electron microscopy of this tumor shows small clusters of cells surrounded by large numbers of collagen fibers in varying states of maturation. Between neighboring cells interdigitating cell membranes and desmosomes can be observed, attesting to the basic meningothelial nature of this tumor. ×12,000.

lipid droplets, and filamentous material in the various compartments (Fig. 204), the same tumor still had some more compact areas in which intracytoplasmic filaments and the presence of desmosomes between neighboring cells helped establish their identity as meningiomas (Fig. 205).

As indicated in the discussion of light microscopy, some meningiomas may very closely imitate fibrous xanthomas, not only by virtue of lipid inclusions in the cytoplasm but also by assuming a storiform pattern in the fascicles of cells comprising the tumor (Figs 94–100). That same tumor, when examined under the electron microscope (Fig. 206), showed sufficient presence of tonofibrils within tumor cells, intricate interdigitations between neighboring cells as well as desmosomes to help establish the diagnosis of meningioma in this particular case.

Scanning Electron Microscopy

Scanning electron microscopy allows the investigator to examine in great detail surfaces and cut surfaces, including those of human and animal tissues and cells. The picture presented by this method is three-dimensional and furthers the understanding of spatial relations only inferred by other methods. Magnification can range from very low power, showing fields similar in size to those seen by light microscopy, to magnifications of 100,000 or more.

After some published studies describing the appearance of tissue cultures of neural cells, of ependyma-lined surfaces and other non-neoplastic tissues using the scanning electron microscope, Arnold and Burrows[61] were the first to examine human brain tumors with this method. They included a meningioma in their study and a malignant meningioma in a later work.[62] Arnold and Burrows[61] found meningioma cells to be quite large and the cells appeared to fuse with each other (undoubtedly a reflection of the syncytial pattern often seen under the light microscope). They believed that a malignant meningioma can be distinguished from a glioblastoma by virtue of different surface characteristics, among others finer microvilli of the surface than those seen on ependymal cells and astrocytes. Virtanen *et al.*[63] were next to use the scanning electron microscope to view meningiomas, and specifically they examined the structure of psammoma bodies, demonstrating in a most picturesque fashion concentrical masses of collagen fibers with beadlike structures, surrounded by a cuplike formation of lining meningothelial cells. The beadlike structures were believed to represent foci of calcification as well as degenerating cellular debris.

Rizzoli *et al.*[64] examined eight psammomatous meningiomas and found, as Virtanen *et al.* before them, collagen fibers forming a ball of twine, which they felt was the immediate precursor of the fully calcified psammoma body.

McKeever and Brissie[65] studied four transitional meningiomas with the scanning electron microscope. All four tumors had whorls of overlapping cells with a conspicuous surface topography resembling thin concave–convex discs tapering into broad, flat processes. The reader is referred to this article for a detailed description of present-day methods in preparing and examining specimens through scanning electron microscopy.

We are including pictures of a meningothelial meningioma that by light microscopy consisted almost exclusively of noncalcified cellular whorls (Fig. 207). By scanning electron microscopy of the same tumor, the resemblance between the spherical masses of layers on layers of flat menin-

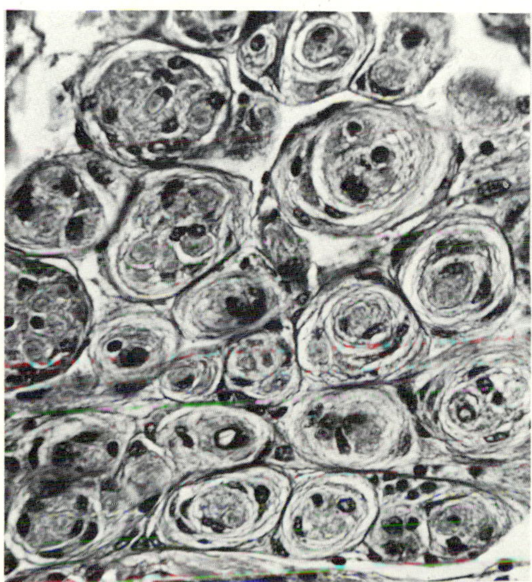

FIGURE 207
Light-microscopic view of a meningothelial meningioma, composed almost exclusively of noncalcified cellular whorls. H&E. ×200.

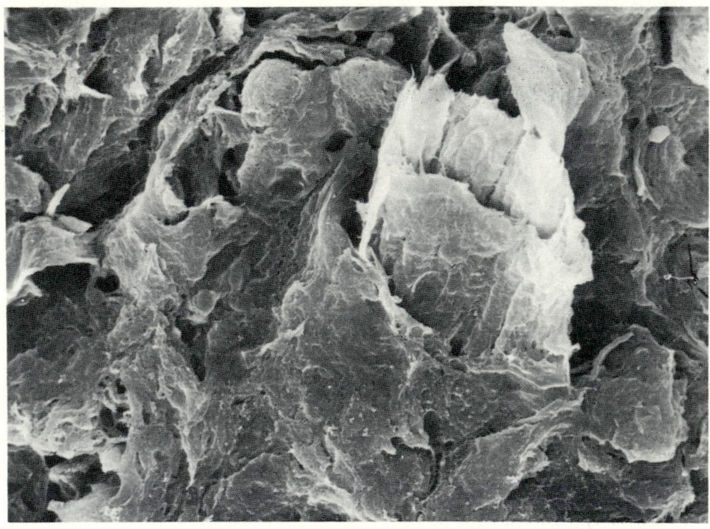

FIGURE 208
Scanning electron microscopic view of the external aspects of one whorl. The individual tumor cells are flat and curved around each other. They have tapering edges and a few short processes rising from their surfaces. ×1,400.

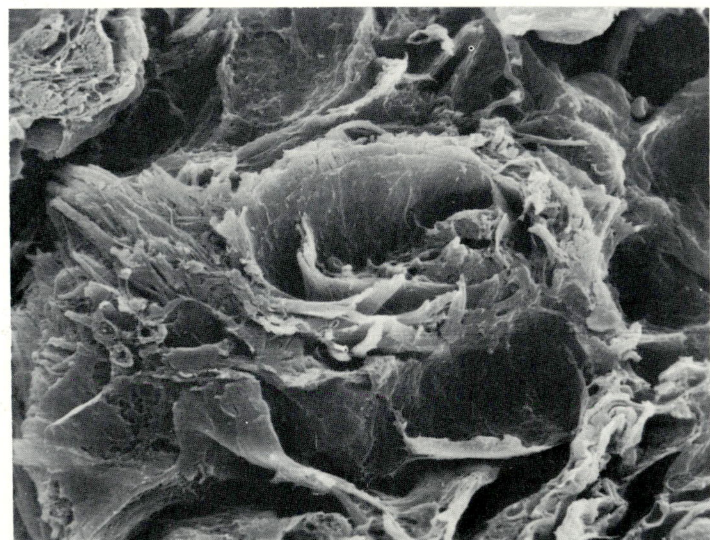

FIGURE 209
Slicing of a whorl removed its upper two-thirds and the central cells. The remaining cells form a cup-shaped structure of concentric leaflike cells. ×1,500.

FIGURE 212
Psammoma body with laminated structure and dense central calcification. (Rizzoli, H.V., *et al.:* Psammoma bodies in meningioma. Appearance by scanning electron microscopy. *Virchows Arch.* [*Pathol. Anat.*] *380: 317–325, 1978.* Reproduced with permission.)

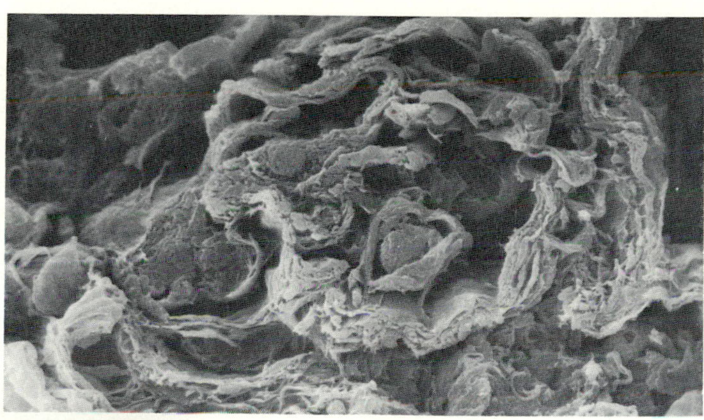

FIGURE 210
This section is from the equator of a whorl showing a central cell as well as others wrapped around it. ×1,200.

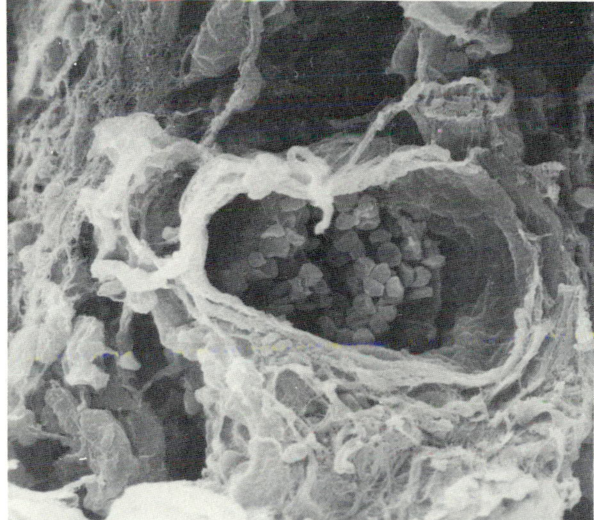

FIGURE 211
The center is occupied by a thin-walled blood vessel containing red blood corpuscles. The vessel is surrounded by concentrical layers of tumor cells. Reduced from ×1,000.

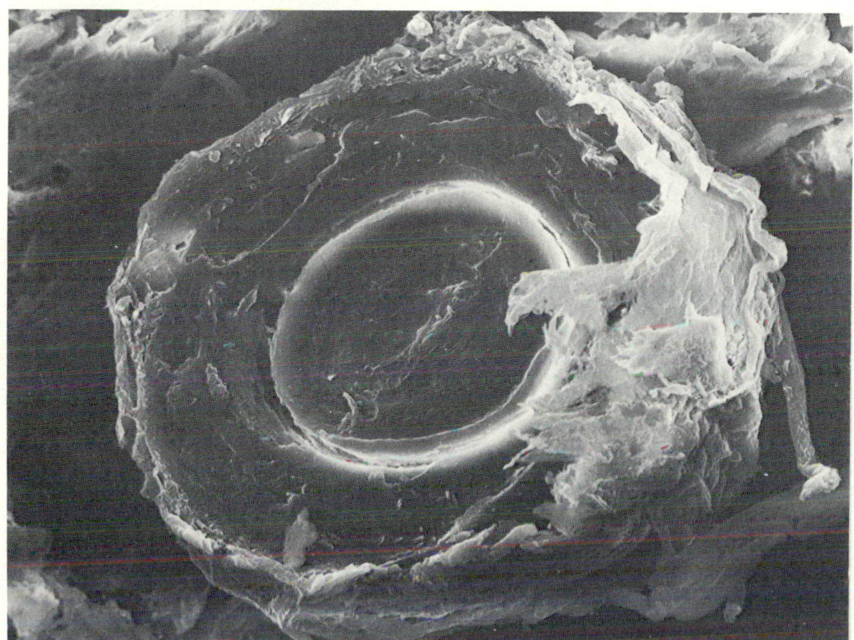

←

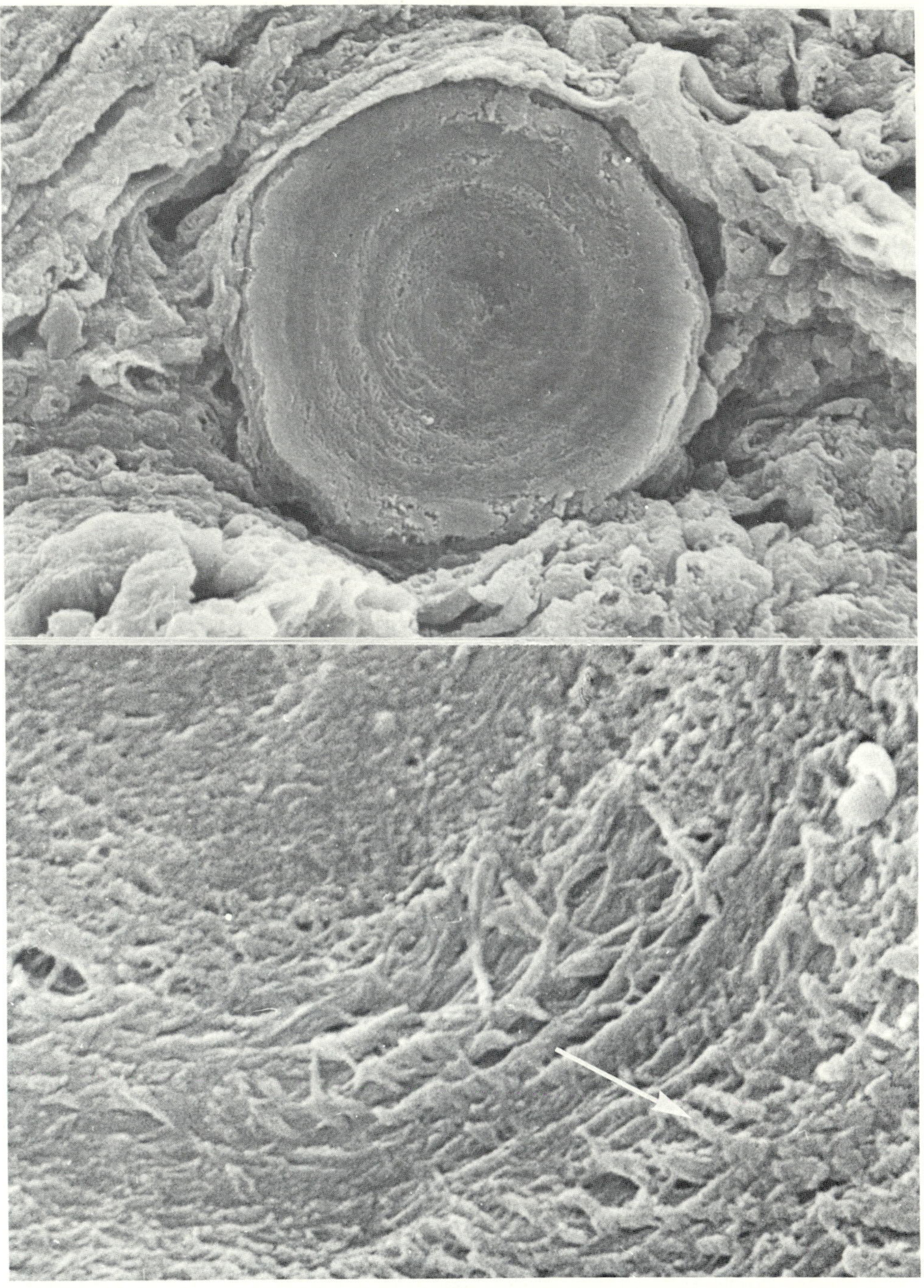

FIGURES 213 and 214
Low- and high-power view of psammoma body with densely interwoven circular masses of collagen fibers. Fig. 213, reduced from ×1,200. Fig. 214, reduced from ×10,000. (Virtanen, I., *et al.*: Structure of psammoma bodies of a meningioma in scanning electron microscopy. *Cancer 38: 824–829, 1976.* Reproduced with permission.)

gothelial cells and a cabbage patch, as envisioned by McKeever and Brissie,[65] is quite striking. Cell bodies and their fine processes are shown in Figures 208–210. Figure 211 shows a blood vessel with a number of doughnut-shaped red blood corpuscles in its lumen, forming the center of a whorl. Pictures of cross sections of psammoma bodies as seen by Rizzoli *et al.*[64] (Fig. 212) and by Virtanen *et al.*[63] (Figs. 213 and 214) are included here.

References

1. Pease, D.C., and Schultz, R.L.: Electron microscopy of rat cranial meninges. *Am. J. Anat. 102: 301–321, 1958.*
2. Waggener, J.D., and Beggs, J.: The membranous coverings of neural tissues: An electron microscopic study. *J. Neuropathol. Exp. Neurol. 26: 412–426, 1967.*
3. Leventhal, M.R.: Electron microscopy of brain tumors. *In Clinical Neurosurgery, Proceedings of the Ninth Congress of Neurosurgery, Miami Beach, Florida, 1959.* Baltimore, William & Wilkins, 1961, Vol. 7.
4. Luse, S.A.: Electron microscopic studies of brain tumors. *Neurology (Minneapolis) 10: 881–905, 1960.*
5. Kepes, J.: Electron microscopic studies of meningiomas. *Am. J. Pathol. 39: 499–510, 1961.*
6. Kepes, J.: Electron microscopic studies of meningiomas. In: *Proceedings of the 4th International Congress of Neuropathology, Munich, 1961*, H. Jacob (ed.). Stuttgart, G. Thieme, 1962.
7. Romhányi, G.: Histopathologic studies on the submicroscopic structure of fibers. *Orv. Lapja 3: 1569–1574.* (In Hungarian.)
8. Koizumi, J.: Electron microscopic studies of brain tumors. *Prog. Res. Nerv. Syst. 7: 61–84, 1963.* (In Japanese.)
9. Rascol, M.: *Microscopie Électronique des Tumeurs de la Méninge. (Méningiomes et Hemangioblastomes).* Paris, Libraire Arnette, 1966.
10. Choux, R., Hassoun, J., Gambarelli, D., Sedan, R., and Toga, M.: Étude ultrastructurale d'un "méningiome humide" de Masson. *Bull. Cancer 62: 125–136, 1975.*
11. Raimondi, A.J., Mullan, S., and Evans, J.P.: Human brain tumors: An electron microscopic study. *J. Neurosurg. 19: 731–753, 1962.*
12. Gonatas, N.K., and Besen, M.: An electron microscopic study of three human psammomatous meningiomas. *J. Neuropathol. Exp. Neurol. 22: 263–273, 1963.*
13. Koinov, R., Boyadjieva, A., and Hadjioloff, A.I.: Reserches en microscopie électronique sus les méningiomes. *Arch. Union Med. Balkan 2: 684–688, 1964.*
14. Gusek, W.: Submikroskopische Untersuchungen als Beitrag zur Struktur und Onkologie der "Meningeome." *Beitr. Pathol. Anat. 127: 274–326, 1962.*
15. Napolitano, L., Kyle, R., and Fischer, E.R.: Ultrastructure of meningiomas and the derivation and nature of their cellular components. *Cancer 17: 233–241, 1963.*
16. Ishida, Y., S., Sato, S., Takayanagi, T., and Kawafuchi, J.-I.: Electron microscopy of meningothelial meningioma. *Gunma J. Med. Sci. 13: 181–197, 1964.*
17. Rascol, M., Izard, J., Jorda, P., and Rascol, A.: Étude ultrastructurale des méningiomes. *Rev. Med. (Toulouse) 1: 621–640, 1965.*
18. Nyström, S.H.M.: A study on supratentorial meningiomas with special reference to gross and fine structure. *Acta Pathol. Microbiol. Scand. [C] Suppl. 176: 1–90, 1965.*
19. Castaigne, P., Escourolle, R., and Poirier, J.: L'ultrastructure des meningiomes. Etude de 4 cas en microscope electronique. *Rev. Neurol. (Paris) 114: 249–261, 1966.*
20. Cervós-Navarro, J.: Zur Feinstruktur endotheliomatöser Meningeome des Menschen. *Acta Neuropathol. (Berl.) 8: 141–148, 1967.*
21. Cervós-Navarro, J., and Vazquez, J.J.: An electron microscopic study of meningiomas. *Acta Neuropathol (Berl.) 13: 301–323, 1969.*
22. Woyke, S., Domagala, W., and Olszewski, W.: Some peculiar ultrastructural features of meningiomas. *Pol. Med. J. 10: 975–1005, 1971.*
23. Humeau, C., Sentein, P., and Vlahovitch, B.: Characteristiques ultrastructurales des cellules de meningiomes. *C.R. Soc. Biol. (Paris) 166: 1728–1730, 1972.*
24. Humeau, C., Vic, P., Sentein, P., and Vlahovitch, B.: The fine structure of meningiomas an attempted classification. *Virchows Arch. [Pathol. Anat.] 382: 201–216, 1979.*
25. Tani, E., Ikeda, K., Yamagata, S., Nishiura, M., and Higashi, N.: Specialized junctional complexes in human meningioma. *Acta Neuropathol. (Berl.) 28: 305–315, 1974.*
26. Tani, E., Nishiura, M., and Higashi, N.: Freeze-fracture studies of gap junctions in human meningioma. *Acta Neuropathol. (Berl.) 30: 305–314, 1974.*
27. Sipe, J.C.: Gap junctions between human meningioma cells maintained in organ culture. *Acta Neuropathol. (Berl.) 35: 69–76, 1976.*
28. Copeland, D.D., Bell, S.W., and Shelburne, J.D.: Hemidesmosome-like intercellular specializations in human meningioma. *Cancer 41: 2242–2249, 1978.*
29. Wolf, A., and Orton, S.T.: Intranuclear inclusions in brain tumors. *Bull. Neurol. Inst. NY 3: 113–123, 1933.*
30. Russell, D.S., Krayenbühl, H., and Cairns, H.: The wet film technique in the histological diagnosis of intracranial tumors; a rapid method. *J. Pathol. Bacteriol. 45: 501–505, 1937.*
31. Bland, J.O.W., and Russell, D.S.: Histological types of meningiomata and a comparison of their behaviour in tissue culture with that of certain normal tissues. *J. Pathol. Bacteriol. 47: 291–309, 1938.*
32. Fischmann, C.F., and Russell, D.S.: The occurrence of intranuclear inclusions in culture of foetal leptomeninges. *J. Pathol. Bacteriol. 50: 53–59, 1940.*
33. Robertson, D.M.: Electron microscopic studies of nuclear inclusions in meningiomas. *Am. J. Pathol. 45: 835–848, 1964.*
34. Cervós-Navarro, J., and Vazquez, J.: Elektronmikroskopische Untersuchungen über das Vorkommen von Cilien in Meningeomen. *Virchows Arch. [Pathol. Anat.] 341: 280–290, 1966.*
35. Peña, C.E.: Intracranial hemangiopericytoma. Ultrastructural evidence of its leiomyoblastic differentiation. *Acta Neuropathol. (Berl.) 33: 279–284, 1975.*
36. Long, D.M.: Vascular ultrastructure in human meningiomas and schwannomas. *J. Neurosurg. 38: 409–419, 1973.*
37. Horten, B.C., Urich, H., Rubinstein, L.J., and Montague, S.R.: The angioblastic meningioma: a reappraisal of a nosological problem. Light-electron-microscopic, tissue and organ culture observations. *J. Neurol. Sci. 31: 387–410, 1977.*

38. Ermel, A.E.: Histogenesis of angiomatous areas in meningiomas. An electron microscopic study. *Pathol. Res. Pract. 9: 217–231, 1974.*
39. Kepes, J.: Observations on the formation of psammoma bodies and pseudopsammoma bodies in meningiomas. *J. Neuropathol. Exp. Neurol. 20: 255–262, 1961.*
40. Nyström, S.: Electron microscopic studies of psammoma bodies in human supratentorial meningioma. *Naturwissenschaften 49: 186, 1962.*
41. Poon, T.P., Hirano, A., and Zimmerman, H.M.: *Electron Microscopic Atlas of Brain Tumors.* New York, Grune & Stratton, 1971, pp. 68–79.
42. Lipper, S., Dalzell, J.C., and Watkins, P.J.: Ultrastructure of psammoma bodies of meningioma in tissue culture. *Arch. Pathol. Lab. Med. 103: 670–675, 1979.*
43. Anderson, H.C.: Vesicles associated with calcification in the matrix of epiphyseal cartilage. *J. Cell Biol. 41: 59–72, 1969.*
44. Mena, H., and Garcia, J.H.: Primary brain sarcomas. Light and electron microscopic features. *Cancer 42: 1298–1307, 1978.*
45. Pietruszka, M., Salazar, H., and Pena, C.: Malignant meningioma: Ultrastructure and observations on histogenesis. *Pathology 10: 169–173, 1978.*
46. Cushing, H., and Eisenhardt, L.: Meningiomas. Their Classification, Regional Behaviour, Life History and Surgical End Results. Springfield, Ill., Charles C. Thomas, 1938, p. 175.
47. Kepes, J.: The fine structure of hyaline inclusions (pseudopsammoma bodies) in meningiomas. *J. Neuropathol. Exp. Neurol. 34:282–295, 1975.*
48. Berard, M., Tripier, M.-F., Choux, R., Chrestian, M.-A., Hassoun, J., and Toga, M.: Étude ultrastructurale des corps hyalins d'un méningiome pseudo-epithelial. *Acta Neuropathol. (Berl.) 42: 59–62, 1978.*
49. Font, R.L., and Croxatto, J.O.: Intracellular inclusions in meningothelial meningioma. A histochemical and ultrastructural study. *J. Neuropathol. Exp. Neurol. 39: 575–583, 1980.*
50. Ferrer, I., and Aceves, J.: Cambios xantomatosos y contenido de melanina en tumores meningeos. Xanthomatous changes and melanin content in meningeal tumors. *Morfol. Normal Patol. B2: 531–539, 1978.*
51. Limas, C., and Tio, F.O.: Meningeal melanocytoma ("Melanotic meningioma") Its melanocytic origin as revealed by electron microscopy. *Cancer 30: 1286–1294, 1972.*
52. Goldman, J.E., Horoupian, D.S., and Johnson, A.B.: Granulofilamentous inclusions in a meningioma. *Cancer 46: 156–161, 1980.*
53. Ramsey, H.J.: Fine structure of hemangiopericytoma and hemangioendothelioma. *Cancer 19: 2005–2018, 1966.*
54. Popoff, N.A., Malinin, T.I., and Rosomoff, H.L.: Fine structure of intracranial hemangiopericytoma and angiomatous meningioma. *Cancer 34: 1187–1197, 1974.*
55. Choux, R., Chrestian, M.A., Tripier, M.F., Gambarelli, D., Hassoun, J., and Toga, M.: Hemangiopericytome cerebral. Étude ultrastructurale d'un cas. *J. Neurol. Sci. 28: 361–371, 1976.*
56. Goellner, J.R., Laws, E.R., Soule, E.H., and Okazaki, H.: Hemangiopericytoma of the meninges. Mayo Clinic experience. *Am. J. Clin. Pathol. 70: 375–380, 1978.*
57. Challa, V.R., Dixon, M.M., Marshall, R.B. and Kelly, D.L., Jr.: The vascular component in meningiomas associated with severe cerebral edema. *Neurosurgery 7: 363–368, 1980.*
58. Mirra, S.S., and Miles, M.L.: Unusual pericytic proliferation in a meningotheliomatous meningioma: An ultrastructural study. *J. Neuropathol. Exp. Neurol. 39: 376, 1980.* (Abstract.)
59. Kleinman, G.M., Liszczak, T., Tarlov, E., and Richardson, E.P., Jr.: Microcystic variant of meningioma. A light-microscopic and ultrastructural study. *Am. J. Surg. Pathol. 4: 383–389, 1980.*
60. Eimoto, T., and Hashimoto, K.: Vacuolated meningioma, a light and electron microscopic study. *Acta Pathol. Jpn. 27: 557–566, 1977.*
61. Arnold, A., and Burrows, D.: Scanning electron microscopy of cerebral tumors and glial cells. *Recent Results Cancer Res. 51: 52–62, 1975.*
62. Arnold, A., and Burrows, D.: Comparative studies of tumors of the central nervous system of man by scanning electron microscopy, phase microscopy, and light microscopy. *Scan. Electron Microsc. 9: 25–30, 1976.*
63. Virtanen, I., Lehtonen, E., and Wartiovaara, J.: Structure of psammoma bodies of a meningioma in scanning electron microscopy. *Cancer 38: 824–829, 1976.*
64. Rizzoli, H.V., Randall, J.D., and Smith, D.R.: Psammoma bodies in meningioma. Appearance by scanning electron microscopy. *Virchows Arch. [Pathol. Anat.] 380: 317–325, 1978.*
65. McKeever, P.E., and Brissie, N.T.: Scanning electron microscopy of neoplasms removed at surgery: Surface topography and comparison of meningioma, colloid cyst, ependymoma, pituitary adenoma, Schwannoma and astrocytoma. *J. Neuropathol. Exp. Neurol. 36: 875–896, 1977.*

CHAPTER 27

Spinal Fluid Cytology in the Diagnosis of Meningiomas

A review of articles and textbooks dealing with cytological studies of the cerebrospinal fluid (CSF) indicates that this modality of examination has relatively little to offer in the preoperative diagnosis of meningiomas. This very technique, which is so helpful in finding evidence for the presence of meningeal involvement by lymphoms, leukemias, metastatic carcinomas, and some neuroectodermal tumors (particularly medulloblastomas, and to a lesser extent ependymomas and other gliomas), does not lend itself too well to show tumor cells exfoliated from meningiomas. Thus, Oehmichen[1] could not report a single positive case from his own material. Having reviewed the combined series of other authors, he found that 525 meningiomas yielded only two positive findings. And Choi and Anderson,[2] examining 775 CSF specimens, did not find a single specimen that was positive for exfoliated meningioma cells. Even in series of clinically known meningiomas, the yield is typically very low, for example, 1 of 13 patients,[3] 2 of 17 cases,[4] and 5%.[5] The reason for this low yield is very likely as suggested by Kline,[6] namely, that "the cells apparently simply do not desquamate into the fluid." An additional difficulty lies in the fact that meningiomas are most often benign tumors. Hence, even if an occasional tumor cell makes its appearance in the spinal fluid sediment, it may be mistaken for a normal meningeal cell. When by chance a whole cluster of meningioma cells is found by the cytologist, this will obviously be easier to recognize, as in the case of McMenemey and Cumings,[7] who apparently were the first to encounter this phenomenon. We have seen two cases in which closely packed clusters of meningioma tumor cells formed whorls, thereby making recognition easy (Figs. 215 and 216).

One can assume that malignant meningiomas will have a greater tendency to seed and metastasize via the spinal fluid.[8,9] In such cases, a positive cytological examination may be expected, but

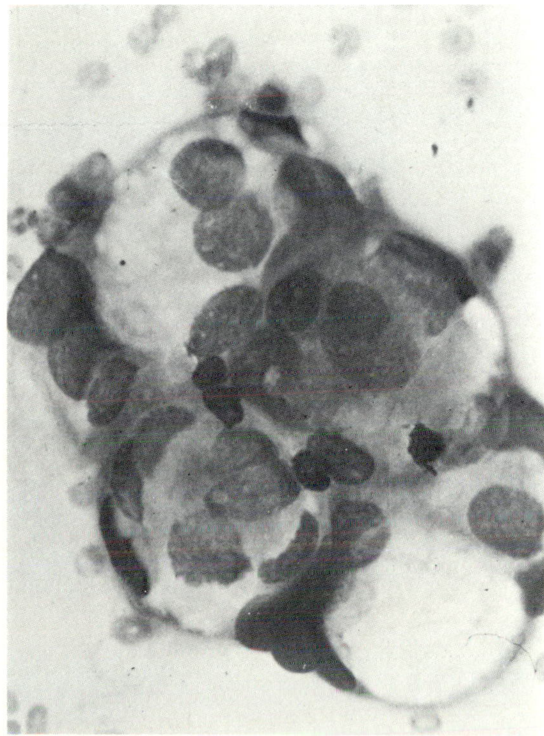

FIGURE 215
Spinal fluid sediment from a middle-aged woman with intracranial meningothelial meningioma. A cluster of meningioma tumor cells shows nuclear and cytoplasmic molding. (Courtesy Dr. A. Barabas.)

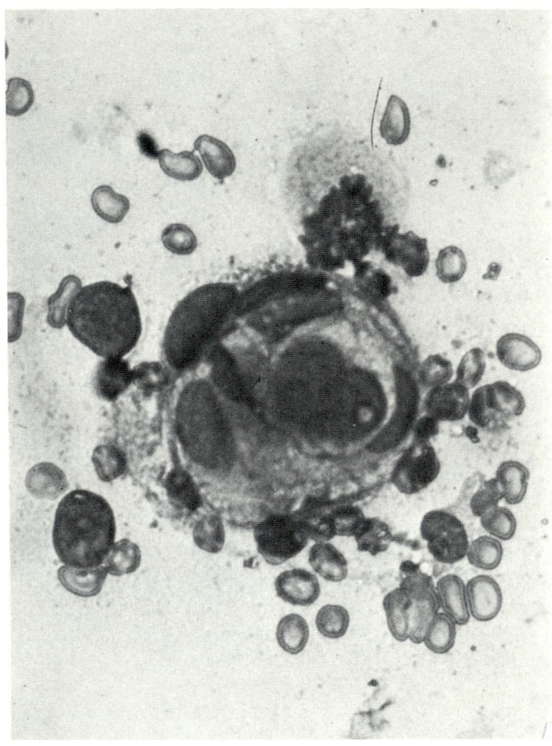

FIGURE 216
Sixty-one-year-old woman with right parasagittal meningioma. Cellular whorl found in spinal fluid sediment. (Courtesy Dr. A. Barabas.)

in these reports no mention was made as to whether the cytology of the spinal fluid was examined.

References

1. Oehmichen, M.: *Cerebrospinal Fluid Cytology*. Saunders–G. Thieme, 1976, p. 155.
2. Choi, H.S.H., and Anderson, P.I.: Diagnostic cytology of cerebrospinal fluid by the cytocentrifuge method. *Am. J. Clin. Pathol. 72: 931–943, 1979.*
3. Watson, C. W., and Hajdu, S.I.: Cytology of primary neoplasms of the central nervous system. *Acta Cytol. (Balt.) 21: 40–47, 1977.*
4. Kajikawa, H., Ohta, T., Ohshiro, H., Harada, K., and Ishikawa, S.: Cerebrospinal fluid cytology in patients with brain tumors: a simple method using the cell culture technique. *Acta Cytol. (Balt.) 21: 162–167, 1977.*
5. Sher, J.H. Cytologic diagnosis of brain tumors, *In Primary Intracranial Neoplasms*, J.H. Sher and D.H. Ford (eds.). New York–London, SP Medical and Scientific Books, 1979, p. 112.
6. Kline, T.S.: Cytological examination of the cerebrospinal fluid. *Cancer 15: 591–597, 1962.*
7. McMenemey, W.H., and Cumings, J.N.: The value of the examinations of the cerebrospinal fluid in the diagnosis of intracranial tumors. *J. Clin. Pathol. 12: 400–411, 1959.*
8. Hoffmann, G.T., and Earle, K.M.: Meningioma with malignant transformation and implantation in the subarachnoid space. *J. Neurosurg. 17: 486–492, 1960.*
9. Ludwin, S.K., and Conley, F.F.: Malignant meningioma metastasizing throughout the cerebrospinal pathways. *J. Neurol. Neurosurg. Psychiatry 38: 136–142, 1975.*

CHAPTER 28

Tissue Culture

Several references have been made with regard to the use of tissue cultures of meningiomas as employed for chromosomal studies of these tumors (Chapter 22), the search for virus-specific tumor antigens in cultures[1] (Chapter 6), and the analysis of tumor cell DNA content by flowthrough cytometry.[2] Tissue cultures also made possible detailed electron microscopic studies of certain cytological details of meningiomas (e.g., of gap junctions[3]), or of matrix vesicles in calcifying psammoma bodies[4] (see Chapter 26).

A review of the early papers dealing with the subject of meningioma tissue cultures shows that, like so many other forms of brain tumor study, this too originated in Harvey Cushing's laboratory. It was in that workshop that Kredel[5] first attempted to explant human meningioma cells into tissue culture, using the hanging drop method with Locke's solution and heparinized human plasma. Out of five meningiomas, Kredel derived satisfactory cultures from three, and these were kept alive as long as 3 weeks. There is some difference of opinion in the literature as to whether the cells of these first cultures were tumor cells or macrophages. The cells did, indeed, have a phagocytic capability, but after 1 week they lost their phagocytic activity and increasingly resembled fibroblasts. As arachnoidal cells are capable of phagocytosis, and meningioma cell cultures often appear as cultures of fibroblasts, it is quite possible that Kredel's explanted cells were *bona fide* meningioma cells. Buckley and Eisenhardt,[6] from the same laboratory, were successful in culturing one case (out of 22 meningiomas). The cultured cells were considered to be true tumor cells and had a reticular arrangement. Cox and Cranage[7] observed good migration of explanted cells in four of nine cases.Some but not all of the cultured cells were phagocytic.

Bland and Russell[8] made some very important contributions through their study of tissue cultures from 14 meningiomas. They observed in the cultured cell population different cell types, such as "flame" cells, flat fusiform cells, spindle cells, and flat polygonal cells forming a carpetlike growth. The tumor cells were observed "to glide forward like slugs" on the cover slips. Macrophages always accompanied the outgrowing tumor cells. Cultures from fetal leptomeninges showed similar features.

Bland and Russell made the important observation that although the meningiomas used for culturing had a variable morphology; that is, the cases included endothelial, fibroblastic, angioblastic, and myxoid forms, the cultures growing out from these tumors were indistinguishable from each other. Thus, these investigators provided an important argument favoring the "unitarian" view of meningiomas. In addition, the nuclei of the cells were closely examined and were found to be vacuolated in older cultures. Intranuclear inclusions were also found and examined. On the basis of the morphology and staining properties of such inclusions, Bland and Russell concluded that they are not of viral origin, as had been surmised earlier. Fischmann and Russell[9] suggested of the same type of intranuclear inclusions found in tissue culture of fetal leptomeninges that they were possibly of cytoplasmic origin.

Time-lapse cinematography and phase-contrast examination of living cell cultures made what Pomerat[10] called *dynamic neuropathology* possible. That author as well as Costero *et al.*,[11-12] who cultured as many as 18 meningiomas, observed rapid cellular migration of cells, which proceeded to form what appeared to be a syncytium. In 12 cases whorls were found during the early days of culture, but the cells became fibroblasts between the 3rd and 42nd days. Such cells were believed to elaborate collagenous bundles actively, although prior to that, reticular precollagenous fibrils appeared. The fact that whorls were present only initially, and meningioma cells changed to fibroblasts, was explained as a sign of simplification or, using their term, nomicoplasia.[11-12]

Two years later, Kersting and Lennarzt[13] took issue with the inevitability of such dedifferentiation, since they observed the process going in the opposite direction. Their findings were based on a modification of the technique of culturing in a

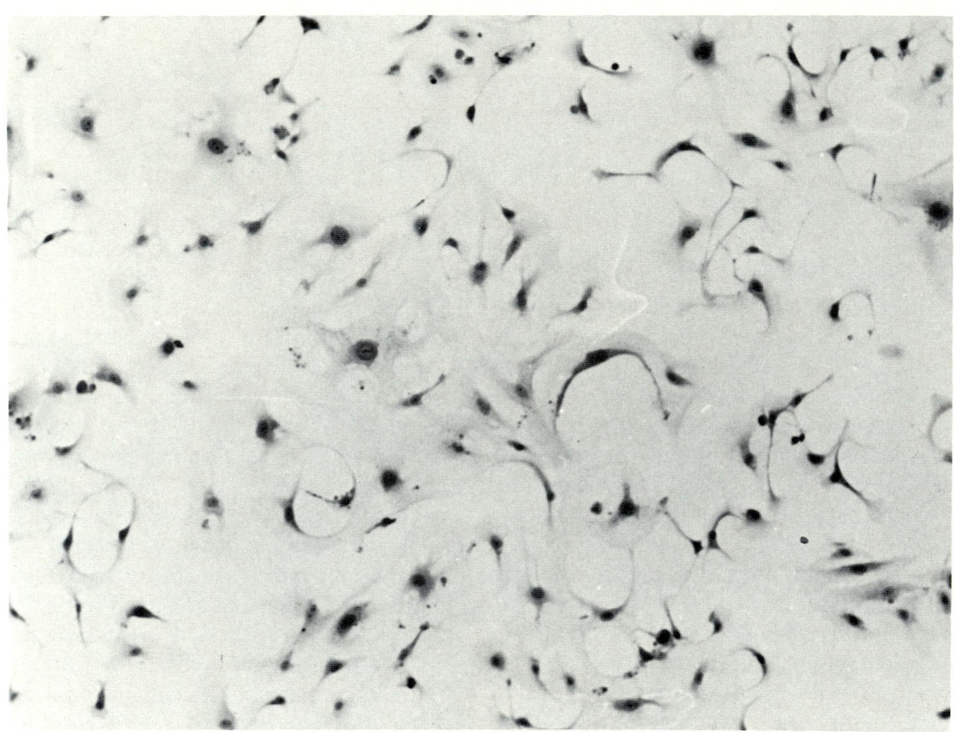

FIGURE 217
Monolayer cell culture of a meningothelial meningioma. The cells appear as fibroblasts with slight winding and curving of the cytoplasm and nuclei. No whorl formation is noted. (Courtesy Dr. B. Liwnicz.)

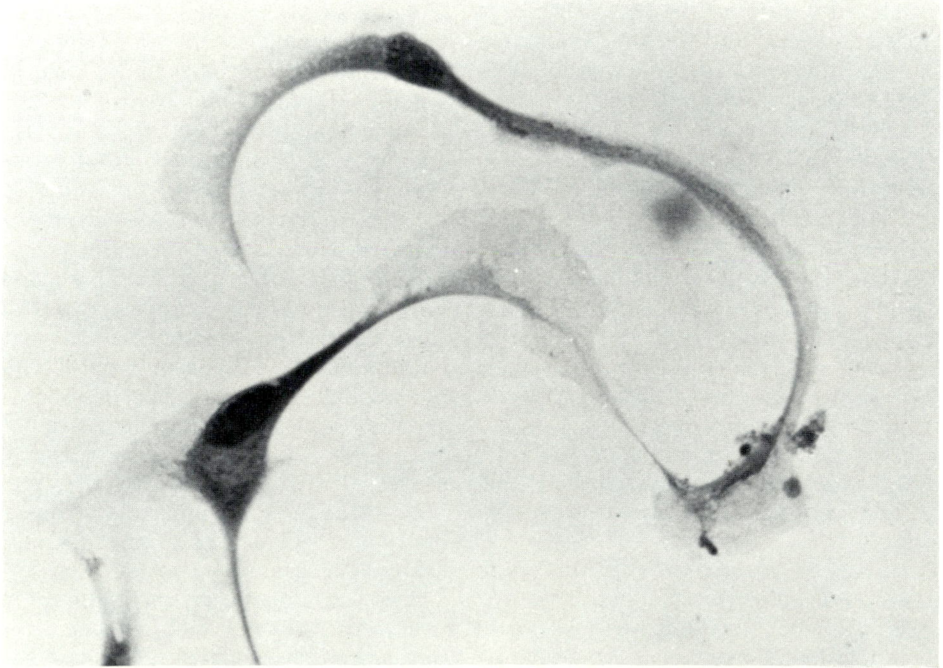

FIGURE 218
Higher-power view of Figure 210 shows curvature of cells. (Courtesy Dr. B. Liwnicz.)

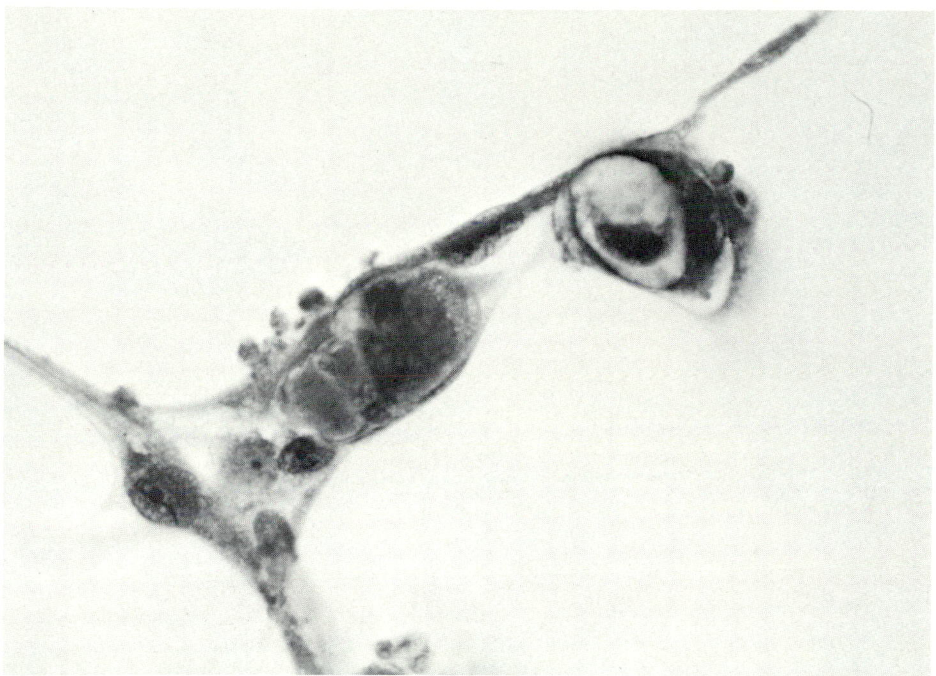

FIGURE 219
Culture of same cell line shown in Figures 211 and 212, with lectin added to culture media. Note early formation of whorls in several foci. (Courtesy Dr. B. Liwnicz.)

way that turned out to be significant. Instead of placing a piece of tissue into the culture medium, waiting for tumor cells to sprout from the periphery of that piece, they cut up their specimens into very fine pieces, then trypsinized them to create suspensions of isolated cells, and it was such suspensions that were explanted directly on a glass surface.

The result was that first a two-dimensional reticulum developed, the cells at 36 hours resembling fibroblasts. At 48 hours, whorls began to form in the culture, and after a while these structures were found in significant numbers. It seemed that one or two cells formed the center and the rest of the cells composing the whorls, joined from the outside.

As observed by Costero et al.,[11] as well, in some of the cellular whorls a basophilic material made its appearance, which was considered to represent early calcification. This was, to some extent, at variance with the observations of Bennington *et al.*,[41] who believed that the collagen bundles of a psammoma body become calcified—and not the cells and their derivates, whereas, Lipper *et al.*[4] (*vide supra*), also using a tissue-culture mode, stressed the role of matrix vesicles in the process of calcification.

Pomerat *et al.*[15] adopted the trypsinization method of Kersting and Lennarzt and, as a result, they too could observe the formation of many whorls in their meningioma cultures. Their time-lapse cinematography method showed the whorls

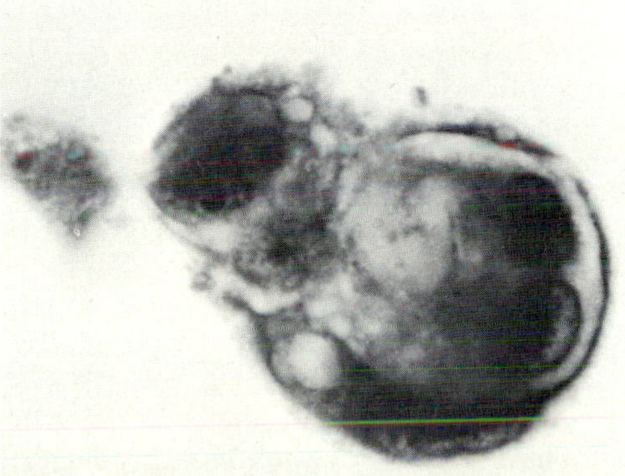

FIGURE 220
Another whorl from the same culture shown in Figure 212. (Courtesy Dr. B. Liwnicz.)

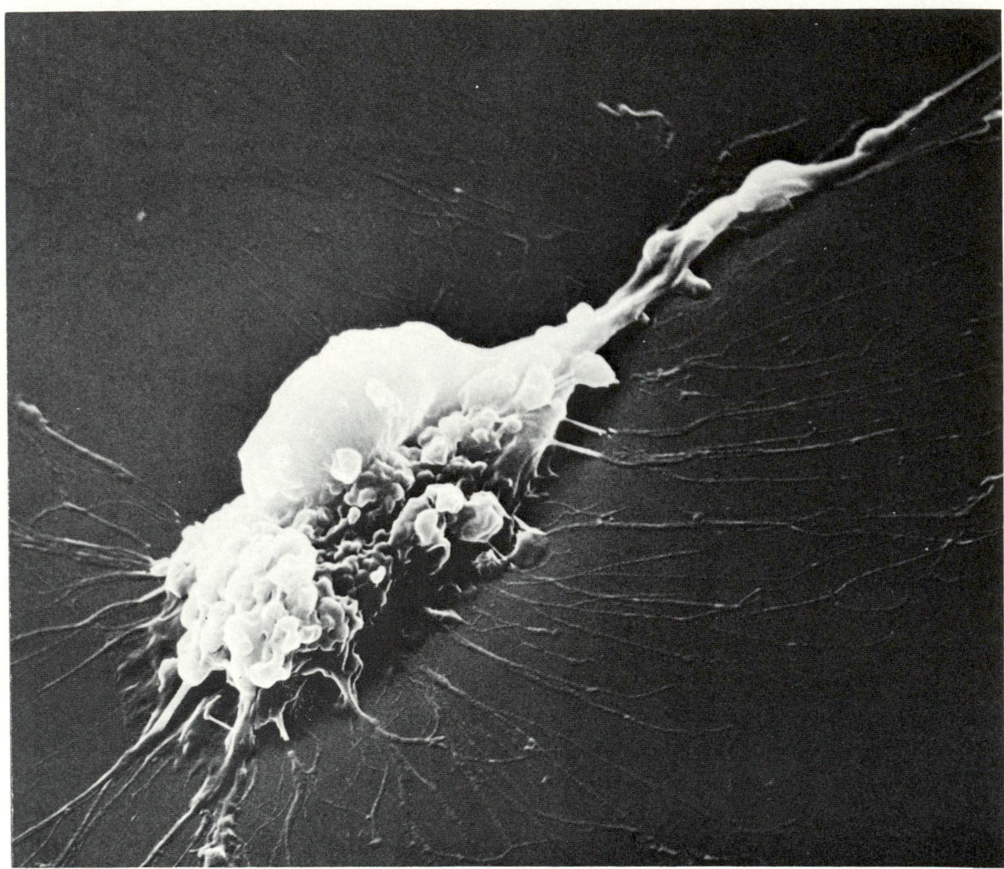

FIGURE 221
Scanning electron micrograph of a single cell from a cell line originating from a meningothelial meningioma. The cell line was kept in culture for three generations, a total of 30 days. The cell is shown migrating from the explant. ×4,500. (Courtesy Dr. B. Liwnicz.)

taking part in a circular motion, which resulted in new cells becoming wrapped onto the outside of whorls. Other complex rhythmic motions of the peristaltic type were observed as well. Pomerat and his group observed fibrils within the cultured meningioma cells, an observation also made by Morley,[16] who called them intracellular desmofibrils having extracellular counterparts in the form of similar fibrils. Both groups stained well with phosphotungstic acid–hematoxylin.

Lumsden[17] dedicated much time and effort to culturing brain tumor cells, and of the meningiomas he observed, "No brain tumor grows with greater technical ease *in vitro*, and no tumor has been considered to display such a poor performance in the sense that its cultural behavior seemed to have so little relevance to its histological structure." In a later work, Lumsden[18] gave a more detailed account of the progress of cell-culture techniques in general, including such refinements as the roller tube method, and the monolayer culture, which made it possible to keep cultures alive for 5 to 6 months. Three-dimensional cultures with close resemblance to the original tissues from which they were derived could be created in *organ cultures*, using the porous substance of cellular sponge matrix, gelatin sponge foam, or tantalum steel gauze to provide growing space for the cultures. Organ cultures were also used by Russell and Rubinstein.[19] Duffy *et al.*[20] found that the addition of polyamines to cell cultures of meningiomas influenced their growth rate. Aminoguanidine and in some cases putrescin caused acceleration of cell growth, whereas adding spermidine or spermine to the cultures had an inhibiting effect. It is still true that in ordinary monolayer cultures the cells may grow out as fibroblasts without evidence of whorl formation. B. H. Liwnicz (personal communication, 1980) found that the addition of lectins to the culture media brings about a striking change in that the same cells will now begin to take part in the formation of cellular whorls (Figs. 217–220). A three-dimensional view by scanning electron microscopy of one such cell in culture is shown in Figure 221.

Tissue cultures occasionally contribute to solving problems of histogenesis of tumors. In the case of meningiomas, this is well exemplified by the important study of Muller and Mealy,[21] who cultured a hemangiopericytoma of the pontocerebellar angle and found numerous cellular whorls in the culture, whereas the original tumor had none. This finding, added to the case of Bland and Russell[8] mentioned earlier, has provided a very forceful argument in favor of considering meningeal hemangiopericytomas a form of meningiomas.

It is very likely that tissue cultures of brain tumors, including meningiomas, will most importantly serve as useful models of the parent tumor, ready to be studied for characteristics that have therapeutic implications for the patient. Such characteristics will probably include *in vitro* responsiveness to sex hormones, to various chemotherapeutic agents, and to other treatment modalities.

References

1. Weiss, A.F., Zang, K.D., Birkmayer, G.D., and Miller, F.: SV 40 related Papova viruses in human meningiomas. *Acta Neuropathol.* (*Berl.*) *34: 171–174, 1976.*
2. Kajikawa, H., Kawamoto, K., Herz, F., Wolley, R.C., Hirano, A., and Koss, L.G.: Flow-through cytometry of meningiomas and cultured meningioma cells. *Acta Neuropathol.* (*Berl.*) *44: 183–187, 1978.*
3. Sipe, J.C.: Gap junctions between human meningioma cells maintained in organ culture. *Acta Neuropathol.* (*Berl.*) *35: 69–76, 1976.*
4. Lipper, S., Dalzell, J.C., and Watkins, P.J.: Ultrastructure of psammoma bodies of meningioma in tissue culture. *Arch. Pathol. Lab. Med. 103: 670–675, 1979.*
5. Kredel, F.E.: Tissue culture of an intracranial tumor. With a note on the meningiomas. *Am. J. Pathol. 4: 337–340, 1928.*
6. Buckley, R.C., and Eisenhardt, L.: Study of meningioma in supravital preparation, tissue culture and paraffin sections. *Am. J. Pathol. 5: 659–664, 1929.*
7. Cox, L.B., and Cranage, M.L.: Studies on the tissue culture of intracranial tumors. *J. Pathol. Bacteriol. 45:477–499, 1937.*
8. Bland, J.O.W., and Russell, D.S.: Histological types of meningiomata and a comparison of their behavior in tissue culture with that of certain normal human tissues. *J. Pathol. Bacateriol. 47:291–309, 1938.*
9. Fischmann, C.F., and Russell, D.S.: The occurrence of intranuclear inclusion in cultures of fetal leptomeninges. *J. Pathol. Bacteriol. 50: 53–59, 1940.*
10. Pomerat, C.M.: Dynamic neuropathology. *J. Neuropathol. Exp. Neurol. 14: 28–38, 1955.*
11. Costero, I., Pomerat, C.M., Jackson, I.J., Barroso-Moguel, R., and Chevez, A.Z.: Tumors of the human nervous system in tissue culture. I. The cultivation and cytology of meningioma cells. *J. Natl. Cancer Inst. 15: 1319–1340, 1955.*
12. Costero, I., Pomerat, C.M., Barroso-Moguel, R., and Chevez, A.Z.: Tumors of the human nervous system in tissue culture. II. Analysis of fibroblastic activity in meningiomas. *J. Natl. Cancer Inst. 15: 1341–1366, 1955.*
13. Kersting, G., and Lennarzt, H.: In vitro cultures of human meningioma tissue. *J. Neuropathol. Exp. Neurol. 16: 507–513, 1957.*
14. Bennington, J.L., Smith, J.V., and Lagunoff, D.: Calcification in psammoma bodies of the human meningioma. *Lab. Invest. 22: 241–244, 1970.*
15. Pomerat, C.M., Todd, E.M., and Goldblatt, D.: Activity of meningiomal whorls in vitro. *In The Biology and Treatment of Intracranial Tumors*, Fields, W. S. and Sharkey, P. C. *et al.* (ed.). Springfield, Ill., Charles C Thomas, 1962, pp. 104–121.
16. Morley, T.P.: The morphology of meningiomas grown in culture. *J. Neuropathol. Exp. Neurol. 17: 635–643, 1958.*
17. Lumsden, C.E.: Tissue culture in relation to tumors of the nervous system. *In Pathology of Tumours of the Nervous System*, D.S. Russell and L.J. Rubinstein (eds.). London, Edward Arnold, 1959, p. 301.
18. Lumsden, C.E.: The study of tissue culture of tumors of the nervous system. *In Pathology of Tumours of the Nervous System*, D.S. Russell and L.J. Rubinstein (eds.), 3rd ed. Baltimore, Williams & Wilkins, 1971, pp. 383–386.
19. Russell, D.S., and Rubinstein, L.J.: *Pathology of Tumours of the Nervous System*, 4th ed. Baltimore, Williams & Wilkins, 1977.
20. Duffy, P. E., Defendini, R., and Kremzner, L. T.: Regulation of meningioma cell growth in vitro by polyamines. *J. Neuropathol. Exp. Neurol.* 30: 698–713, 1971.
21. Muller, J., and Mealey, J., Jr.: The use of tissue culture in differentiation between angioblastic meningioma and hemangiopericytoma. *J. Neurosurg. 34: 341–348, 1971.*

CHAPTER 29

Metastases of Meningiomas

Considering the fact that meningiomas make up about 15% of primary intracranial and intraspinal neoplasms in this and many other countries, the number of instances in which these tumors metastasize to distant sites is quite small. In the case of an intracranial neoplasm, the term *metastasis* implies both seeding via the cerebrospinal fluid to other points of the neural axis, and the more conventional notion of the formation of secondary tumor deposits in distant extraneural organs.

Both types of metastases are distinctly rare. Among the 313 cases of Cushing and Eisenhardt,[1] only one, the famous patient Dorothy May Russell, had a meningioma that metastasized to the lungs after numerous local recurrences and 17 operations. Many other large series (e.g., the 243 meningiomas of the Frazier-Grant Collection of Tumors, reviewed by Earle and Richany[2]) do not contain any instances of distant metastases. (Strang *et al.*[3] estimated the incidence of distant metastases to be about 0.1%, and metastases within the neural axis are even less commonly encountered.) That this should be so is probably more a function of the biologic potential of the tumor cells than of the lack of access to transport routes leading to distant sites. Certainly, most meningiomas are quite close to the cerebrospinal pathways, whether they occur on the surface of the brain or intraventricularly. Individual cells of meningiomas, however, do not seem to have any great tendency to detach themselves from the main tumor mass and exfoliate (see Chapter 27 for discussion of the rare, almost exceptional, appearance of meningioma tumor cells in spinal fluid specimens examined by cytologists.)

For meningioma cells to gain access to the bloodstream should not be difficult either. After all, even the normal arachnoidal cells of the Pachionian granulations are separated by only a thin layer of endothelium from the blood current in the large venous sinuses, and meningiomas—particularly parasagittal forms—frequently invade the lumen of the dural sinuses, thereby exposing themselves directly to the bloodstream without in many instances producing metastatic deposits elsewhere. No doubt this is partly because of the cohesive nature of these tumors—quite understandable, if one considers the intricate junctions between tumor cells as revealed by electron microscopy—allowing few tumor cells to break off from the main mass. With by far most meningiomas being biologically benign, it follows that even if occasional cells or clusters of the cells do get swept away by the bloodstream, they do not as a rule have the ability to colonize and form metastatic nodules in distant organs. Thus, by far most meningiomas in the literature that did metastasize had histological hallmarks of malignancy, although a few of them appeared histologically benign both in the primary tumor and its metastases. Yet even among those meningeal tumors that have clear-cut histological and cytological features of malignancy, distant metastases are quite rare and the malignant biological potential of the tumor is much more likely expressed in local recurrences. Indeed, as the study of metastasizing meningiomas collected from the literature (Table 2) shows, many of these tumors had one or several local recurrences before they metastasized to distant organs.

MENINGIOMAS SEEDING THROUGH THE CEREBROSPINAL FLUID

The seeding of meningioma cells through CSF pathways with the establishment of metastatic implants in the subarachnoid space or in distant areas of the nervous parenchyma itself, is very rare. Only 11 cases have been reported in the literature (Table 1) to which we have added one of our own cases (case 10).

Twelve cases, of course, represent a very small number to analyze, but it is perhaps worth mentioning that all patients were adults, six men and six women. The primary tumors were found in various intracranial locations, both supra- and infratentorially. Seven tumors were described as meningothelial (syncytial, psammomatous) and three as fibroblastic or fibrous; two simply as sar-

TABLE 1

Meningiomas with Metastases to Distant areas of the Cerebral Nervous System, via Cerebrospinal Fluid

No.	Author(s)	Year	Patient Age	Sex	Location	Histology	Surg.	Local Rec.	Re-op.	Site of Metastases	Comments
1	Kalm[39]	1950	48	M	Tentorium	Transitional, with signs of malignancy	No	—	—	Med. oblongata spinal cord. Spinal nerve roots.	—
2	Schöpe[40]	1951	56	F	Left pterion	Psammomatous	No	—	—	Multiple intracerebral	Histologically benign
3	Winkelman[41]	1954	60	F	Sphenoidal ridge	Meningothelial; no signs of malignancy	Yes	—	—	Multiple cerebral and cerebellar	Histologically benign
4	Hoffmann and Earle[42]	1960	39	F	Left frontal	Fibroblastic with pleomorphism; in metastases more like fibrosarcoma	Yes	Yes	2	Spinal subarachnoid space. Cauda equina	
5	Kantorovich[65]	1964	23	F	Parasagittal	Arachnoendothelial sarcoma	Yes	—	—	Dura, brain	Extracranial metastases
6	Shuangshoti *et* al.[43]	1970	21	F	Occipital	Malignant syncytial	No	—	—	Lower cervical, upper thoracic spinal canal, subdural	Many extracranial metastases
7	Riley[25]	1971	38	F	Occipital	Fibroblastic	Yes	Yes	5	Spinal canal	Extraneural metastases
8	Guszowski *et* al.[72]	1971	47	M		Meningeal sarcoma	Yes	—	—	Spinal meninges	Submandibular lymph-nodes (scalp was involved)
9	Miller and Ramsden[26]	1972	45	M	Parasagittal	Malignant syncytial (many mitoses, prominent nucleoli)	Yes	Yes	1	Cranial and spinal nerves	Extraneural metastases
10	McGregor and Kepes[27]	1974	49	M	Foramen magnum	Atypical fibrous; in metastases fibrosarcoma	Yes	Yes	1	Multiple subdural and subarachnoidal	Extraneural metastases
11	Ludwin and Conley[44]	1975	53	M	Parasagittal	Syncytial, occasionally transitional; metastases partly papillary	Yes	—	—	Ventral medulla cerebellopontine angle	
12	Russell and Rubinstein[38]	1977	78	M	Foramen magnum	Benign endotheliomatous	No	—	—	Metastasis over a lateral orbital gyrus.	Histologically benign

TABLE 2

Distant Metastases of Meningiomas

No.	Author(s)	Year	Patient Age	Sex	Location	Histology	Surg.	Local Rec.	Reop.	Site of Metastases	Comments
1	Power[4]	1886	25	F	Left parietal	Fibrosarcoma	—	—	—	Lung	—
2	Klebs[5]	1889	—	—	—	Pial endothelioma	—	—	—	Lung	Arachnoid and lung involved. Primary? cit. Russell and Sachs
3	Lindner[6]	1902	63	M	—	Endothelioma	—	—	—	Urinary bladder	—
4	Olivecrona[7]	1914	57	M	Diffuse meningeal infiltrate	Endothelioma sarcoma	—	—	—	Liver kidney	Cells resembling large cell lymphoma
5	Towne[45]	1926	54	F	Falx	Meningioma	Yes	—	—	Invasion of jugular vein sup. vena. cava. Cerv. mass.	No pictures. Text mentions glandlike structures (ca.?)
6	Pendergass and Wilbur[46]	1928	41	F	Post. fossa	Endothelioma	Yes	Yes 1	2	Lungs (by x-ray film)	No autopsy performed
7	Brandt[47]	1934	62	M	Parasellar, sphenoid ridge	Spindle-cell sarcoma	—	—	—	Liver	—
8	Derevici *et al.*[48]	1937	—	—	—	—	—	—	—	—	—
9	Cushing and Eisenhardt[1]	1938	35	F	Left frontotemporal	Angioblastic, with whorls in the end papillary	Yes	Yes	16	Lungs	Papillary
10	Jurow[49]	1941	22	F	Left parasagittal	Psammomatous meningioma	—	—	—	Lungs	—
11	Russell and Sachs,[11] Case 1	1942	33	F	Right parietooccipital	Malignant arachnoidal fibroblastoma	Yes	Yes	2	Lungs, tracheobronch. nodes vertebrae, retroperit. nodes	Described as moderately cellular with numerous mitoses
12	Russell and Sachs,[11] Case 2	1942	38	F	Left temporal	Highly cellular fibroblastic, called fibrosarcoma	Yes	—	—	Liver, mediastinum, lung	—
13	Russell and Sachs,[11] Case 3	1942	12	F	Right occipital	Fibrosarcoma	Yes	Yes	1	Pleura	—
14	Abbott and Love[13]	1943	32	M	Right, frontal parasagittal; invaded sup. sag. sinus	Hemangiopericytoma	Yes	Yes	1		Superior sagittal sinus invaded and completely filled
15	Dublin[12]	1944	83	M	Right parietooccipital	Low-grade meningeal fibrosarcoma	—	—	—	Lung, pleura	—
16	Hamblet[50]	1944	41	M	Anterior fossa	Meningothelial	Yes	—	—	Liver	
17	Laymon and Becker[17]	1949	72	M	Right frontoparietal with scalp involvement	Meningothelial	—	—	—	Cervical lymph nodes	Scalp was involved
18	Christensen *et al.*[32] Case 1	1949	21	M	Right motor region	Cellular meningioma, later fibrosarcoma	Yes	Yes	—	Liver, kidney	—
19	Christensen *et al*[32] Case 2	1949	31	M	Left paramed.	Psammomatous meningioma	Yes	—	Pulmonectomy for meta.	Lung	Metastasis operated

20	Swingle[51]	1949	40	M	Right falx	Malignant meningioma with mitoses, called sarcoma	Yes	Yes	1	Lung	—
21	Lima[18]	1951	55	M	Parasagittal	Meningioma	Yes	Yes	4	Cervical lymph nodes	Scalp involved in recurrences
22	Winkelman *et al.*[52]	1952	50	M	Right temporoparietal	Undifferentiated, somewhat perithelial fibrous meningioma	Yes	Yes	2	Lung Pleura	—
23	Cross and Cooper[53]	1952	45	M	Left parietal parasagittal	Malignant meningioma with many psammoma bodies	Yes	Yes	2	Lung	—
24	Shozawa[54]	1953	35	F	Falx	Sarcomatous meningioma	Yes, incomplete removal	—	—	Liver Portal and mesenteric lymph nodes	Nodes secondary to liver metastases?
25	Zülch *et al.*[55]	1954	47	F	Right temporal (started with bone defect)	Fibroblastic-hemangio-pericytic	Yes	—	—	Lungs, kidney, liver, scalp, finger	—
26	Rosen and Branch[56]	1954	44	M	Right temporal	Meningosarcoma	Yes	—	—	Liver, bones	—
27	Paparo and Pasetti[10]	1955	5	M	Frontal parasagittal	—				Cervical nodes	—
28	Simpson,[57] Case 1	1957	Not given	Not given	Parasagittal	Syncytial	Yes	—	—	Lungs, liver, kidney and elsewhere	—
29	Simpson,[57] Case 2	1957	56	F	Parasagittal frontal	Anaplastic meningioma with many mitoses	Yes	Yes	1	Lung, pleura	—
30	Baumann[58]	1958	65	F	Right parietal	Meningioma, rich in mitoses with psammomatous and sarcomatous component				Kidney (with fat cells!)	Could be angiolipoma in kidney
31	Ringsted[21]	1958	37	M	Bilateral	Meningothelial meningioma without sarcomatous character	Yes	—	—	Lung, pleura	Nonmalignant histologically
32	Vlachos and Prose[14]	1958	63	M	Right orbitotemporal, spb. ridge, invasion of cavernous sinus	Meningothelial with necroses and mitoses	—	—	—	Mediastinal lymph nodes	Invasion of cavernous sinus
33	Gibbs[59]	1958	23	F	Left parasagittal	Meningothelial with psammoma bodies and necrosis	Only negative biopsies	—	—	Lung	Tumor was attached to superior sagittal sinus; no surgery of tumor proper
34	Shtern[60]	1958	39	M	Left frontal	Meningothelial meningioma—mature and differentiated	—	—	—	Lungs	—
35	Meredith and Belter[61]	1959	31	F	Right occipital	Benign, later revised; many mitoses; fibrous and hemangiopericytic	Yes	Yes	1	Ribs, vertebrae sacrum, clavicle, lungs, liver, kidney, pancreas, mediastinum	—
36	Haberich and Zülch[8]	1959	7 days	F	Subfrontal	Angiomatous	Yes	—	—	Lungs, thyroid, thymus, heart, liver, pancreas, stomach, colon, skin	Liver metastasis surgically removed

TABLE 2 (Continued)

No.	Author(s)	Year	Patient Age	Sex	Location	Histology	Surg.	Local Rec.	Reop.	Site of Metastases	Comments
37	Hukill and Lowman[34]	1960	31	F	Left frontal	Hemangiopericytic	Yes	—	—	Liver and neighboring lymph nodes	Liver metastasis surgically removed
38	Robertson[15]	1960	44	M	Left frontal parasagittal with invasion of sup. sag. sinus	Moderately cellular nonmalignant meningioma, later, malignant fibrous meningioma	Yes	Yes	4	Lung	Sagittal sinus invaded
39	Rossman[9]	1960	16 mo.	—	Hemispheric	Sarcomatous	—	—	4	Lung	—
40	Kruse,[16] Case 1	1960	19	M	Right parasagittal; sinus invaded	Meningioma with whorls	Yes	Yes	1	Lungs	—
41	Kruse,[11] Case 2	1960	55	M	Frontomedial	Transitional meningioma with psammoma bodies	—	—	—	Lungs	Neither primary nor metastasis appeared histologically malignant
42	Arnould *et al.*[22]	1961	34	M	C_6–C_7; spinal extradural	Meningotheliomatous; no mitoses	Yes	Yes	2	Lungs (by x-ray film)	Primary tumor appeared histologically benign
43	Kruse[62]	1961	22	F	Right frontal parasagittal	Hemangiopericytoma	Yes	—	—	Vertebra, femur	—
44	Noto and Györi[63]	1961	47	F	Left frontal	Malignant meningothelial; later, fibroblastic	Yes	Yes	4	Pleura, lungs	—
45	Kernohan and Uihlein,[31] Case 1	1962	—	—	—	Hemangiopericytoma	—	—	—	Lung	—
46	Kernohan and Uihlein,[31] Case 2	1962	—	—	—	Hemangiopericytoma	—	—	—	Lung	—
47	Kernohan and Uihlein,[31] Case 3	1962	—	—	—	Hemangiopericytoma	—	—	—	Humerus	Pathological fracture
48	Steinke and Eder[33]	1964	—	—	—	—	Yes	Yes	4	Lung	Metastasis in lung excised
49	Zambo[64]	1964	59	F	Left parietal	Meningothelial, highly cellular	No	—	—	Left lung	—
50	Kantorovich[65]	1964	23	F	Parasagittal	Arachnoendothelial sarcoma	Yes	Yes	2	Kidney	Also metastasized to distant areas within brain
51	Strang *et al.*[3]	1964	57	M	Postparietal	Meningothelial very cellular with mitoses	Yes	—	—	Cerebrum cerebellum ('57) liver, lungs	Both intra- and extraaxial metastases
52	Young[66]	1965	48	F	Right occipital	Fibroblastic	Yes	Yes	3	Lung	—
53	Opsahl and Löken[19]	1965	70	M	Left frontal temporal and scalp	Meningothelial cellular meningioma with some atypical signs (a few mitoses)	Yes	Yes	No	Cervical lymph nodes	Scalp involved
54	Gordon and Maloney[29]	1965	42	M	Left parietal falx	Hemangiopericytoma	Yes	Yes	1	Thyroid, lungs	—
55	Samotkin and Civkin[67]	1965	—	—	—	—	—	—	—	Lungs	—

56	Postma[68]	1967	32	M	Left occipital subcortial	Meningothelical meningioma; few mitoses; areas of necrosis	Yes	Yes	2	Cervical lymph node, vertebrae femur, rib, para-aortic nodes	—
57	Gessaga[69]	1968	56	F	Bifrontal	Transitional meningioma with atypism of cells and nuclei and invasion of brain	No	—	—	Liver, bones, lungs	—
58	Agrawal and Junnakar[70]	1968	50	M	Spinal Th_{11}–L_2 (infiltrated)	Fibrous	—	—	—	Tracheobronchial lymph nodes	No metastases found in lungs
59	Shuangshoti[43]	1970	21	F	Occipital	Angioblastic (hemangioperi-cytic)	Yes	—	—	Thyroid, breast, right vulva, pleura, lung, pancreas, abdomen, lymph nodes	—
60–63	Pitkethly[71] Four cases	1970	—	—	—	Hemangiopericytic	All four oper-ated	Yes One or more	—	Lungs, liver, kidney, pancreas, adrenal	—
64	Guszowski *et al.*[72]	1971	47	M	—	Meningeal sarcoma with many mitoses	Yes	—	—	Submandibular lymph nodes	Also had spinal meningeal metastases
65	Riley[25]	1971	38	F	Occipital	Fibroblastic	Yes	Yes	3 plus 2 spinal lami-necto-mies and excision of lung metas-tasis	Lung	Metastasis excised from lung
66	Fekas and Economo-poulos[73]	1971	35	M	Right parietal, parasagittal	Meningioma, pleomorphic with many mitoses	Yes	—	—	Lung, axillary lymph nodes	Metastases in lymph nodes and lungs verified by biopsy
67	Kepes *et al.*[30]	1971	40	M	Tentorium–sigmoid sinus	Fibroblastic, hemangiopericytic, later papillary	Yes	Yes	1	Lungs, pleura, kidneys, liver	High alkaline phosphate in tumor and in serum
68	Petito and Porro[36]	1971	59	F	Tentorium	Hemangiopericytic	Yes	Yes	3	Liver	—
69	Fényes and Slowik,[35] Case 1	1972	51	F	Confluens sinuum	Fibroblastic-hemangioper-icytic	Yes	Yes	3	Lungs, pleura, liver, vertebrae, ocular fundus	Metastasis to fundus unique
70	Fényes and Slowik,[35] Case 2	1972	51	F	Right occipital	Malignant meningothelial	Of thigh metas-tasis only	—	—	Right thigh	Thigh metastasis was found 2 years before intracranial symptoms
71	Miller and Ramsden[26]	1972	45	M	Parasagittal	Cellular meningioma	—	—	—	Lungs, tracheobronchial and mediastinal lymph nodes, and subarachnoid metastases	Both CNS and extraneural metastases present

TABLE 2 (Continued)

No.	Author(s)	Year	Patient Age	Sex	Location	Histology	Surg.	Local Rec.	Reop.	Site of Metastases	Comments
72	Karasich and Mullan,[37] Case 1	1974	39	M	Right parieto-occipital parasagittal	Hemangiopericytoma	Yes	Yes	1	Rib, vertebra	—
73	Karasich and Mullan,[37] Case 2	1974	30	F	Left convexity	Fibroblastic	Yes	Yes	—	Right femur	—
74	Lowden and Taylor[74]	1974	39	F	Postparasagittal	Hemangiopericytoma	Yes	Yes	1	Breast	—
75	Palacios and Azar-Kia,[75] Case 1	1975	63	F	Left parasagittal	Angioblastic	Yes	Yes	1	Lung	—
76	Palacios and Azar-kia,[75] Case 2	1975	30	F	Spinal cervical intra- and extradural	Angioblastic	Yes	Yes	—	Lung, liver, left femur	For Case 3 of Palacios and Azar-Kia, see Kepes *et al.*[67]
77	Ludwin *et al.*[24] Case 3	1975	33	M	Left parieto-occipital, attached to falx and transverse sinus	Papillary	Yes	Yes	1	Femur	Case 1, Ludwin *et al.*[80] (Russell and Rubinstein)
78	Ludwin *et al.*[24] Case 8	1975	28	F	Clivus	Papillary	Yes	Yes	1	Spinal intradural and lungs (by x-ray film)	Both neural (spinal intradural) and extraneural metastases.
79	Jestico and Lantos[28]	1976	47	—	Right parasagittal	Angioblastic	Yes	Yes	1	Liver, kidneys, pancreas, abdomen, lymph nodes	Liver metastases weighed 9 kg; massive hypoglycemia
80	Repola and Weatherbee[23]	1976	72	M	Frontal, with invasion of skull and temporalis muscle	Transitional	Yes	Yes (orbit)	1	Liver	—
81	Russell and Rubinstein[38]	1977	41	M	Occipital	Syncytial, more mitoses in recurrence, later papillary	Yes	Yes	1	Lungs, liver	—
82	Mignot *et al.*[76]	1978	32	M	Left pontocerebellar	Transitional big nucleoli, some mitoses	Yes	Yes	1	Lungs	Elevated sedimentation rate, high serum alkaline phosphatase levels
83–85	Goellner *et al.*,[77] 3 patients	1978	—	—	—	Hemangiopericytoma	—	—	—	Bone, lung, liver, retroperitoneum	Reports on six patients, two with metastases, three of them previously described by Kernohan and Uihlein[45–47].

comas. It would appear that histological malignancy is related to metastatic potential through the CSF, because nine of the 12 cases were considered histologically malignant, or at least markedly atypical from the outset (with case 11 having a papillary pattern in the metastases), but in cases 2, 3, and 12, the tumors were regarded as histologically and cytologically benign, both at the primary sites and in the metastatic deposits. Conceivably, surgical intervention might mobilize clusters of meningioma tumor cells leading to future subarachnoid deposits and, indeed, eight patients of the series underwent operative removal of their respective tumors, but in four patients (cases 1, 2, 6, and 12) intracerebral or subarachnoid metastases developed in the absence of prior surgery, and one of the operated patients (11) already had metastatic implants in the walls of his lateral ventricle when first operated. Also, considering that of the thousands of operated meningioma cases all over the world, only six were reported to have developed metastases of the neural axis postoperatively, the role of surgical mobilization of tumor cells cannot be all that important in the pathogenesis of such metastases. It is more likely that the basic biologic character of the given tumor predisposes to the development of metastatic deposits. This is also supported by the fact that no fewer than six of the 12 cases having neural axis metastases (cases 5–10) also had a few or many extraneural metastases as well. For this reason, they are also included in Table 2, which lists the much larger group of reported cases of meningioma with extraneural metastases.

EXTRANEURAL METASTASES OF MENINGIOMAS

Table 2 attempts to summarize all the previously reported cases known to this author of primary meningeal tumors metastasizing to other organs. Several difficulties were encountered during the compilation of this table. One is that in some case reports—particularly the earlier ones—no adequate illustrations were presented to allow the present-day reviewer to establish the histological character of the tumor in case. Thus, the first case of Power,[4] reported to the Pathological Society of London, and printed in their *Transactions* in 1886, was described both in its primary site and in its pulmonary metastasis as a fibrosarcoma, but no illustrations were provided. In retrospect, it is also difficult to establish whether in the case of a lung tumor and multiple pial endotheliomas of the meninges, described by Klebs,[5] the meningeal or the pulmonary neoplasm should be regarded as the primary.

The same question arises when one considers the highly unusual metastatic site: the urinary bladder of the meningeal endothelioma of Lindner,[6] Olivecrona[7] published drawings of the meningeal tumor he called endothelioma/sarcoma with metastases to the liver and kidney, but so little cohesiveness is seen between the tumor cells in the drawings, that the picture reminds one more of a large cell histiocytic lymphoma than of a meningioma. A second problem derives from the fact that even today there is disagreement as to what constitutes a malignant meningioma, as opposed to a primary sarcoma of the meninges. Table 2 excludes some forms of reported malignant mesenchymal tumors, such as the various forms of primary meningeal lymphomas and mesenchymal chondrosarcomas, but tumors regarded as leptomeningeal fibrosarcomas by their investigators were retained, as it is very difficult to differentiate, particularly by light microscopy, a malignant meningioma of the fibroblastic type from a fibrosarcoma. The controversy over hemangiopericytic tumors of the meninges also creates a problem. Those who do not regard these neoplasms as true meningiomas would not, of course, include them in a list of metastasizing malignant meningiomas. Nevertheless, the table was considered more useful by including hemangiopericytic tumors. Their histology, when known, has been designated as such, and any future user of this table who is unwilling to count them among meningiomas can always delete them from the group if so wished.

Age

Most meningiomas occur in adults. It is therefore not surprising that few childhood cases were found among the metastasizing forms. The youngest patient with widespread metastases was 7 days old, as reported by Haberich and Zülch,[8] followed by the 16-month-old girl described by Rossman,[9] but other children, such as the 5-year-old boy of Paparo and Pasetti[10] and the 12-year-old girl of Russell and Sachs,[11] were also found in this series. The oldest patient, an 83-year-old man with pulmonary and pleural metastases, was reported by Dublin.[12]

Sex

Of the 78 cases in which the patient's gender was known to us, most (41) were males, as opposed to 37 females, quite unlike the sex distribution of meningiomas in general.

Location of Primary Tumor

The location of the primary tumor was perhaps of limited significance, as metastases developed from meningiomas located in various and sundry areas. The proximity to a major venous sinus might have played a role in some of the cases. Abbott and Love,[13] Dublin,[12] Vlachos and Prose,[14] Robertson,[15] and Kruse[16] (case 1) specifically cite the invasion of a large dural sinus by the primary tumor. It also seems that invasion of the scalp by the primary tumor may facilitate metastases to cervical lymph nodes, as in the cases of Laymon and Becker,[17] Lima,[18] and Opsahl and Löken.[19]

It is not known to what extent surgical intervention (removal of the primary tumor) will increase the likelihood of future distant metastases. In 59 cases of the series, such surgery did take place, but no surgery on the primary tumor was performed in at least 13 of the patients listed, who nevertheless did suffer from distant metastases.

Histology of Primary Tumor

The histology of the primary tumor showed at least some hallmarks of malignancy (high cellularity, mitotic figures, necroses, invasion of underlying brain)[20] in almost all cases, with four notable exceptions. Ringsted[21] specifically stated that in his 37-year-old male patient neither the bilateral parasagittal primary meningothelial meningioma nor its metastases to lung and pleura showed histological signs of malignancy. The same was true for case 2 of Kruse[16] (55 M, frontomedial psammomatous meningioma with pulmonary metastases), that of Arnould *et al.*[22] (34-year-old male with spinal extradural meningotheliomatous meningioma that has metastasized, at least by testimony of x-ray examination, to the lungs.) Finally, Repola and Weatherbee[23] reported a benign appearing meningioma that metastasized to the liver of their 72-year-old male patient.

Aside from the general signs of histological malignancy, the basic pattern of the primary tumors was also of interest. The largest group of tumors (34 cases) were of the meningothelial (e.g., syncytial, endothelial, meningotheliomatous, psammomatous) type. Fifteen cases were malignant fibrous meningiomas (spindle cell sarcomas, leptomeningeal fibrosarcomas), four were angioblastic without further specification (some of them may have been of the hemangiopericytic type), and a strikingly large number, 22, were designated as being of the hemangiopericytic type of meningiomas, or simply called hemangiopericytomas. Thus, the highly malignant potential of this particular subgroup of meningiomas is confirmed when observing their high rate (28.9%) among metastasizing meningeal tumors. Ludwin *et al.*[24] called attention to the malignant potential of that rare variant among meningiomas, the papillary type. The fact that five such tumors were found in this series attests to the seriousness of finding a papillary pattern in any meningioma. The above figures refer to the principal histological pattern described in any of the listed tumors, but in at least six of the above, the pattern was mixed, so that for example hemangiopericytic and fibrous, or meningothelial and papillary patterns coexisted in the same tumor.

Location of Metastases

Perhaps not surprisingly, the most common sites for metastases were the lungs (46 cases), followed by the liver (23 cases), lymph nodes (16), bones (12), pleura (10, some of these may have been surface extensions of lung metastases), kidney (8), pancreas (6), thyroid (3), mediastinum (2), breast (2), and one each of urinary bladder, thymus, wall of superior vena cava, heart, stomach, colon, skin, vulva, thigh, finger, ocular fundus, and adrenal gland.

In seven cases distant metastases coexisted with secondary tumor deposits within the neural axis, that is, seeding via the CSF.[3,24–27,65,72] Given the fact that many, although not all, patients with distant metastases of meningiomas also suffered from local recurrences of their tumor, the metastases were often just incidental findings at autopsy or had otherwise only limited role in bringing about the patient's demise. But there were cases in which the metastases were responsible for significant morbidity and mortality. In the patient of Jestico and Lantos,[28] a huge (9-kg) metastasis developed in the liver and probably as a consequence, the patient suffered massive attacks of hypoglycemia. Gordon and Maloney[29] described their patient's lungs as being full of metastases, and the unusually extensive bilateral pulmonary metastases in the case of Kepes *et al.*[30] virtually caused the patient's suffocation owing to the large areas of pulmonary parenchyma replaced by metastatic tumor nodules. One of Kernohan and Uihlein's[31] patients, with a metastasis to the humerus, suffered a pathologic fracture.

In rare instances, metastatic meningiomas were surgically attacked and removed, particularly those occurring in the lung,[25,32,33] while a liver metastasis was removed in the patient of Hukill and Lowman.[34] In the remarkable case reported by Fenyes and Slowik,[35] a metastatic meningioma was removed from the patient's thigh 2 years before the primary intracranial tumor made its presence known clinically.

The clinical course (length of time between discovery and surgery of the primary tumor and the appearance of distant metastases) varied greatly from patient to patient in this series, but in some instances it was rather extensive. (Cushing and Eisenhardt,[1] 18 years; Petito and Porro,[36] 17 years; Lima[18]; Christensen *et al.*[32]; Karasich and Mullan[37] Russell and Rubinstein,[38] each 16 years; and several others with a clinical history of more than 10 years duration.)

Thus, it appears that meningiomas, even in their malignant forms, rarely metastasize to distant organs. Even if they do, this often happens only after repeated recurrences and reoperations, and even then sometimes only long years after the primary tumor was first discovered and treated.

References

1. Cushing, H., and Eisenhardt, L.: *Meningiomas. Their Classification, Regional Behaviour, Life History and Surgical End Results.* The story of Dorothy May Russell. New York, Hafner, 1962, pp. 692–719.
2. Earle, K.M., and Richany, S.F.: Meningiomas. A study of histology, incidence, and biologic behavior of 243 cases from the Frazier-Grant collection of brain tumors. *Med. Ann. D.C. 38: 353–357, 1969.*
3. Strang, R.R., Tovi, D., and Nordenstam, H.: Meningioma with intracerebral, cerebrellar and visceral metastases. *J. Neurosurg. 21: 1098–1107, 1964.*
4. Power, D'Arcy: Fibro-sarcoma of the dura mater (card specimen). *Trans. Pathol. Soc. Lond. 37: 12, 1886.*
5. Klebs, E.: *Die Allgemeine Pathologie.* Jena, G. Fisher, 1889, Vol. II, p. 628.
6. Lindner, E.: Ein Fall von Endotheliom der Dura Mater mit Metastase in der Harnblase. Beitrag zur Histogenese und Differentialdiagnose der Endotheliome. Inaugural Dissertation. München 59, 1902.
7. Olivecrona, H.: Ein Fall von Geschwulstbildung in den weichen Häuten des Zentralnervensystems. *Virchows Arch. [Pathol. Anat.] 217: 161–173, 1914.*
8. Haberich, J., and Zülch, K.J.: Über die "Fernmetastasen" der Hirngeschwülste (unter besonderer Berücksichtigung der Mesodermalen Tumoren). *Zentralbl. Neurochir. 19: 213–219, 1959.*
9. Rossman, P.S.: Extracranial metastases of tumor of the meninges (meningioma). (In Russian.) *Arkh. Patol. 22: 74–79, 1960.*
10. Paparo, F., and Pasetti, A.: Le metastasi extracraniche de meningiomi. *Lav. Neuropsichiat. 17: 317–330, 1955.*
11. Russell, W.O., and Sachs, E.: Fibrosarcoma of arachnoidal origin with metastases. Report of four cases with necropsy. *Arch. Pathol. 34: 240–261, 1942.*
12. Dublin, W.B.: metastasizing intracranial tumors. *Northwest. Med. (Seattle) 43: 83–84, 1944.*
13. Abbott, K.H., and Love, J.G.: Metastasizing intracranial tumors. *Ann. Surg. 118: 343–352, 1943.*
14. Vlachos, J., and Prose, P.H.: Meningioma with extracranial metastases: report of a case. *Cancer 11: 439–445, 1958.*
15. Robertson, B.: A case of meningioma with extracranial metastasis. *Acta Pathol. Microbiol. Scand. [C] 48: 335–340, 1960.*
16. Kruse, F., Jr.: Meningeal tumor with extracranial metastasis. A clinicopathological report of 2 cases. *Neurology (Minneapolis) 10: 197–201, 1960.*
17. Laymon, C.W., and Becker, F.T.: Massive metastasizing meningioma involving the scalp. *Arch. Dermatol. Syphil. NY 59: 626–635, 1949.*
18. Lima, A.P.: Metastase cervical de um meningioma parassagital. *Rev. Esp. Oto-Neuro-Oftalmol. Neurocir. 57: 313–316, 1951.*
19. Opsahl, R., and Löken, A.C.: Meningioma with metastases to cervical lymph nodes. Case report. *Acta Pathol. Microbiol. Scand. [C] 64: 294–298, 1967.*
20. Tytus, J.S., Lasersohn, J.T., and Reifel, E.: The problem of malignancy in meningiomas. *J. Neurosurg. 27: 551–557, 1967.*
21. Ringsted, J.: Meningeal tumor with extracranial metastasis. *Acta Pathol. Microbiol. Scand [C] 43: 9–20, 1958.*
22. Arnould, G., Lepoire, J., Pierson, B., and Barrucand, D.: Les meningiomes malins. (A propos d'une observation.) *Rev. Neurol. (Paris) 105: 469–479, 1961.*
23. Repola, D., and Weatherbee, L.: Meningioma with sarcomatous changes and hepatic metastasis. *Arch. Pathol. Lab. Med. 100: 667–669, 1976.*
24. Ludwin, S.K., Rubinstein, L.J., and Russell, D.S.: Papillary meningioma: A malignant variant of meningioma. *Cancer 36: 1363–1373, 1975.*
25. Riley, C.G.: Metastasizing meningeal tumor: Case report. *NZ Med. J. 73: 210–214, 1971.*
26. Miller, A.A., and Ramsden, F.: Malignant meningioma with extracranial metastases and seeding of the subarachnoid space and the ventricles. *Pathol. Eur. 7: 167–175, 1972.*
27. McGregor, D., and Kepes, J. J.: Personal observation, 1974.
28. Jestico, J.V., and Lantos, P.C.: Malignant meningioma with liver metastasis and hypoglycemia. A case report. *Acta Neuropathol. (Berl.) 35: 357–361, 1976.*
29. Gordon, A., and Maloney, F.J.: A case of metastasizing meningioma. *J. Neurol. Neurosurg. Psychiatry 28: 159–162, 1965.*
30. Kepes, J.J., MacGee, E.E., Vergara, G., and Sil, R.: Malignant meningioma with extensive pulmonary metastases. A case report. *J. Kans. Med. Soc. 72: 312–316, 1971.*
31. Kernohan, J.W., and Uihlein, A.: *Sarcomas of the Brain.* Springfield, Ill., Charles C Thomas, 1962, p. 25.
32. Christensen, E., Kiaer, W., and Winblad, S.: Meningeal tumors with extracerebral metastases. *Br. J. Cancer 3: 485–493, 1949.*
33. Steinke, H.J., and Eder, M.: Rezidiverendes parasagittales Meningeom mit Lungenmetastase—ein Fallbericht. *Zentralbl. Neurochir. 25: 89–98, 1964.*
34. Hukill, P.B., and Lowman, R.M.: Visceral metastasis from a meningioma. Report of a case. *Ann. Surg. 152: 804–808, 1960.*
35. Fenyes, G., and Slowik, F.: Über extrakraniell metastasierende Meningiome. *Zentralbl. Neurochir. 33: 131–135, 1972.*

36. Petito, C.K., and Porro, R.S.: Angioblastic meningioma with hepatic metastasis.
J. Neurol. Neurosurg. Psychiatry 34: 541–545, 1971.
37. Karasich, J., and Mullan, S.: A survey of metastatic meningiomas.
J. Neurosurg. 40: 206–212, 1974.
38. Russell, D.S., and Rubinstein, L.J.: *Pathology of Tumours of the Nervous System*, 4th ed. Baltimore, Williams & Wilkins, 1977, p. 91.
39. Kalm, H.: Ein malignes Tentoriummeningeom mit Metastasierung in die Medulla oblongata und in die subarachnoidalen Liquorräume.
Dtsch.. Z. Nervenheilkd. 163: 131–140, 1950.
40. Schöpe, M.: Zur Frage der multiplen Meningiome und der Metastasierung von Meningiomen.
Arch Psychiatr Nervenkr. 186: 623–640, 1951.
41. Winkelman, N.W.: Post-operative seeding of the subarachnoid space and ventricles from a meningioma.
J. Neuropathol. Exp. Neurol. 13: 260–266, 1954.
42. Hoffmann, G.T., and Earle, K.M.: Meningioma with malignant transformation and implantation in the subarachnoid space.
J. Neurosurg. 17: 486–492, 1960.
43. Shuangshoti, S., Hongsaprabhas, C., and Netsky, M.G.: Metastasizing meningioma.
Cancer 26: 832–841, 1970.
44. Ludwin, S.K., and Conley, F.K.: Malignant meningioma metastasizing through the cerebrospinal pathways.
J. Neurol. Neurosurg. Psychiatry 38: 138–142, 1975.
45. Towne, E.B.: Invasion of the intracranial venous sinuses by meningioma (Dural endothelioma).
Ann. Surg. 83: 321–327, 1926.
46. Pendergass, E.P., and Wilbur, D.L.: Tumor of the brain with widespread metastases. A report of two cases.
Arch. Neurol. Psychiatry 19: 437–445, 1928.
47. Brandt, M.: Fünf Fälle mehrfacher Gliome im Grosshirn.
Verh. Dtsch. Ges. Pathol. 27: 39–42, 1934.
48. Derevici, M., Ionescu, E.I., and Smilovici, L.: Étude anatomopathologique d'un méningoblastome avec métastases.
Bull. Soc. Rom. Neurol. 18: 14–18, 1937.
49. Jurow, H.N.: Psammomatous dural endothelioma (meningioma) with pulmonary metastasis.
Arch. Pathol. 32: 222–226, 1941.
50. Hamblet, J.B.: Arachnoidal fibroblastoma (meningioma) with metastases to liver.
Arch. Pathol. 37: 216–218, 1944.
51. Swingle, A.: Meningiosarcoma with pulmonary metastasis. Report of a case.
Arch Neurol. Psychiatry 61: 65–72, 1949.
52. Winkelman, N.W., Cassel, C., and Schlesinger, B.: Intracranial tumours with extracranial metastases.
J. Neuropathol. Exp. Neurol. 11: 149–168, 1952.
53. Cross, K.R., and Cooper, T.J.: Intracranial tumors with extracranial metastases. Report of two cases.
J. Neuropathol. Exp. Neurol. 11: 200–208, 1952.
54. Shozawa, T.: Meningioma with metastases to liver and lymph nodes. Gann
43: 345–347, 1952.
55. Zülch, K.J., Pompeu, F., and Pinto, F.: Über die Metastasierung der Meningeome.
Zentralbl. Neurochir. 14: 253–260, 1954.
56. Rosen, H.J., and Branch, A.: Meningeal sarcoma with extracranial metastasis.
Can. Serv. Med. J. 10: 153–158, 1954.
57. Simpson, D.: The recurrence of intracranial meningiomas after surgical treatment.
J. Neurol. Neurosurg. Psychiatry 20: 22–39, 1957.
58. Baumann, J.: A contribution to the problem of extracranial metastasis in meningiomas.
Confin. Neurol. (Basel) 18: 394–397, 1958.
59. Gibbs, N.M.: Meningioma with extracranial metastasis.
J. Pathol. Bacteriol. 76: 285–288, 1958.
60. Shtern, R.D.: Metastatic spread of arachnoid endotheliomas. (In Russian.)
Arkh. Patol. 20: 72–83, 1958.
61. Meredith, J.M., and Belter, L.F.: Malignant meningioma. Case report of a parasagittal meningioma of the right cerebral hemisphere with multiple extracranial metastases to the vertebrae, sacrum, ribs, clavicle, lungs, liver, left kidney, mediastinum and pancreas.
South. Med. J. 52: 1035–1040, 1959.
62. Kruse, F.: Hemangiopericytoma of the meninges (angioblastic meningioma of Cushing and Eisenhardt). Clinicopathologic aspects and follow-up studies in 8 cases.
Neurology (Minneapolis) 11: 771–777, 1961.
63. Noto, T.A., and Györi, E.: Malignant metastasizing meningioma. Report of a case.
Arch. Pathol. 72: 191–196, 1961.
64. Zambo, Z.: Intracranialis tumor (meningeoma) extracranialis metastasisa.
Ideggy. Szle. 17: 371–374, 1964.
65. Kantorovich, V.I.: Arachnoid endotheliosarcoma with intra- and extracranial metastases. (In Russian.)
Arkh. Patol. 26: 77–80, 1964.
66. Young, R.G.: Meningeal tumors with extracranial metastases: Report of a case.
NZ Med J. 64: 204–209, 1964.
67. Samotkin, B.A., and Civkin, M.V.: Metastasis of arachnoendothelioma to lung. (In Russian.)
Vopr. Nejrochir. 30: 57–58, 1966.
68. Postma, J.N.: A case of metastasizing meningioma.
Psychiatr. Neurol. Neurochir. 70:245–259, 1967.
69. Gessaga, E.: Ueber einen fall eines malignen Meningeomes mit extrakranialen Metastasen.
Sist. Nerv. 20: 258–270, 1968.
70. Agrawal, R.V., and Junnarkar, R.V.: Spinal meningioma with lymph node metastasis. An autopsy report.
Neurology (India) 16: 81–82, 1968.
71. Pitkethly, D.T., Hardman, J.M., Kempe, L.G., and Earle, K.M.: Angioblastic meningiomas. Clinicopathologic study of 81 cases.
J. Neurosurg. 32: 539–544, 1970.
72. Guzowski, K., Gruszka, A., and Sosnik, H.: Primary meningeal sarcoma with extracranial metastases. (In Polish.)
Neurol. Neurochir. Pol. 5: 753–757, 1971.
73. Fekas, L., and Economopoulos, A.: Hirnmeningiom mit Lungen- und Achsellymphdrüsen-Metastasen.
Neurochirurgia (Stuttg.) 14: 28–33, 1971.
74. Lowden, R.G., and Taylor, H.B.: Angioblastic meningioma with metastasis to the breast.
Arch. Pathol. Lab. Med. 98: 373–375, 1974.
75. Palacios, E., and Azar-Kia, B.: Malignant metastasizing angioblastic meningiomas.
J. Neurosurg. 42: 185–188, 1975.
76. Mignot, B., Hauw, J.J., Pasquier, P., de Sigalony, J.P.H., and Bricaire, F.: Perturbations biologiques reversibles evoluant parallelement à un méningiome recidivant et avec métastases.
Sem. Hop. Paris. 54: 1231–1237, 1978.
77. Goellner, J.R., Laws, E.R., Soule, E.H., and Okazaki, H.: Hemangiopericytoma of the meninges. Mayo Clinic experience.
Am. J. Clin. Pathol. 70: 375–380, 1978.

Index